Contents

3rd Edition

PRIORITIZATION, DELEGATION, and ASSIGNMENT

Practice Exercises for the NCLEX® Examination

Linda A. LaCharity, PhD, RN
Formerly, Accelerated Program Director
Assistant Professor
College of Nursing
University of Cincinnati
Cincinnati, Ohio

Candice K. Kumagai, RN, MSN
Formerly, Instructor in Clinical Nursing
School of Nursing
University of Texas at Austin
Austin, Texas

Barbara Bartz, MN, ARNP, CCRN
Nursing Instructor
Yakima Valley Community College
Yakima, Washington

With an introduction by
Ruth Hansten, RN, MBA, PhD, FACHE
Principal
Hansten Healthcare PLLC
Port Ludlow, Washington

ELSEVIER
MOSBY

3251 Riverport Lane
St. Louis, Missouri 63043

PRIORITIZATION, DELEGATION, AND ASSIGNMENT: PRACTICE
EXERCISES FOR THE NCLEX® EXAMINATION, THIRD EDITION   ISBN: 978-0-323-11343-4

Library of Congress Cataloging-in-Publication Data

LaCharity, Linda A., author.
 Prioritization, delegation, and assignment : practice exercises for the NCLEX examination / Linda A. LaCharity, Candice K. Kumagai, Barbara Bartz ; with an introduction by Ruth Hansten.—Third edition.
   p. ; cm.
 Includes biographical references.
 ISBN 978-0-323-11343-4 (pbk.)
 I. Kumagai, Candice K., author. II. Bartz, Barbara, author. III. Title.
 [DNLM: 1. Nursing Care—organization & administration—Case Reports. 2. Nursing Care—organization & administration—Examination Questions. 3. Decision Making—Case Reports. 4. Decision Making—Examination Questions. 5. Delegation, Professional—Case Reports. 6. Delegation, Professional—Examination Questions. 7. Nurse's Role—Case Reports. 8. Nurse's Role—Examination Questions. WY18.2]
 RT55
 610.73076—dc23

                                                                        2013024837

Executive Content Strategist: Lee Henderson
Senior Content Development Specialist: Rae Robertson
Publishing Services Manager: Deborah L. Vogel
Project Manager: Pat Costigan
Book Designer: Margaret Reid

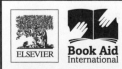
Printed in the United States of America

Last digit is the print number: 9 8 7 6 5 4 3 2 1

Preface

Prioritization, Delegation, and Assignment: Practice Exercises for the NCLEX® Examination has evolved since its first edition from a medical-surgical nursing–focused test preparation workbook to a resource that spans general nursing knowledge while emphasizing management of care to assist students in preparing for the NCLEX® Examination. A second and equally important purpose of the book is to assist novice as well as seasoned nurses in applying concepts of prioritization, delegation, and assignment to nursing practice in today's patient care settings.

Patient care acuity is higher than ever, while staffing shortages remain very real. Nurses must use all available patient care personnel and resources competently and efficiently, and be familiar with variations in state laws governing the practice of nursing, as well as differences in scopes of practice and facility-specific job descriptions. Nurses must also be aware of the different skill and experience levels of the health care providers with whom they work on a daily basis. Which nursing actions can be delegated to an experienced versus a new graduate RN or LPN/LVN? What forms of patient care can the nurse delegate to a certified nursing assistant? Who should help the postoperative patient who has had a total hip replacement get out of bed and ambulate to the bathroom? Can the nurse ask unlicensed assistive personnel (UAPs) such as nursing assistants to check a patient's oxygen saturation using pulse oximetry? What reporting parameters should the nurse give to the LPN/LVN who is monitoring a patient after cardiac catheterization or to the UAP checking patients' vital signs? What patient care interventions and actions should not be delegated by the nurse? The answers to these and many other questions should be much clearer after completion of the exercises in this book.

Prioritization, delegation, and assignment are essential concepts and skills for nursing practice. Our students and graduate nurses have repeatedly told us of their difficulties with the application of these principles when taking program exit and licensure examinations. Nurse managers have told us many times that novice nurses and even some experienced nurses lack the expertise to effectively and safely practice these skills in real-world settings.

Although several excellent resources deal with these issues, there is still a need for a book that incorporates management of care concepts into real-world practice scenarios. Our goal in writing the third edition of *Prioritization, Delegation, and Assignment: Practice Exercises for the NCLEX® Examination* is to provide a resource that challenges nursing students, as well as novice and experienced nurses, to develop the knowledge and understanding necessary to effectively apply these important nursing skills. Since publication of the first edition, we continue to receive many letters and e-mails from students, faculty, and novice nurse educators telling us about the value of this book as a resource for successful NCLEX® Examination preparation and real-world practice. In the third edition, we continue making changes that reflect the current focus on evidence-based best practices. For the second edition, our readers requested expansion of the book to include pediatrics, labor and delivery, psychiatric nursing, and long-term care. For the third edition, our readers requested more focus on fundamentals of safe practice, expansion of diabetes care, and separate chapters focused on pediatric and psychiatric nursing care. New chapters and questions were added to respond to the need to broaden comprehension of these key concepts and knowledge areas.

The exercises in this book range from simple to complex and use various patient care scenarios. The purpose of these chapters and case studies is to encourage the student or practicing nurse to conceptualize using the skills of prioritization, delegation, and assignment in many different settings. Our goal is to make these concepts tangible to our readers.

The questions are written in NCLEX® Examination style to help student nurses prepare for licensure examination. The chapters and case studies focus on real and hypothetical patient care situations to challenge nurses and nursing students to develop the skills necessary to apply these concepts in practice. The exercises are also useful to nurse educators as they discuss, teach, and test their students and nurses for understanding and application of these concepts in nursing programs, examination preparations, and facility orientations. Correct answers, along with in-depth rationales, are provided at the end of the book to facilitate the learning process.

Each new copy of the book comes with a fully interactive version of the book content, with scoring, on Evolve at http://evolve.elsevier.com/LaCharity/prioritization/. This interactive version of the book helps to simulate the experience of taking the NCLEX® Examination.

We would like to thank the many people whose support and assistance made the creation of the third edition of this book possible. Thanks to our families, colleagues, and friends for listening, reading, encouraging, and making sure we had the time to research, write, and review this book. Special thanks to Ruth Hansten, whose expertise in the area of clinical delegation skills continues to keep us on track. Many thanks to the clinical reviewers listed on the following page, whose expertise helped us keep the scenarios accurate and realistic. Finally, we wish to acknowledge our students, graduates, and readers who have taken the time to keep in touch and let us know about their need for additional assistance in developing the skills to practice the arts of delegation, prioritization, and assignment.

Linda A. LaCharity
Candice K. Kumagai
Barbara Bartz

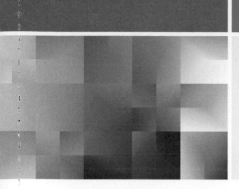

Contributor and Reviewers

CONTRIBUTOR

Martha Barry, MS, RN, APN, CNM
Adjunct Clinical Instructor
Department of Women, Children and Family Health
Science
College of Nursing
University of Illinois at Chicago
Chicago, Illinois

NURSING FACULTY REVIEWERS

Sophia Beydoun, RN, MSN
Nursing Instructor
School of Nursing
Henry Ford Community College
Dearborn, Michigan

Diane L. Cooper-McLean, RN, MSN
Instructor of Nursing
Department of Nursing
Faulkner State Community College
Bay Minette, Alabama

Margie L. Francisco, EdD(c), MSN, RN
Nursing Professor
Department of Nursing
Illinois Valley Community College
Oglesby, Illinois

Jamie Lynn Jones, MSN, RN, CNE
Assistant Professor
Department of Nursing
University of Arkansas at Little Rock
Little Rock, Arkansas

Kathleen S. Jordan, RN, MS, FNP-BC, SANE-P
Lecturer
School of Nursing
University of North Carolina at Charlotte;
Nurse Practitioner
Mid-Atlantic Emergency Medicine Associates
Charlotte, North Carolina

Mary Ann Kolis, MSN, RN, ANP-PC
Nurse Practitioner
Lake City VA Medical Center
Lake City, Florida

Melissa McNulty, PhD, ARNP
Professor of Nursing
Department of Nursing
Pasco-Hernando Community College
New Port Richey, Florida

Jenny L. Sauls, DSN, MSN, RN, CNE
Professor
School of Nursing
Middle Tennessee State University
Murfreesboro, Tennessee

STUDENT REVIEWERS

Carly Decker
Des Moines Area Community College
Ankeny, Iowa

Abby Wohl, RN
SUNY Empire State College
Saratoga Springs, New York;
Staff Nurse, Adult Emergency Department
Lincoln Medical and Mental Health Center
Bronx, New York

Contents

Guidelines for Prioritization, Delegation, and Assignment Decisions

Ruth Hansten, RN, PhD, FACHE

OUTCOMES FOCUS

Expert nurses have discovered that the most successful method of approaching their practice is to maintain a laser-like focus on the outcomes that the patients and their families want to achieve. To attempt to prioritize, delegate, or assign care without understanding the patient's preferred results is like trying to put together a jigsaw puzzle without the top of the puzzle box that shows the puzzle picture. Not only does the puzzle player pick up random pieces that don't fit well together, wasting time and increasing frustration, but also the process of puzzle assembly is fraught with inefficiencies and wrong choices. In the same way, the nurse who scurries haphazardly without a plan, unsure of what could be the most important, lifesaving task to be done first, or which person should do which tasks for this group of patients, is not fulfilling his or her potential to be a channel for healing.

Let's visit a change-of-shift report in which a group of nurses receives information about two patients whose blood pressure is plummeting at the same rate. How would one determine which nurse would be best to assign to care for these patients, which patient needs to be seen first, and which tasks could be delegated to assistive personnel, if none of the nurses is aware of each patient's preferred outcomes? Patient Apple is a young mother who has been receiving chemotherapy for breast cancer; she has been admitted this shift because of dehydration from uncontrolled emesis. She is expecting to regain her normally robust good health and watch her children graduate from college. Everyone on the health care team would concur with her long-term goals. Patient Orange is an elderly gentleman of 92 whose wife recently died from complications of repeated cerebrovascular events and dementia. Yesterday while in the emergency department, he was given the diagnosis of acute myocardial infarction and preexisting severe heart failure. He would like to die and join his wife, has requested a "do not resuscitate" (DNR) order, and is awaiting transfer to a hospice. These two patients are as different as apples and oranges. A savvy charge RN would make the obvious decisions: to assign the most skilled RN to the young mother and to ask assistive personnel to function in a supportive role to the primary care RN.

The elderly gentleman needs palliative care and would be best cared for by an RN and care team with excellent people skills. Even a novice nursing assistant could be delegated tasks to help keep Mr. Orange and his family comfortable and emotionally supported. The big picture on the puzzle box for these two patients ranges from long-term "robust good health" requiring immediate emergency assessment and treatment to "a supported and comfortable death" requiring timely palliative care, including supportive emotional and physical care. Without envisioning these patients' pictures and knowing their preferred outcomes, the RNs cannot prioritize, delegate, or assign appropriately.

There are a few times in nursing practice, however, when correct choices are not so apparent. All cases in acute care settings today are complex. Many patients have preexisting comorbidities that stump expert practitioners and clinical specialists planning their care. Care delivery systems must flex on a moment's notice as a nursing assistant arrives in place of a scheduled LPN/LVN, and agency, float, or traveling nurses fill vacancies, while new patients, waiting to be admitted, accumulate in the emergency department. Assistive personnel arrive with varying educational preparation and dissimilar levels of motivation and skill. Critical thinking and complex clinical judgment are required from the minute the shift begins until the nurse clocks out.

In this book, the authors have filled an educational need for students and practicing nurses who wish to hone their skills in prioritizing, assigning, and delegating. The scenarios and patient problems presented in this workbook are practical, challenging, and complex learning tools. The patient stories will stimulate thought and discussion and help polish the higher-order intellectual skills necessary to practice as a successful, safe, and effective nurse.

DEFINITION OF TERMS

The intellectual functions of prioritization, delegation, and assignment engage the nurse in projecting into the future from the present state. Thinking about what might occur if competing decisions are chosen, weighing options, and making split-second decisions, given the available data, is not an easy process. Unless resources in terms of staffing, budget, time, or supplies are unlimited, nurses must relentlessly focus on choosing which issues or concerns must take precedence.

Prioritization

Prioritization is defined as **"deciding which needs or problems require immediate action and which ones could be delayed until a later time because they are not urgent"** (Silvestri, 2011). Prioritization in a clinical setting is a process that includes envisioning clearly patient outcomes but also includes predicting possible problems if another task is performed first. One also must weigh potential future events if the task is not completed, the time it would take to accomplish it, and the relationship of the tasks and outcomes. New nurses often struggle with prioritization because they have not yet worked with typical patient progressions through care pathways and have not experienced the complications that may emerge in association with a particular clinical condition. In short, knowing the patient's **purpose for care, current clinical picture,** and **picture of the outcome or result** is necessary to be able to plan priorities. The part played by each team member is designated as the RN assigns or delegates. The "Four Ps"—purpose, picture, plan, and part—become a guidepost for appropriately navigating these processes (Hansten, 2008a, 2011; Hansten and Jackson, 2009). The Four Ps will be referred to throughout this introduction because these concepts are the framework on which RNs base decisions about supporting the patient and family toward their preferred outcomes, whether RNs provide the care themselves or work closely with assistive team members.

Prioritization includes evaluating and weighing each competing task or process using the following criteria (Hansten and Jackson, 2009, pp. 194-196):

- Is it life threatening or potentially life threatening if the task is not done? Would another patient be endangered if this task is done now or the task is left for later?
- Is this task or process essential to patient or staff safety?
- Is this task or process essential to the medical or nursing plan of care?

In each case, an understanding of the overall patient goals and the context and setting is essential.

In her book on critical thinking and clinical judgment, Rosalinda Alfaro-Lefevre (2013) suggests three levels of priority setting:

1. The first level is airway, breathing, cardiac status and circulation, and vital signs ("ABCs plus V").
2. The second level is immediately subsequent to the first level and includes concerns such as mental status changes, untreated medical issues, acute pain, acute elimination problems, abnormal laboratory results, and risks.

3. The third level is health problems other than those at the first two levels, such as more long-term issues in health education, rest, coping, and so on (p. 201).

Maslow's hierarchy of needs can be used to prioritize from the most crucial survival needs to needs related to safety and security, affiliation (love, relationships), self-esteem, and self-actualization (Alfaro-Lefevre, 2013, p. 199).

Delegation and Assignment

The official definitions of *assignment* have been altered through ongoing discussion among nursing leaders, and terminology distinctions such as *observation* versus *assessment, critical thinking* versus *clinical reasoning,* and *delegation* versus *assignment* continue to be contentious as nursing leaders attempt to describe complex thinking processes that occur in various levels of nursing practice. Historically, the definition of **assignment** was **"designating nursing activities to be performed by another nurse or assistive personnel that are consistent with his/her scope of practice (licensed person) or role description (unlicensed person)"** (National Council of State Boards of Nursing [NCSBN], 2004). **Delegation** was defined as **"transferring to a competent individual the authority to perform a selected nursing task in a selected situation"** (NCSBN, 1995). This definition of delegation remains the current definition. Both the American Nurses Association (ANA) and the NCSBN describe delegation as "the process for a nurse to direct another person to perform nursing tasks and activities." The ANA specifies that delegation is a transfer of responsibility rather than authority (ANA and NCSBN, 2006, p. 1).

Some state boards have argued that "assignment" is the process of directing a nursing assistant to perform a task such as taking blood pressure, a task on which nursing assistants are tested in the certified nursing assistant examination and that would commonly appear in a job description. Others contend that all nursing care is a part of the RN scope of practice and therefore that such a task would be "delegated" rather than "assigned." Other nursing leaders argue that only when a task is clearly within the RN's scope of practice, and not included in the role of the assistive personnel, is the task delegated. However, this differentiation is confusing to nurses. Because both processes are identical in terms of the actions and thinking processes of the RN from a practical standpoint, the distinctions are irrelevant. Therefore, in its 2005 White Paper, the NCSBN states that "using the verb *assign* in this manner [as in the above 2004 definition] is a variation of delegation. Since the process for both is the same, this Paper uses the verb 'delegate' to describe the process of working through others and the noun 'assignment' to describe what a person is directed to do (reflecting the common usage of language among nurses working in clinical settings)" (NCSBN, 2005, p. 174).

In 2006, the ANA and the NCSBN collaborated in their Joint Statement on Delegation and altered the definition of **assignment** to **"describes the distribution of work that each staff member is responsible for during a given shift or work period"** (ANA and NCSBN, 2006, p. 1). This "work plan" terminology is the definition of assignment used in this workbook, and it connotes the nursing leadership role of human resources deployment in a manner that most wisely promotes the patient's/family's preferred outcome.

Although states vary in their definitions of the functions and processes in professional nursing practice, including that of delegation, the authors use the NCSBN definition, including the caveat present in the sentence following the definition: **delegation** is **"transferring to a competent individual the authority to perform a selected nursing task in a selected situation. The nurse retains the accountability for the delegation"** (NCSBN, 1995, p. 2). Assignments are work plans; the nurse "assigns" or distributes work and also "delegates" nursing care as she or he works through others.

Delegation and Supervision

The definition of delegation alone offers some important clues to nursing practice and to the composition of an effective patient care team. The person who makes the decision to ask a person to do something (a task or assignment) must know that the chosen person is competent to perform that task. The RN selects the particular task, given his or her knowledge of the individual patient's condition and that particular circumstance. Because of the nurse's preparation, knowledge, and skill, the RN chooses to render judgments of this kind and stands by the choices made. According to licensure and statute, the nurse is obligated to delegate based on the unique situation, patients, and personnel involved, and to provide ongoing follow-up.

Supervision

Whenever a nurse delegates, he or she must also supervise. **Supervision** is defined by the NCSBN as **"the provision of guidance and direction, oversight, evaluation and follow up by the licensed nurse for accomplishment of a nursing task delegated to nursing assistive personnel"** (NCSBN, 2005, p. 194). The act of delegating is just the beginning of the RN's responsibility. As for the accountability of the delegatees (or persons given the task duty), these individuals are accountable for "[accepting] the delegation and for their own actions in carrying out the act" (NCSBN, 1995, p. 3). For example, nursing assistants who are unprepared or untrained to complete a task should say as much when asked and can then decline to perform that particular duty. In such a situation, the RN would determine whether to allocate time to train the assistive personnel and review the skill as it is learned, to delegate the task to another competent person, to do it herself or himself, or to make arrangements for later skill training. The ANA defines supervision as "the provision of guidance or direction, guiding, and influencing the outcome of an individual's performance of a task" (ANA and NCSBN, 2006, p. 1). In either definition, it is clear that the RN's job continues throughout the performance and results of task completion.

Scope of Practice for RNs, LPNs/LVNs, Unlicensed Assistive Personnel

Heretofore this text has discussed national recommendations for definitions. National trends suggest that nursing is moving toward standardized licensure through mutual recognition compacts and multistate licensure, and as of June 2013, 24 states had adopted the nurse license compact allowing a nurse in a member state to possess one state's license and practice in another member state, with six states pending (NCSBN, 2013). Standardized and multistate licensure supports electronic practice and promotes improved practice flexibility during the current nurse shortage. However, each RN must know his or her own state's regulations. Except for the 24 licensure compact participants, definitions still differ from state to state, as do regulations about the tasks that nursing assistants or other assistive personnel are allowed to perform in various settings.

For example, unlicensed assistive personnel (UAPs) are delegated tasks for which they have been trained and that they are currently competent to perform for stable patients in uncomplicated circumstances; these are routine, simple, repetitive, common activities not requiring nursing judgment, for example, activities of daily living, hygiene, feeding, and ambulation. Some states have generated statutes and/or rules that list specific tasks that can or cannot be delegated (NCSBN, 2005, pp. 178-179). However, trends indicate that more tasks will be delegated as research supports such delegation through evidence of positive outcomes. Nursing assistants in hospitals do not administer medications, whereas in some states, specially certified medication assistants administer oral medications in the community (group homes) and in some long-term care facilities. More states are employing specially trained nursing assistants as CMAs (Certified Medication Assistants) or MA-Cs (Medication Assistants-Certified) to administer routine, nonparenteral medications in long-term care or community settings with training as recommended by the NCSBN's Model Curriculum (NCSBN, 2007). In Washington State in 2008, a process was initiated to alter the statute and related administrative codes to allow trained nursing assistants in home or community-based settings, such as boarding homes or adult family homes, to administer insulin if the patient is an appropriate candidate (in a stable and predictable condition) and if the nursing assistant has been appropriately trained and supervised for the first 4 weeks of performing this task (Revised Code of Washington, 2012). In all states, nursing judgment is used to delegate tasks that fall within, but never exceed, the nurse's legal scope of practice, and an RN always makes decisions based on the individual patient situation. An RN may decide not to delegate the task of feeding a patient if the patient is dysphagic and the nursing assistant is not familiar with feeding techniques.

The scope of practice for LPNs (licensed practical nurses) or LVNs (licensed vocational nurses) also differs from state to state and is continually evolving. For example, in Texas and Colorado, LPNs have been prohibited from delegating nursing tasks; only RNs are allowed to delegate (Hansten and Jackson, 2009, p. 91). In 23 states in 2004 and in 28 states in 2005, LPNs were allowed to delegate, while in 33 states they were allowed to assign (NCSBN, 2005, pp. 112, 178-179). Although practicing nurses know that LPNs often review a patient's condition and perform data-gathering tasks such as observation and auscultation, RNs remain accountable for the total assessment of a patient, including synthesis and analysis of reported and reviewed information to lead care planning based on the nursing diagnosis. A large majority of 48 state board respondents (46 to 2) indicated that LPNs/LVNs were not allowed to develop plans of care independently, but many (14) commented that the LPN could contribute to the care plan (NCSBN, 2005, pp. 108-109). In their periodic review of actual practice by recent PN (practical nurse) test participants employed in hospitals, long-term care, and home health, in 2006 the NCSBN discovered that over three fourths of recent graduates contributed to development of the plan of care, almost 90% took verbal or telephone orders from physicians, approximately half administered or monitored IV piggyback medications, about 40% inserted nasogastric tubes, and about 30% had monitored blood transfusions (NCSBN, 2008, pp. 30-38). In an updated 2009 NCSBN survey of 1400 practicing LPNs, 85.4% assigned client care or related tasks to other LPNs or assistive personnel, and 81.2% supervised or evaluated activities of assistive personnel, with 65.8% working in long-term care settings (NCSBN, 2010, p. 35). IV therapy and administration of blood products or total parenteral nutrition (TPN) by LPNs/LVNs also vary widely. Even in states whose laws allow LPNs/LVNs to administer blood products, a given health care organization's policies or job descriptions may limit practice and place additional safeguards because of the life-threatening risk involved in the administration of blood products and other medications. The RN must know the job descriptions as well as the state regulations.

LPN/LVN practice continues to change rapidly, and in any state, tasks to support the assessment, planning, intervention, and evaluation phases of the nursing process can be allocated. However, the nursing process remains the responsibility of the RN. Also, the total nursing care of the patient rests squarely on the RN's shoulders, no matter

who is asked to perform care activities. To obtain more information about the statute and rules in a given state and to access decision trees and other helpful aides to delegation and supervision, visit the NCSBN website at http://www.ncsbn.org. The state practice act for each state is linked at that site.

ASSIGNMENT PROCESS

In current hospital environments, the process of assigning or creating a work plan is dependent on who is available, present, and accounted for, and what their roles and competencies are, for each shift. Assignment **"describes the distribution of work that each staff member is responsible for during a given shift or work period"** (ANA and NCSBN, 2006, p. 1). Classical care delivery models once known as *total patient care* have been transformed into a combination of team, functional, and primary care nursing, depending on the projected patient outcomes, the present state, and the available staff. Assignments must be created with knowledge of the following issues (Hansten and Jackson, 2009, pp. 207-208):

- How complex is the patients' required care?
- What are the dynamics of patients' status and their stability?
- How complex is the assessment and ongoing evaluation?
- What kind of infection control is necessary?
- Are there any individual safety precautions?
- Is there special technology involved in the care, and who is skilled in its use?
- How much supervision and oversight will be needed based on the staff's numbers and expertise?
- How available are the supervising RNs?
- How will the physical location of patients affect the time and availability of care?
- Can continuity of care be maintained?
- Are there any personal reasons to allocate duties for a particular patient, or are there nurse or patient preferences that should be taken into account? Factors such as staff difficulties with a particular diagnosis, patient preferences for an employee's care on a previous admission, or a staff member's need for a particular learning experience will be taken into account.
- Is there an acuity rating system that will help distribute care based on a point or number system?

For more information on care delivery modalities, refer to the texts by Hansten and Jackson (2009) and Alfaro-LeFevre (2013) listed in the References section. Whichever type of care delivery plan is chosen for each particular shift, the relationship with the patient and the results that the patient wants to achieve must be foremost, followed by the placing together of the right pieces in the form of competent team members, to compose the complete picture (Hansten, 2005a, 2008a).

DELEGATION AND ASSIGNMENT: THE FIVE RIGHTS

As you contemplate the questions in this workbook, you can use mnemonic devices to order your thinking process, such as the "Five Rights." The right task is assigned to the right person in the right circumstances. The RN then offers the right direction and communication, and the right supervision (Hansten and Jackson, 2009, pp. 205-206; NCSBN, 1995, pp. 2-3).

Right Circumstances

Recall the importance of the context in clinical decision making. Not only do rules and regulations adjust based on the area of practice (i.e., home health care, acute care, long-term care), but patient conditions and the preferred patient results must also be considered. If information is not available, a best judgment must be made. Often RNs must balance the need to know as much as possible and the time available to obtain the information. The instability of patients immediately postoperatively or in the intensive care unit (ICU) means that a student nurse will have to be closely supervised and partnered with an experienced RN. The questions in this workbook give direction as to context and offer hints to the circumstances.

For example, in long-term care skilled nursing facilities, LPNs/LVNs often function as "team leaders" with ongoing care planning and oversight by a smaller number of on-site RNs. Some emergency departments use paramedics, who may be regulated by the state emergency system statutes, in different roles in hospitals. Medical clinics often employ "medical assistants" who function under the direction and supervision of physicians. Community group homes, assisted living facilities, and other health care providers beyond acute care hospitals seek to create safe and effective care delivery systems for the growing number of older adults. Whatever the setting or circumstance, the nurse is accountable to know the laws and regulations that apply.

Right Task

Returning to the guideposts for navigating care, the patient's Four Ps (purpose, picture, plan, and part), the right task is a task that, in the nurse's best judgment, is one that can be safely delegated for this patient, given the patient's current condition (picture) and future preferred outcomes (purpose, picture), if the nurse has a competent individual to perform it. Although the RN may believe that he or she personally would be the best person to accomplish this task, the nurse must prioritize the best use of his or her time given a myriad of factors. "What other tasks and processes must I do because I am the only RN on this team? Which tasks can be delegated based on state

regulations and my thorough knowledge of job descriptions here in this facility? How skilled are the personnel working here today? Who else could be available to help if necessary?"

In its draft model language for nursing assistive personnel, the NCSBN lists criteria for determining nursing activities that can be delegated. The following are recommended for the nurse's consideration. It should be kept in mind that the nursing process and nursing judgment cannot be delegated.

- Knowledge and skills of the delegatee
- Verification of clinical competence by the employer
- Stability of the patient's condition
- Service setting variables such as available resources (including the nurse's accessibility) and methods of communication, complexity and frequency of care, and proximity and numbers of patients relative to staff

Assistive personnel are not to be allocated the duties of "ongoing assessment, interpretation, or decision making that cannot be logically separated from the procedures" (NCSBN, 2005, p. 197).

Right Person

Licensure, Certification, and Role Description

One of the most commonly voiced concerns during workshops with staff nurses across the nation is, "How can I trust the delegatees?" Knowing the licensure, role, and preparation of each member of the team is the first step in determining competency. What tasks does a PCT (patient care technician) perform in this facility? What is the role of an LPN/LVN? Are different levels of LPN/LVN designated here (LPN I or II)? Nearly 100 different titles for assistive personnel have been developed in care settings across the country. To effectively assign or delegate, the RN must know the role descriptions of co-workers as well as his or her own.

Strengths and Weaknesses

The personal strengths and weaknesses of usual team members are no mystery. Their skills are discovered through practice, positive and negative experiences, and an ever-present but unreliable rumor mill. An expert RN helps create better team results by using strengths in assigning personnel to exploit their gifts. The most compassionate team will work with the hospice patient and his or her family. The supervising nurse helps identify performance flaws and develops staff by providing judicious use of learning assignments. For example, a novice nursing assistant can be partnered with an experienced oncology RN during the assistant's first experiences with a terminally ill patient.

When working with students, float nurses, or other temporary personnel, nurses sometimes forget that the assigning RN has the duty to determine competency. Asking personnel about their previous experiences and about their understanding of the work duties, as well as pairing them with a strong unit staff member, is as essential as providing the ongoing support and supervision needed throughout the shift. If your mother was an ICU patient and her nurse was an inexperienced float from the rehabilitation unit, what level of leadership and direction would that nurse need from an experienced ICU RN? Many hospitals delegate only tasks, a functional form of assignment, to temporary personnel who are unfamiliar with the clinical area.

Right Direction and Communication

Now that the right staff member is being delegated the right task for each particular situation and setting, team members must find out what they need to do and how the tasks must be done. Relaying instructions about the plan for the shift or even for a specific task is not as simple as it seems. Some RNs believe that a written assignment board provides enough information to proceed because "everyone knows his or her job," whereas others spend copious amounts of time giving overly detailed directions to bored staff. The "Four Cs" of initial direction will help clarify the salient points of this process (Hansten and Jackson, 2009, pp. 287-288; 2012, pp. 299-300). Instructions and ongoing direction must be clear, concise, correct, and complete.

Clear communication is information that is understood by the listener. An ambiguous question such as "Can you get the new patient?" is not helpful when there are several new patients and returning surgical patients, and "getting" could mean transporting, admitting, or taking full responsibility for the care of the patient. Asking the delegatee to restate the instructions and work plan can be helpful to determine whether the communication is clear.

Concise statements are those that give enough but not too much additional information. The student nurse who merely wants to know how to turn on the chemical strip analyzer machine does not need a full treatise on the transit of potassium and glucose through the cell membrane. Too much or irrelevant information confuses the listener and wastes precious time.

Correct communication is that which is accurate and is aligned to rules, regulations, or job descriptions. Are the room number, patient name, and other identifiers correct? Are there two patients with similar last names? Can this task be delegated to this individual? Correct communication is not cloudy or confusing (Hansten and Jackson, 2009, pp. 287-288; 2012, p. 299).

Complete communication leaves no room for doubt on the part of supervisor or delegatees. Staff members often say, "I would do whatever the RNs want if they would just tell me what they want me to do and how to do it." Incomplete communication wins the top prize for creating team strife and substandard work. Assuming that staff "know" what to do and how to do it, along with what information to report and when, creates havoc, rework, and

frustration for patients and staff alike. Each staff member should have in mind a clear map or plan for the day, what to do and why, and what and when to report to the team leader. Parameters for reporting and the results that should be expected are often left in the team leader's brain rather than being discussed and spelled out in sufficient detail. RNs are accountable for clear, concise, correct, and complete initial and ongoing direction.

Right Supervision

Once prioritization, assignment, and delegation have been considered, determined, and communicated, the RN remains accountable for the total care of the patients throughout the tour of duty. Recall that the definition of **supervision** includes not only initial direction but also that "supervision is the active process of directing, guiding, and influencing the outcome of an individual's performance of a task. Similarly, NCSBN defines supervision as the provision of guidance or direction, oversight, evaluation and follow-up by the licensed nurse for the accomplishment of a delegated nursing task by assistive personnel" (ANA and NCSBN, 2006, p. 1). RNs may not actually perform each task of care, but they must oversee the ongoing progress and results obtained, reviewing staff performance. In a typical medical-surgical unit in an acute care facility, the RN can ensure optimal performance as the RN begins the shift by holding a short "second report" meeting with assistive personnel, outlining the day's plan and the plan for each patient, and giving initial direction at that time. Subsequent short team update or "checkpoint" meetings should be held before and after breaks and meals and before the end of the shift (Hansten, 2005b, 2008a, 2008b). During each short update, feedback is often offered and plans are altered. The last checkpoint presents all team members with an opportunity to give feedback to one another using the step-by-step feedback process (Hansten, 2008a, pp. 79-84; Hansten and Jackson, 2012, pp. 301-302). This step is often called the "debriefing" checkpoint or huddle, in which the team's processes are also examined. Questions such as "What would you recommend I do differently if we worked together tomorrow on the same group of patients? What can we do better as a team to help us navigate the patients toward their preferred results?" will help the team function more effectively in the future.

1. **The team member's input should be solicited first.** "I noted that the vital signs for the first four patients aren't yet on the electronic record. Do you know what's been done?" rather than "WHY haven't those vital signs been recorded yet?" At the end of the shift, the questions might be global, as in "How did we do today?" "What would you do differently if we had it to do over?" "What should I do differently tomorrow?"

2. **Credit should be given for all that has been accomplished.** "Oh, so you have the vital signs done but

they aren't recorded? Great, I'm so glad they are done so I can find out about Ms. Johnson's temperature before I call Dr. Smith." "You did a fantastic job with cleaning Mr. Orange after his incontinence episodes; his family is very appreciative of our respect for his dignity."

3. **Observations or concerns should be offered.** "The vital signs are routinely recorded on the EMR [electronic medical record] before patients are sent for surgery and procedures and before the doctor's round so that we can see the big picture of patients' progress before they leave the unit and to make sure they are stable for their procedures." Or, "I think I should have assigned another RN to Ms. Apple. I had no idea that your mother recently died of breast cancer."

4. **The delegatee should be asked for ideas on how to resolve the issue.** "What are your thoughts on how you could order your work to get the vital signs on the EMR before 8:30 AM?" Or, "What would you like to do with your work plan for tomorrow? Should we change Ms. Apple's team?"

5. **A course of action and plan for the future should be agreed upon.** "That sounds great. Practice use of the handheld computers today before you leave and that should resolve the issue. When we work together tomorrow, let me know whether that resolves the time issue for recording; if not, we will go to another plan." Or, "If you still feel that you want to stay with this assignment tomorrow after you've slept on it, we will keep it as is. If not, please let me know first thing tomorrow morning when you awaken so we can change all the assignments before the staff arrive."

PRACTICE BASED ON RESEARCH EVIDENCE

Rationale for Maximizing Nursing Leadership Skills at the Point of Care

If the skills presented in this book are used to save lives by providing care prioritized to attend to the most unstable patients first, optimally delegated to be delivered by the right personnel, and assigned using appropriate language with the most motivational and conscientious supervisory follow-up, then clinical outcomes should be optimal and work satisfaction should flourish. As stated in a 2008 article in *Nurse Leader*, "at this juncture we lack research evidence about the best use of personnel to multiply the RN's ability to remain vigilant over patient progress and avoid failures to rescue, but common sense would advise that better delegation and supervision skills would prevent errors and omissions as well as unobserved patient decline" (Hansten, 2008b).

In an era of value-based purchasing and health care reimbursement based on clinical results, an RN's accountability has irrevocably moved beyond task orientation to leadership practices that ensure better outcomes for patients, families, and populations. The necessity of efficiency and effectiveness in health care means that RNs must delegate and supervise appropriately so that all tasks that can be safely assigned to UAPs are completed flawlessly. Nurses are accountable for processes as well as outcomes measures so that insurers will reimburse health care organizations. If hospital-acquired conditions (HACs) occur, such as pressure ulcers, falls with injury, and some infections, reimbursement for the care of that condition will be negatively impacted.

- Nurses spend from 10% to 25% of their shifts looking for other staff members (Tucker and Spear, 2006). Better initial direction and a plan for supervision during the day decreases time wasted in attempting to connect with team members. At one facility in the Midwest, shift hand-offs were reduced to 10 to 15 minutes per shift per RN as a result of a planned approach to initial direction and care planning, which thus saved each RN 30 to 45 minutes per day (Hansten, 2008a, p. 34). Better use of nursing and UAP time can result in more time to care for patients, giving RNs the opportunity to teach patients self-care or to maintain functional status.
- When nurses did not appropriately implement the Five Rights of delegation and supervision with assistive personnel, errors occurred that potentially could have been avoided with better RN leadership behaviors. About 14% of task errors or care omissions related to teamwork were due to lack of RN direction or communication, and approximately 12% of the issues stemmed from lack of supervision or follow-up (Standing, Anthony, and Hertz, 2001). Errors can result in uncompensated conditions or readmissions, unhappy patients and providers, disgruntled health care purchasers, and a disloyal, anxious patient community.
- Teamwork and job satisfaction have been found to be negatively correlated with over-delegation and a hierarchical relationship between nurses and assistive personnel (Kalisch and Begeny, 2005), whereas offering feedback effectively has been shown to improve team thinking and performance (Kozlowski and Ilgen, 2007). When staff in a long-term care facility were able to connect their work with personal purposes and patient results, there was a 23% increase in teamwork, a 10% jump in job satisfaction, a 17% increase in morale, and a $12,000 drop in absenteeism costs (Kinjerski and Skrypnek, 2008). Best practices for deployment of personnel include a connection to patient outcomes, which can occur during initial direction and debriefing supervision checkpoints.
- Unplanned readmissions to acute care within 30 days of discharge are linked to potential penalties and reduced reimbursement. Inadequate RN initial direction and

supervision of UAPs can lead to missed mobilization, hydration, and nutrition of patients, thereby discharging deconditioned patients, and can be traced to emergency department visits and subsequent readmissions.

- As public quality transparency and competition for best value becomes the norm, ineffective delegation has been a significant source of missed care, such as lack of care planning, lack of turning or ambulation, delayed or missed nutrition, and lack of hygiene (Bittner et al., 2011; Kalisch, 2006). These care omissions can be contributing factors for the occurrence of unreimbursed "never events" (events that should never occur) such as pressure ulcers and pneumonia, as well as prolonged lengths of stay. Other nurse-sensitive quality indicators such as catheter-associated urinary tract infections (CAUTIs) could be correlated to omitted perineal hygiene and inattention to discontinuation of catheters.

Evidence does indicate that appropriate nursing judgment in prioritization, delegation, and supervision can save time and improve communication, and thereby improve care, clinical outcomes, and job satisfaction, potentially saving patient-days and absenteeism and recruitment costs. Patient satisfaction, staff satisfaction, and clinical results decline when nursing care is poor. Potential reimbursement is lost, patients and families suffer, and the health of our communities decays when RNs do not assume the leadership necessary to work effectively with all team members (Bittner et al., 2011.)

PRINCIPLES FOR IMPLEMENTATION OF PRIORITIZATION, DELEGATION, AND ASSIGNMENT

Return to our goalposts of the Four Ps (purpose, picture, plan, and part) as a framework as you answer the questions in this workbook and further develop your own expertise, and recall the following principles:

- The RN should always start with the patient's and family's preferred outcomes in mind. The RN is first clear about the patient's purpose for accessing care and his or her picture for a successful outcome.
- The RN should refer to the applicable state nursing practice statute and rules as well as the organization's job descriptions for current information about roles and responsibilities of RNs, LPNs/LVNs, and UAPs. (These are the roles or the part that people play.)
- Student nurses, novices, float nurses, and other infrequent workers will also require variable levels of supervision, guidance, or support. (The workers' abilities and roles become a piece of the plan [Hansten and Jackson, 2009, pp. 52-55].)
- The RN is accountable for nursing judgment decisions and for ongoing supervision of any care that is delegated or assigned.

- The RN cannot delegate the nursing process (in particular the assessment, planning, and evaluation phases) or clinical judgment to a non-RN. Some interventions or data-gathering activities may be delegated based on the circumstances.
- The RN must know as much as practical about the patients and their conditions, as well as the skills and competency of team members, to prioritize, delegate, and assign. Decisions must be specifically individualized to the patient, the delegatees, and the situation.
- In a clinical situation, everything is fluid and shifting. No priority, assignment, or delegation is written indelibly and cannot be altered. The RN in charge of a unit, a team, or one patient is accountable to choose the best course to achieve the patient's and family's preferred results.

Good luck in completing the workbook! The authors invite you to use the questions as an exercise in assembling the pieces to the puzzle that will become a picture of health-promoting practice.

REFERENCES

Alfaro-Lefevre R: *Critical thinking, clinical reasoning, and clinical judgment: a practical approach,* ed 5, St Louis, 2013, Saunders.

American Nurses Association, National Council of State Boards of Nursing: *Joint statement on delegation,* 2006, retrieved May 31, 2012, from http://www.ncsbn.org/joint_statement/pdf.

Bittner N, Gravlin G, Hansten R, Kalisch B: Unraveling care omissions, *J Nurs Adm* 41(12):510–512, 2011.

Hansten R: Relationships and results: solid patient relationships can improve clinical outcomes, *Healthc Exec* 20(4):34–35, 2005a.

Hansten R: Relationship and results-oriented healthcare: evaluate the basics, *J Nurs Adm* 35(12):522–524, 2005b.

Hansten R: *Leadership at the point of care: nursing delegation,* 2011, retrieved May 31, 2012, from http://www.MyFreeCE.com.

Hansten R: *Relationship and results oriented healthcare™ planning and implementation manual,* Port Ludlow, Wash, 2008a, Hansten Healthcare PLLC.

Hansten R: Why nurses still must learn to delegate, *Nurse Leader* 6(5):19–26, 2008b.

Hansten R, Jackson M: *Clinical delegation skills: a handbook for professional practice,* ed 4, Sudbury, Mass, 2009, Jones & Bartlett.

Hansten R, Jackson M: Delegation in the clinical setting. In Zerwekh J, Claborn J, editors: *Nursing today: transitions and trends,* ed 7, St Louis, 2012, Elsevier.

Kalisch B: Missed nursing care, *J Nurs Care Qual* 21(4):306–313, 2006.

Kalisch B, Begeny S: Improving nursing unit teamwork, *J Nurs Adm* 35(12):550–556, 2005.

Kinjerski V, Skrypnek B: The promise of spirit at work, *J Gerontol Nurs* 34(10):17–25, 2008.

Kozlowski S, Ilgen D: The science of team success, *Sci Am Mind,* June-July:54–61, 2007.

National Council of State Boards of Nursing: Delegation: concepts and decision-making process, *Issues,* December:1–4, 1995.

National Council of State Boards of Nursing: *NCSBN Model Nurse Practice Act*, 2004, Article III, Section 4C, retrieved August 8, 2005, from http://www.ncsbn.org/regulation/nursing.

National Council of State Boards of Nursing: *Business book: NCSBN annual meeting: mission possible: building a safer nursing workforce through regulatory excellence*, 2005, retrieved August 12, 2005, from http://www.ncsbn.org/pdfs/V_Business_Book_Section_I.pdf.

National Council of State Boards of Nursing: *Medication assistant model curriculum*, 2007, retrieved May 31, 2012, from https://www.ncsbn.org/07_Final_MAC.pdf.

National Council of State Boards of Nursing: Report of findings from the 2006 LPN/VN practice analysis comparability of survey administration methods, *Research Brief* (Vol 33), Chicago, 2008, The Council.

National Council of State Boards of Nursing: 2009 LPN/VN practice analysis: linking the NCLEX-PN® examination to practice, March 2010, *Research Brief* (Vol 44), retrieved May 31, 2012, from https://www.ncsbn.org/10_LPN_VN_PracticeAnalysis_Vol44_web.pdf.

National Council of State Boards of Nursing: *Participating states in the nurse licensure compact implementation*, 2013, retrieved June 24, 2013, from https://www.ncsbn.org/2538.htm.

Revised Code of Washington, Title 18, Chapter 18.79, Section 18.79.260, Registered nurse—activities allowed—delegation of tasks, 2008, retrieved May 31, 2012, from http://apps.leg.wa.gov/RCW/default.aspx?cite=18.79.260.

Silvestri L: *Saunders comprehensive review for the NCLEX-RN® Examination*, ed 5, St Louis, 2011, Saunders.

Standing T, Anthony M, Hertz J: Nurses' narratives of outcomes after delegation to unlicensed assistive personnel, *Outcomes Manag Nurs Pract* 5(1):18–23, 2001.

Tucker A, Spear S: Operational failures and interruptions in hospital nursing, *Health Serv Res* 41(3 Pt 1):643–662, 2006.

RECOMMENDED RESOURCES

Alfaro-Lefevre R: *Critical thinking, clinical reasoning, and clinical judgment: a practical approach*, ed 5, St Louis, 2013, Saunders.

Hansten R: *Relationship and results oriented healthcare™ planning and implementation manual*, Port Ludlow, Wash, 2008, Hansten Healthcare PLLC.

Hansten R, Jackson M: *Clinical delegation skills: a handbook for professional practice*, ed 4, Sudbury, Mass, 2009, Jones & Bartlett.

Hansten Healthcare PLLC website, http://www.Hansten.com or www.RROHC.com. Check for new delegation/supervision resources.

National Council of State Boards of Nursing website, http://www.ncsbn.org. Contains links to state boards and abundant resources relating to delegation and supervision. Also download the ANA and NCSBN Joint Statement on Delegation. The decision trees and step-by-step process through the Five Rights is exceptionally clear and a great review to prepare for the NCLEX.

CHAPTER 1

Pain

20/29 68%

1. You are the charge nurse. A client with chronic pain reports to you that the nurses have not been responding to requests for pain medication. What is your initial action?
   1. Check the medication administration records (MARs) for the past several days.
   2. Ask the nurse educator to provide in-service training about pain management.
   3. Perform a complete pain assessment on the client and take a pain history.
   4. Have a conference with the nurses responsible for the care of this client.

2. Family members are encouraging your client to "tough out the pain" rather than risk drug addiction to narcotics. The client is stoically abiding. You recognize that the sociocultural dimension of pain is the current priority for the client. Which question will you ask?
   1. "Where is the pain located, and does it radiate to other parts of your body?"
   2. "How would you describe the pain, and how is it affecting you?"
   3. "What do you believe about pain medication and drug addiction?"
   4. "How is the pain affecting your activity level and your ability to function?"
   5. "What information do you need about pain, healing, and addiction?"

3. A client with diabetic neuropathy reports a burning, electrical-type pain in the lower extremities that is worse at night and not responding to nonsteroidal anti-inflammatory drugs. Which medication will you advocate for first?
   1. Gabapentin (Neurontin) *for diabetic neuro pathy.*
   2. Corticosteroids
   3. Hydromorphone (Dilaudid)
   4. Lorazepam (Ativan)

4. Which client is most likely to receive opioids for extended periods of time?
   1. A client with fibromyalgia *non opioid*
   2. A client with phantom limb pain in the leg *Anti sz*
   3. A client with progressive pancreatic cancer
   4. A client with trigeminal neuralgia *Anti sz*

5. As the charge nurse, you are reviewing the charts of clients who were assigned to the care of a newly graduated RN. The RN has correctly charted dose and time of medication, but there is no documentation regarding nonpharmaceutical measures. What action should you take first?
   1. Make a note in the nurse's file and continue to observe clinical performance.
   2. Refer the new nurse to the in-service education department.
   3. Quiz the nurse about knowledge of pain management and pharmacology.
   4. Give praise for correctly charting the dose and time and discuss the deficits in charting.

6. Which clients must be assigned to an experienced RN? *(Select all that apply.)*
   1. Client who was in an automobile crash and sustained multiple injuries
   2. Client with chronic back pain related to a workplace injury
   3. Client who has returned from surgery and has a chest tube in place
   4. Client with abdominal cramps related to food poisoning
   5. Client with a severe headache of unknown origin
   6. Client with chest pain who has a history of arteriosclerosis

7. In application of the principles of pain treatment, what is the first consideration?
   1. Treatment is based on client goals.
   2. A multidisciplinary approach is needed.
   3. The client's perception of pain must be accepted.
   4. Drug side effects must be prevented and managed.

8. Which client has the most immediate need for IV access to deliver immediate analgesia with rapid titration?
   1. Client who has sharp chest pain that increases with cough and shortness of breath
   2. Client who reports excruciating lower back pain with hematuria
   3. Client who is having an acute myocardial infarction with severe chest pain
   4. Client who is having a severe migraine with an elevated blood pressure

Common Health Scenarios

PART 2

9. When an analgesic is titrated to manage pain, what is the priority goal?
   1. Titrate to the smallest dose that provides relief with the fewest side effects.
   2. Titrate upward until the client is pain free.
   3. Titrate downward to prevent toxicity.
   4. Titrate to a dosage that is adequate to meet the client's subjective needs.

10. For client education about nonpharmaceutical alternatives, which topic could you delegate to an experienced LPN/LVN, who will function with your continued support and supervision?
   1. Therapeutic touch
   2. Application of heat and cold
   3. Meditation
   4. Transcutaneous electrical nerve stimulation (TENS)

11. A client received "as needed" (PRN) morphine, lorazepam (Ativan), and cyclobenzaprine (Flexeril). The UAP reports that the client has a respiratory rate of 10/min. What is the priority action?
   1. Call the physician to obtain an order for naloxone (Narcan).
   2. Assess the client's responsiveness and respiratory status.
   3. Obtain a bag-valve mask and deliver breaths at 20/min.
   4. Double-check the drug order to see what the client should have received.

12. Which client is at greatest risk for respiratory depression while receiving opioids for analgesia?
   1. Elderly client with chronic pain who has a hip fracture
   2. Client with a heroin addiction and back pain
   3. Young female client with advanced multiple myeloma
   4. Child with an arm fracture and cystic fibrosis

13. A client is crying and grimacing but denies pain and refuses pain medication, because "my sibling is a drug addict and has ruined our lives." What is the priority intervention for this client?
   1. Encourage expression of fears and past experiences.
   2. Provide accurate information about the use of pain medication.
   3. Explain that addiction is unlikely among acute care clients.
   4. Seek family assistance in resolving this problem.

14. A client's opioid therapy is being tapered off, and the nurse is watchful for signs of withdrawal. What is one of the first signs of withdrawal?
   1. Fever
   2. Nausea
   3. Diaphoresis
   4. Abdominal cramps

15. In the care of clients with pain and discomfort, which task is most appropriate to delegate to the UAP?
   1. Assisting the client with preparation of a sitz bath
   2. Monitoring the client for signs of discomfort while ambulating
   3. Coaching the client to deep breathe during painful procedures
   4. Evaluating relief after applying a cold compress

16. The physician has ordered a placebo for a client with chronic pain. You are a newly hired nurse and you feel very uncomfortable administering the medication. What is the first action that you should take?
   1. Prepare the medication and hand it to the physician.
   2. Check the hospital policy regarding the use of a placebo.
   3. Follow a personal code of ethics and refuse to participate.
   4. Contact the charge nurse for advice.

17. For a cognitively impaired client who cannot accurately report pain, what is the first action that you should take?
   1. Closely assess for nonverbal signs such as grimacing or rocking.
   2. Obtain baseline behavioral indicators from family members.
   3. Look at the MAR and chart to note the time of the last dose of analgesic and the client's response.
   4. Give the maximum PRN dose within the minimum time frame for relief.

18. You have received the shift report from the night nurse. Prioritize the order in which you will check on the following clients.
   1. Adolescent who is alert and oriented. He was admitted 2 days ago for treatment of meningitis. He reports a continuous headache that is partially relieved by medication.
   2. Elderly man who underwent total knee replacement surgery 2 days ago. He is using the patient-controlled analgesia (PCA) pump frequently with good relief and occasionally asks for bolus doses.
   3. Middle-aged woman who is demanding and needy. She was admitted for investigation of functional abdominal pain and is scheduled for diagnostic testing this morning.
   4. Elderly woman with advanced Alzheimer disease who requires total care for all activities of daily living (ADLs). She struggles during any type of nursing care and it is difficult to assess her subjective symptoms. She is awaiting transfer to a long-term care facility.
   5. Young man who was admitted with chest pain secondary to a spontaneous pneumothorax. His chest tube will be removed and his PCA pump discontinued today. ____, ____, ____, ____, ____

19. On the first day after surgery, a client receiving an analgesic via PCA pump reports that the pain control is inadequate. What is the first action you should take?
    1. Deliver the bolus dose per standing order.
    2. Contact the physician to increase the dose.
    3. Try nonpharmacologic comfort measures.
    4. Assess the pain for location, quality, and intensity.

20. The team is providing emergency care to a client who received an excessive dose of narcotic pain medication. Which task is best to delegate to the LPN/LVN?
    1. Calling the physician and reporting the situation using the SBAR (situation, background, assessment, recommendation) format
    2. Giving the ordered dose of Narcan and evaluating the response to therapy
    3. Monitoring the respiratory status for the first 30 minutes
    4. Applying oxygen per nasal cannula as ordered

21. What is the best way to schedule medication for a client with constant pain?
    1. PRN at the client's request
    2. Before painful procedures
    3. IV bolus after pain assessment
    4. Around the clock

22. Which clients can be appropriately assigned to an LPN/LVN who will function under the supervision of an RN or team leader? *(Select all that apply.)*
    1. Client who needs preoperative teaching for the use of a PCA pump
    2. Client with a leg cast who needs neurologic and circulatory checks and PRN hydrocodone
    3. Client who underwent a toe amputation and has diabetic neuropathic pain
    4. Client with terminal cancer and severe pain who is refusing medication
    5. Client who reports abdominal pain after being kicked, punched, and beaten
    6. Client with arthritis who needs scheduled pain medications and heat applications

23. You are caring for a client who had abdominal surgery yesterday. The client is restless and anxious and tells you that the pain is getting worse despite the pain medication. Physical assessment findings include the following: temperature, 100.3° F (38° C); pulse rate, 110 beats/min; respiratory rate, 24 breaths/min; and blood pressure, 140/90 mm Hg. The abdomen is rigid and tender to the touch. You decide to notify the client's provider. Place the following report information in the correct order according to the SBAR format.
    1. "He is restless and anxious: temperature is 100.3° F (38° C); pulse is 110 beats/min; respiratory rate is 24 breaths/min; blood pressure is 140/90 mm Hg. Abdomen is rigid and tender to touch with hypoactive bowel sounds."
    2. "He had abdominal surgery yesterday. He is on PCA morphine, but he says the pain is getting progressively worse."
    3. "I have tried to make him comfortable and he is willing to wait until the next scheduled dose of pain medication, but I think his pain warrants evaluation."
    4. "Would you like to give me an order for any laboratory tests or additional therapies at this time?"
    5. "Dr. S, this is Nurse J. I'm calling about Mr. D, who is reporting severe abdominal pain." 5, 2, 1, 3, 4

24. Which clients can be appropriately assigned to a newly graduated RN who has recently completed orientation? *(Select all that apply.)*
    1. Anxious client with chronic pain who frequently uses the call button
    2. Client on the second postoperative day who needs pain medication before dressing changes
    3. Client with human immunodeficiency virus (HIV) infection who reports headache and abdominal and pleuritic chest pain
    4. Client with chronic pain who is to be discharged with a new surgically-implanted catheter
    5. Client who is reporting pain at the site of a peripheral IV line
    6. Client with a kidney stone who needs frequent PRN pain medication

PART 2 Common Health Scenarios

25. A client's family member says to you, "He needs more pain medicine. He is still having a lot of pain." What is your best response?
    1. "The physician ordered the medicine to be given every 4 hours."
    2. "If the medication is given too frequently, he could experience ill effects."
    3. "Please tell him that I will be right there to check on him."
    4. "Let's wait about 30 to 40 minutes. If there is no relief, I'll call the physician."

26. Pain disorder and depression have been diagnosed for a client. He reports chronic low back pain and states, "None of these doctors has done anything to help." Which client statement concerns you the most?
    1. "I twisted my back last night, and now the pain is a lot worse."
    2. "I'm so sick of this pain. I think I'm going to find a way to end it."
    3. "Occasionally I buy pain killers from a guy in my neighborhood."
    4. "I'm going to sue you and the doctor; you aren't doing anything for me."

27. A client has severe pain and bladder distention related to urinary retention and possible obstruction. An experienced UAP states that she received training in Foley catheter insertion at a previous job. What task can be delegated to this UAP?
    1. Assessing the bladder distention and the pain associated with urinary retention
    2. Inserting the Foley catheter, once you ascertain that she knows sterile technique
    3. Evaluating the relief of pain and bladder distention after the catheter is inserted
    4. Measuring the urine output after the catheter is inserted and obtaining a urine specimen

28. You are caring for a young man with a history of substance abuse who had exploratory abdominal surgery 4 days ago for a knife wound. There is an order to discontinue the PCA-delivered morphine and to start oral pain medication. The client begs, "Please don't stop the morphine. My pain is really a lot worse today than it was yesterday." What is the best response?
    1. "Let me stop the pump and we can try oral pain medication to see if it relieves the pain."
    2. "I realize that you are scared of the pain, but we must try to wean you off the pump."
    3. "Show me where your pain is and describe how it feels compared to yesterday."
    4. "Let me take your vital signs, and then I will call the physician and explain your concerns."

29. You are caring for a young client with diabetes who has sustained injuries when she tried to commit suicide by crashing her car. Her blood glucose level is 650 mg/dL, but she refuses insulin; however, she wants the pain medication. What is the best action?
    1. Notify the charge nurse and obtain an order for a transfer to intensive care.
    2. Explain that insulin is a priority and inform the health care provider.
    3. Withhold the pain medication until she agrees to accept the insulin.
    4. Give her the pain medication and document the refusal of the insulin.

Answer Key for this chapter begins on p. 167.

CHAPTER 2

Cancer

1. You are caring for a patient with esophageal cancer. Which task could be delegated to a UAP?
   1. Assisting the patient with oral hygiene
   2. Observing the patient's response to feedings
   3. Facilitating expression of grief or anxiety
   4. Initiating daily weighings

2. A 56-year-old patient comes to the walk-in clinic reporting scant rectal bleeding and intermittent diarrhea and constipation for the past several months. There is a history of polyps and a family history of colorectal cancer. While you are trying to teach about colonoscopy, the patient becomes angry and threatens to leave. What is the priority diagnosis?
   1. Diarrhea/Constipation related to altered bowel patterns
   2. Deficient Knowledge related to the disease process and diagnostic procedure
   3. Risk for Deficient Fluid Volume related to rectal bleeding and diarrhea
   4. Anxiety related to unknown outcomes and perceived threats to body integrity

3. Which patient is at greatest risk for pancreatic cancer?
   1. An elderly African-American man who smokes
   2. A young white obese woman with gallbladder disease
   3. A young African-American man with type 1 diabetes
   4. An elderly white woman who has pancreatitis

4. Patients receiving chemotherapy are at risk for thrombocytopenia related to chemotherapy or disease processes. Which actions are needed for patients who must be placed on bleeding precautions? *(Select all that apply.)*
   1. Provide mouthwash with alcohol for oral rinsing.
   2. Use paper tape on fragile skin.
   3. Provide a soft toothbrush or oral sponge.
   4. Gently insert rectal suppositories.
   5. Avoid aspirin or aspirin-containing products.
   6. Avoid overinflation of blood pressure cuffs.
   7. Pad sharp corners of furniture.

5. When care assignments are being made for patients with alterations related to gastrointestinal (GI) cancer, which patient would be the most appropriate to assign to an LPN/LVN under the supervision of a team leader RN?
   1. A patient with severe anemia secondary to GI bleeding
   2. A patient who needs enemas and antibiotics to control GI bacteria
   3. A patient who needs preoperative teaching for bowel resection surgery
   4. A patient who needs central line insertion for chemotherapy

6. A community health center is preparing a presentation on the prevention and detection of cancer. Which health care professional (RN, LPN/LVN, nurse practitioner, nutritionist) should be assigned responsibility for the following tasks?
   1. Explain screening examinations and diagnostic testing for common cancers. ___RN___ NP
   2. Discuss how to plan a balanced diet and reduce fats and preservatives. ___nutr___ nut
   3. Prepare a poster on the seven warning signs of cancer. ___LPN___ LPN
   4. Discuss how to perform breast or testicular self-examinations. ___RN___ NP
   5. Describe strategies for reducing risk factors such as smoking and obesity. ___RN___

7. The physician tells the patient with cancer that there will be an initial course of treatment with continued maintenance treatments and ongoing observation for signs and symptoms over a prolonged period of time. Which patient statement would concern you the most?
   1. "My symptoms will eventually be cured; I'm so happy that I don't have to worry any longer."
   2. "My doctor is trying to help me control the symptoms; I am grateful for the extension of time with my family."
   3. "My pain will be relieved, but I am going to die soon; I would like to have control over my own life and death."
   4. "Initially, I may have to take some time off of work for my treatments; I can probably work full time in the future."

8. For a patient who is experiencing side effects of radiation therapy, which task would be the most appropriate to delegate to the UAP?
   1. Helping the patient to identify patterns of fatigue
   2. Recommending participation in a walking program
   3. Reporting the amount and type of food consumed from the tray
   4. Checking the skin for redness and irritation after the treatment

9. For a patient receiving the chemotherapeutic drug vincristine (Oncovin), which side effects should be reported to the physician?
   1. Fatigue
   2. Nausea and vomiting
   3. Paresthesia
   4. Anorexia

10. For a patient who is receiving chemotherapy, which laboratory result is of particular importance?
   1. White blood cell (WBC) count
   2. Prothrombin time and partial thromboplastin time
   3. Electrolyte levels
   4. Blood urea nitrogen level

11. For care of a patient who has oral cancer, which task would be appropriate to delegate to an LPN/LVN?
   1. Assisting the patient to brush and floss
   2. Explaining when brushing and flossing are contraindicated
   3. Giving antacids and sucralfate suspension as ordered
   4. Recommending saliva substitutes

12. When staff assignments are made for the care of patients who are receiving chemotherapy, what is the major consideration regarding chemotherapeutic drugs?
   1. During preparation, drugs may be absorbed through the skin or inhaled.
   2. Many chemotherapeutic drugs are vesicants.
   3. Chemotherapeutic drugs are frequently given through central venous access devices.
   4. Oral and venous routes of administration are the most common.

13. You have just received the morning report from the night shift nurse. List the order of priority for assessing and caring for the following patients.
   1. A patient who developed tumor lysis syndrome around 5:00 AM
   2. A patient with frequent reports of breakthrough pain over the past 24 hours
   3. A patient scheduled for exploratory laparotomy this morning
   4. A patient with anticipatory nausea and vomiting for the past 24 hours _____, _____, _____, _____

14. You are monitoring your patient who is at risk for spinal cord compression related to tumor growth. Which patient statement is most likely to suggest an early manifestation?
   1. "Last night my back really hurt, and I had trouble sleeping."
   2. "My leg has been giving out when I try to stand."
   3. "My bowels are just not moving like they usually do."
   4. "When I try to pass urine, I have difficulty starting the stream."

15. You are caring for an older woman with hepatic cancer. The UAP informs you that the patient's level of consciousness is diminished compared to earlier in the shift. Prioritize the steps of assessment and intervention related to this patient's change of mental status.
   1. Take vital signs, including pulse, respirations, blood pressure, and temperature.
   2. Check responsiveness and level of consciousness.
   3. Obtain a blood glucose reading.
   4. Check electrolyte values.
   5. Check ammonia level.
   6. Check the patency of existing IV lines.
   7. Administer oxygen if needed and check pulse oximeter readings. _____, _____, _____, _____, _____, _____, _____

16. Which members of the health care team (advanced practice nurse, MD, RN, LPN/LVN) should perform the tasks related to care of patients who are at risk for breast cancer? *(There may be more than one professional who could complete the task.)*
   1. Perform the clinical breast examination. _____

   2. Teach about breast self-examination. _____

   3. Make a nursing diagnosis based on the assessment data. _____

   4. Assess the patient's belief about and use of complementary and alternative therapies. _____

   5. Reinforce the importance of a baseline screening mammogram starting at age 40. _____

   6. Explain the results of the mammogram to the patient. _____

17. For a patient with osteogenic sarcoma, which laboratory value causes you the most concern?
   1. Sodium level of 135 mEq/L
   2. Calcium level of 13 mg/dL
   3. Potassium level of 4.9 mEq/L
   4. Hematocrit of 40%

18. Which two cancer patients could potentially be placed together as roommates?
    1. A patient with a neutrophil count of 1000/mm³
    2. A patient who underwent debulking of a tumor to relieve pressure
    3. A patient who just underwent a bone marrow transplantation
    4. A patient who has undergone laminectomy for spinal cord compression _____, _____

19. An athletic young man was recently diagnosed with Ewing sarcoma. He has pain, low-grade fever, and anemia. The surgeon recommends amputation of the right lower leg for an operable tumor. The patient tells you he is leaving the hospital to go on a long hiking trip. What is the priority nursing diagnosis?
    1. Acute Pain related to tumor invasion of soft tissue
    2. Fatigue related to anemia
    3. Ineffective Coping related to loss of body image
    4. Noncompliance related to personal values

20. Following chemotherapy, a patient is being closely monitored for tumor lysis syndrome. Which laboratory value requires particular attention?
    1. Platelet count
    2. Electrolyte levels
    3. Hemoglobin level
    4. Hematocrit

21. People at risk are the target populations for cancer screening programs. Which of these asymptomatic patients need extra encouragement to participate in cancer screening? *(Select all that apply.)*
    1. A 21-year-old white American woman who is sexually inactive, for a Pap test
    2. A 30-year-old Asian-American woman, for an annual mammogram
    3. A 45-year-old African-American man, for a prostate-specific antigen test
    4. A 50-year-old African-American man, for a fecal occult blood test
    5. A 50-year-old white American woman, for a colonoscopy
    6. A 70-year-old Asian-American woman with normal results on three previous Pap tests, for a Pap test

22. A patient with lung cancer develops syndrome of inappropriate antidiuretic hormone secretion (SIADH). After reporting symptoms of weight gain, weakness, and nausea and vomiting to the physician, you would anticipate which initial order for the treatment of this patient?
    1. A fluid bolus
    2. Fluid restrictions
    3. Urinalysis
    4. Sodium-restricted diet

23. In the care of a patient with neutropenia, what tasks can be delegated to a UAP? *(Select all that apply.)*
    1. Taking vital signs every 4 hours
    2. Reporting temperature of more than 100.4° F (38° C)
    3. Assessing for sore throat, cough, or burning with urination
    4. Gathering the supplies to prepare the room for protective isolation
    5. Reporting superinfections, such as candidiasis
    6. Practicing good hand-washing technique

24. A primary nursing responsibility is the prevention of lung cancer by assisting patients in cessation of smoking or other tobacco use. Which task would be appropriate to delegate to an LPN/LVN?
    1. Development of a "quit plan"
    2. Explanation of how to apply a nicotine patch
    3. Discussion of strategies to avoid relapse
    4. Suggestion of ways to deal with urges for tobacco

25. You are providing end-of-life-care for a patient with terminal liver cancer. The patient is weak and restless. Her skin is cool and mottled. Dyspnea develops and the patient appears anxious and frightened. What should you do?
    1. Obtain an order for morphine elixir.
    2. Alert the rapid response team and call the physician for orders.
    3. Deliver breaths at 20/min with a bag-valve mask and prepare for intubation.
    4. Sit quietly with the patient and offer emotional support and comfort.

26. You are asked to float to a different nursing unit. During report, you are told that the patient is receiving IV administration of vincristine (Oncovin) that should be completed within the next 15 minutes. The IV site is intact, and the patient is not having any problems with the infusion. You are not certified in chemotherapy administration. What is your priority action?
    1. Ask the nurse to stay until the infusion is finished, because you are not certified.
    2. Assess the IV site; check the progress of the infusion and the patient's condition.
    3. Contact the charge nurse and explain that you are not chemotherapy certified.
    4. Look up drug side effects and monitor, because the infusion is almost complete.

PART 2 Common Health Scenarios

27. You are caring for a patient with uterine cancer who is being treated with intracavitary radiation therapy. The UAP reports that the patient insisted on ambulating to the bathroom and now "something feels like it is coming out." What is the priority action?
    1. Assess the UAP's knowledge; explain the rationale for strict bed rest.
    2. Assess for dislodgment; use forceps to retrieve and a lead container to store as needed.
    3. Assess the patient's knowledge of the treatment plan and her willingness to participate.
    4. Notify the physician about the potential or confirmed dislodgment of the radiation implant.

28. You are the charge nurse. Two hours into the shift you discover that two nurses have switched patients because Nurse A does "not like to take care of patients with prostate cancer." Which action should you take first?
    1. Insist that they switch back to the original patient assignments and talk to each of them at the end of the shift.
    2. Allow them this flexibility; as long as the patients are well cared for it doesn't matter if the assignments are changed.
    3. Ask Nurse A to explain her position regarding prostate cancer patients and seek alternatives to prevent future issues.
    4. Explain to Nurse A and B that all patients deserve kindness and care regardless of their condition or the nurses' personal feelings.

Answer Key for this chapter begins on p. 169.

CHAPTER 3

Immunologic Problems

1. A few minutes after you have given an intradermal injection of an allergen to a patient who is undergoing skin testing for allergies, the patient reports feeling anxious, short of breath, and dizzy. Which action included in the emergency protocol should you take first?
   1. Start oxygen at 4 L/min using a nasal cannula.
   2. Obtain IV access with a large-bore IV catheter.
   3. Give epinephrine (Adrenalin) 0.3 mL intramuscularly.
   4. Administer 3 mL of nebulized albuterol (Proventil) 0.083%.

2. As the nurse manager in a public health department, you are implementing a plan to reduce the incidence of infection with human immunodeficiency virus (HIV) in the community. Which nursing action will you delegate to health assistants working for the agency?
   1. Supplying injection drug users with sterile injection equipment such as needles and syringes
   2. Interviewing patients about behaviors that indicate a need for annual HIV testing
   3. Teaching high-risk community members about the use of condoms in preventing HIV infection
   4. Assessing the community to determine which population groups to target for education

3. You are working with a student nurse to care for an HIV-positive patient with severe esophagitis caused by *Candida albicans*. Which action by the student indicates that you need to intervene most quickly?
   1. Putting on a mask and gown before entering the patient's room
   2. Giving the patient a glass of water after administering the ordered oral nystatin (Mycostatin) suspension
   3. Suggesting that the patient should order chile con carne or chicken soup for the next meal
   4. Placing a "No Visitors" sign on the door of the patient's room

4. You are evaluating an HIV-positive patient who is receiving IV pentamidine (Pentam) as a treatment for *Pneumocystis jiroveci* (PCP) pneumonia. Which information is most important to communicate to the physician?
   1. The patient is reporting pain at the site of the infusion.
   2. The patient is not taking in an adequate amount of oral fluids.
   3. Blood pressure is 104/76 mm Hg after pentamidine administration.
   4. Blood glucose level is 55 mg/dL after medication administration.

5. After interviewing an HIV-positive patient who is considering starting highly active antiretroviral therapy (HAART), which patient information concerns you the most?
   1. The patient has been HIV positive for 8 years and has never taken any drug therapy for the HIV infection.
   2. The patient tells you, "I have never been very consistent about taking medications."
   3. The patient is sexually active with multiple partners and says "I always use a condom."
   4. The patient has many questions and concerns regarding the effectiveness and safety of the medications.

6. A patient with newly diagnosed acquired immunodeficiency syndrome (AIDS) has a negative result on a skin test for tuberculosis (TB). Which action will you anticipate taking next?
   1. Obtain a chest radiograph and sputum smear.
   2. Tell the patient that the TB test results are negative.
   3. Teach the patient about the anti-TB drug isoniazid.
   4. Schedule TB testing again in 12 months.

7. You are working in an AIDS hospice facility that is also staffed with LPNs/LVNs and UAPs. Which nursing action will you delegate to the LPN/LVN you are supervising?
   1. Assessing patients' nutritional needs and individualizing diet plans to improve nutrition
   2. Collecting data about the patients' responses to medications used for pain and anorexia
   3. Teaching the UAPs about how to lower the risk for spreading infections
   4. Assisting patients with personal hygiene and other activities of daily living as needed

8. A patient who has received a kidney transplant has been admitted to the medical unit with acute rejection and is receiving IV cyclosporine (Sandimmune) and methylprednisolone (Solu-Medrol). Which staff member is best to assign to care for this patient?
   1. RN who floated to the medical unit from the coronary care unit for the day
   2. RN with 3 years of experience in the operating room who is orienting to the medical unit
   3. RN who has worked on the medical unit for 5 years and is working a double shift today
   4. Newly graduated RN who needs experience with IV medication administration

9. Your patient with rheumatoid arthritis (RA) is taking prednisone (Deltasone) and naproxen (Aleve) to reduce inflammation and joint pain. Which symptom is most important to communicate to the health care provider?
   1. RA symptoms are worst in the morning
   2. Dry eyes
   3. Round and moveable nodules just under the skin
   4. Dark-colored stools

10. A patient with chronic hepatitis C has been receiving interferon alfa-2a (Roferon-A) injections for the last month. Which information gathered during a home visit is most important to communicate to the physician?
    1. The patient has persistent nausea and vomiting.
    2. The patient injects the medication into the thigh by the intramuscular route.
    3. The patient's temperature is 99.7° F (37.6° C) orally.
    4. The patient reports chronic fatigue, muscle aches, and anorexia.

11. A patient with a history of liver transplantation is receiving cyclosporine (Sandimmune), prednisone (Deltasone), and mycophenolate (CellCept). Which finding is of most concern?
    1. Gums that appear very pink and swollen
    2. A blood glucose level that is increased to 162 mg/dL
    3. A nontender lump above the clavicle
    4. Grade 1+ pitting edema in the feet and ankles

12. An HIV-positive patient who has been started on HAART is seen in the clinic for follow-up. Which test will be most helpful in determining the response to therapy?
    1. CD4 level
    2. Complete blood count
    3. Total lymphocyte percent
    4. Viral load

13. A hospitalized patient with AIDS has a nursing diagnosis of Imbalanced Nutrition: Less than Body Requirements related to nausea and anorexia. Which nursing action is most appropriate to delegate to an LPN/LVN who is providing care to this patient?
    1. Administering oxandrolone (Oxandrin) 5 mg daily
    2. Assessing the patient for other nutritional risk factors
    3. Developing a plan of care to improve the patient's appetite
    4. Providing instructions about a high-calorie, high-protein diet

14. You assess a 24-year-old patient with RA who is considering using methotrexate (Rheumatrex) for treatment. Which patient information is most important to communicate to the health care provider?
    1. The patient has many concerns about the safety of the drug.
    2. The patient has been trying to get pregnant.
    3. The patient takes a daily multivitamin tablet.
    4. The patient says that she has taken methotrexate in the past.

15. An 18-year-old college student with an exacerbation of systemic lupus erythematosus (SLE) has been receiving prednisone (Deltasone) 20 mg daily for 4 days. Which medical order should you question?
    1. Discontinue prednisone after today's dose.
    2. Give a "catch-up" dose of varicella vaccine.
    3. Check the patient's C-reactive protein level.
    4. Administer ibuprofen (Advil) 800 mg PO.

16. A patient with wheezing and coughing caused by an allergic reaction to penicillin is admitted to the emergency department. Which medication do you anticipate administering first?
    1. Methylprednisolone (Solu-Medrol) 100 mg IV
    2. Cromolyn (Intal) 20 mg via nebulizer
    3. Albuterol (Proventil) 3 mL via nebulizer
    4. Aminophylline (Theophylline) 500 mg IV

17. A patient with SLE is admitted to the hospital for evaluation and management of acute joint inflammation. Which information obtained in the admission laboratory testing concerns you most?
    1. Elevated blood urea nitrogen level
    2. Increased C-reactive protein level
    3. Positive antinuclear antibody test result
    4. Positive lupus erythematosus cell preparation

18. As the hospital employee health nurse, you are completing a health history for a newly-hired staff member. Which information given by the new employee most indicates the need for further nursing action before he or she begins orientation to patient care?
    1. The employee takes enalapril (Vasotec) for hypertension.
    2. The employee has an allergy to bananas, avocados, and papayas.
    3. The employee received a tetanus vaccination 3 years ago.
    4. TB skin test site has a 5-mm induration at 48 hours.

19. A patient who is HIV-positive and is taking nucleoside reverse transcriptase inhibitors and a protease inhibitor is admitted to the psychiatric unit with a panic attack. Which information about the patient is most important to discuss with the health care provider?
    1. The patient states, "I'm afraid I'm going to die right here!"
    2. The patient has an order for midazolam (Versed) 2 mg IV immediately (STAT).
    3. The patient is diaphoretic and tremulous, and reports dizziness.
    4. The patient's symptoms occurred suddenly while she was driving to work.

20. A patient seen in the sexually-transmitted disease clinic has just tested positive for HIV with a rapid HIV test. Which action will you take next?
    1. Ask about patient risk factors for HIV infection.
    2. Send a blood specimen for Western blot testing.
    3. Provide information about antiretroviral therapy.
    4. Discuss the positive test results with the patient.

Answer Key for this chapter begins on p. 171.

CHAPTER 4

Fluid, Electrolyte, and Acid-Base Balance Problems

1. The client's nursing diagnosis is Deficient Fluid Volume related to excessive fluid loss. Which action related to fluid management should be delegated to a UAP?
   1. Administering IV fluids as prescribed by the physician
   2. Providing straws and offering fluids between meals
   3. Developing a plan for added fluid intake over 24 hours
   4. Teaching family members to assist the client with fluid intake

2. The client also has the nursing diagnosis Decreased Cardiac Output related to decreased plasma volume. Which assessment finding supports this nursing diagnosis?
   1. Flattened neck veins when the client is in the supine position
   2. Full and bounding pedal and post-tibial pulses
   3. Pitting edema located in the feet, ankles, and calves
   4. Shallow respirations with crackles on auscultation

3. The nursing care plan for the client with dehydration includes interventions for oral health. Which interventions are within the scope of practice for an LPN/LVN being supervised by a nurse? *(Select all that apply.)*
   1. Reminding the client to avoid commercial mouthwashes
   2. Encouraging mouth rinsing with warm saline
   3. Observing the lips, tongue, and mucous membranes
   4. Providing mouth care every 2 hours while the client is awake
   5. Seeking a dietary consult to increase fluids on meal trays

4. The health care provider has written all of these orders for a client with a diagnosis of Excess Fluid Volume. The client's morning assessment reveals bounding peripheral pulses, weight gain of 2 lb, pitting ankle edema, and moist crackles bilaterally. Which order takes priority at this time?
   1. Weigh the client every morning.
   2. Maintain accurate intake and output records.
   3. Restrict fluids to 1500 mL/day.
   4. Administer furosemide (Lasix) 40 mg IV push.

5. You have been floated to the telemetry unit for the day. The monitor watcher informs you that the client has developed prominent U waves. Which laboratory value should you check immediately?
   1. Sodium
   2. Potassium
   3. Magnesium
   4. Calcium

6. A client's potassium level is 6.7 mEq/L. Which intervention should you delegate to the first-year student nurse whom you are supervising?
   1. Administer sodium polystyrene sulfonate (Kayexalate) 15 g orally.
   2. Administer spironolactone (Aldactone) 25 mg orally.
   3. Assess the electrocardiogram (ECG) strip for tall T waves.
   4. Administer potassium 10 mEq orally.

7. A client is admitted to the unit with a diagnosis of syndrome of inappropriate antidiuretic hormone secretion (SIADH). For which electrolyte abnormality would you be sure to monitor?
   1. Hypokalemia
   2. Hyperkalemia
   3. Hyponatremia
   4. Hypernatremia

8. The charge nurse assigned the care of a client with acute kidney failure and hypernatremia to you, a newly-graduated RN. Which action can you delegate to the UAP?
   1. Providing oral care every 3 to 4 hours
   2. Monitoring for indications of dehydration
   3. Administering 0.45% saline by IV line
   4. Assessing daily weights for trends

9. An experienced LPN/LVN reports to you that a client's blood pressure and heart rate have decreased, and when his face is assessed, one side twitches. What action should you take at this time?
   1. Reassess the client's blood pressure and heart rate.
   2. Review the client's morning calcium level.
   3. Request a neurologic consult today.
   4. Check the client's pupillary reaction to light.

10. You are preparing to discharge a client whose calcium level was low but is now just barely within the normal range (9 to 10.5 mg/dL). Which statement by the client indicates to you the need for additional teaching?
    1. "I will call my doctor if I experience muscle twitching or seizures."
    2. "I will make sure to take my vitamin D with my calcium each day."
    3. "I will take my calcium citrate pill every morning before breakfast."
    4. "I will avoid dairy products, broccoli, and spinach when I eat."

11. The UAP asks you why the client with a chronically low phosphorus level needs so much assistance with activities of daily living. What is your best response?
    1. "The client's low phosphorus is probably due to malnutrition."
    2. "The client is just worn out from not getting enough rest."
    3. "The client's skeletal muscles are weak because of the low phosphorus."
    4. "The client will do more for himself when his phosphorus level is normal."

12. You are reviewing the client's morning laboratory results. Which of these results is of most concern to you?
    1. Serum potassium level of 5.2 mEq/L
    2. Serum sodium level of 134 mEq/L
    3. Serum calcium level of 10.6 mg/dL
    4. Serum magnesium level of 0.8 mEq/L

13. As the charge nurse, you would assign which client to the step-down unit nurse floated to the intensive care unit for the day?
    1. 68-year-old on a ventilator with acute respiratory failure and respiratory acidosis
    2. 72-year-old with chronic obstructive pulmonary disease (COPD) and normal blood gas values who is ventilator dependent
    3. Newly-admitted 56-year-old with diabetic keto-acidosis receiving an insulin drip
    4. 38-year-old on a ventilator with narcotic overdose and respiratory alkalosis

14. The client with respiratory failure is receiving mechanical ventilation and continues to produce arterial blood gas results indicating respiratory acidosis. Which change in ventilator setting should you expect to correct this problem?
    1. Increase in ventilator rate from 6 to 10 breaths/min
    2. Decrease in ventilator rate from 10 to 6 breaths/min
    3. Increase in oxygen concentration from 30% to 40%
    4. Decrease in oxygen concentration from 40% to 30%

15. Which action should you delegate to a UAP for the client with diabetic ketoacidosis? *(Select all that apply.)*
    1. Checking fingerstick glucose results every hour
    2. Recording intake and output every hour
    3. Measuring vital signs every 15 minutes
    4. Assessing for indicators of fluid imbalance
    5. Notifying the provider of changes in glucose level

16. You are admitting an older adult client to the medical unit. Which assessment factor alerts you that this client has a risk for acid-base imbalances?
    1. History of myocardial infarction 1 year ago
    2. Antacid use for occasional indigestion
    3. Shortness of breath with extreme exertion
    4. Chronic renal insufficiency

17. A client with lung cancer has received oxycodone (Roxicodone) 10 mg orally for pain. When the student nurse assesses the client, which finding would you instruct the student to report immediately?
    1. Respiratory rate of 8 to 10 breaths/min
    2. Decrease in pain level from 6 to 2 (on a scale of 10)
    3. Request by the client that the room door be closed
    4. Heart rate of 90 to 100 beats/min

18. The UAP reports to you that a client seems very anxious, and vital sign measurement included a respiratory rate of 38 breaths/min. Which acid-base imbalance should you suspect?
    1. Respiratory acidosis
    2. Respiratory alkalosis
    3. Metabolic acidosis
    4. Metabolic alkalosis

19. A client is admitted to your unit for chemotherapy. To prevent an acid-base problem, which finding would you instruct the UAP to report?
    1. Repeated episodes of nausea and vomiting
    2. Reports of pain associated with exertion
    3. Failure to eat all the food on the breakfast tray
    4. Client hair loss during the morning bath

20. The client has a nasogastric (NG) tube connected to intermittent wall suction. The student nurse asks why the client's respiratory rate has decreased. What is your best response?
    1. "It's common for clients with uncomfortable equipment such as NG tubes to have a lower rate of breathing."
    2. "The client may have a metabolic alkalosis due to the NG suctioning, and the decreased respiratory rate is a compensatory mechanism."
    3. "Whenever a client develops a respiratory acid-base problem, decreasing the respiratory rate helps correct the problem."
    4. "The client is hypoventilating because of anxiety, and we will have to stay alert for the development of respiratory acidosis."

21. The client has an order for hydrochlorothiazide (HCTZ, Microzide) 10 mg orally every day. What should you be sure to include in a teaching plan for this drug? *(Select all that apply.)*
    1. "Take this medication in the morning."
    2. "This medication should be taken in 2 divided doses when you get up and when you go to bed."
    3. "Eat foods with extra sodium every day."
    4. "Inform your prescriber if you notice weight gain or increased swelling."
    5. "You should expect your urine output to increase."

22. Which blood test result would you be sure to monitor for the client taking HCTZ?
    1. Sodium level
    2. Potassium level
    3. Chloride level
    4. Calcium level

23. The RN is providing care for a patient diagnosed with dehydration and hypovolemic shock. Which order should the RN question?
    1. Blood pressure every 15 minutes
    2. Place two 18-gauge IV lines
    3. Oxygen at 3 L via nasal cannula
    4. D_5W to run at 250 mL/hr

Answer Key for this chapter begins on p. 172.

CHAPTER 5

Safety and Infection Control

1. A client who has recently traveled to China comes to the emergency department (ED) with increasing shortness of breath and is strongly suspected of having severe acute respiratory syndrome (SARS). Which of these prescribed actions will you take first?
   1. Infuse normal saline at 75 mL/hr.
   2. Obtain blood, urine, and sputum for cultures.
   3. Place the client on airborne and contact precautions.
   4. Give methylprednisolone (Solu-Medrol) 1 g IV.

2. You are caring for a newly admitted client with increasing dyspnea, hypoxia, and dehydration who has possible avian influenza ("bird flu"). Which of these prescribed actions will you implement first?
   1. Start oxygen using a nonrebreather mask.
   2. Infuse 5% dextrose in water at 100 mL/hr.
   3. Administer first dose of oseltamivir (Tamiflu).
   4. Obtain blood and sputum specimens for testing.

3. You are preparing to leave the room after performing oral suctioning on a client who is on contact and airborne precautions. In which order will you perform the following actions?
   1. Remove N95 respirator.
   2. Take off goggles.
   3. Remove gloves.
   4. Take off gown.
   5. Perform hand hygiene.

   _____, _____, _____, _____, _____

4. A client has been diagnosed with disseminated herpes zoster. Which personal protective equipment (PPE) will you need to put on when preparing to assess the client? *(Select all that apply.)*
   1. Surgical face mask
   2. N95 respirator
   3. Gown
   4. Gloves
   5. Goggles
   6. Shoe covers

5. You are working as the triage nurse in the ED when the following four clients arrive. Which client requires the most rapid action to protect other clients in the ED from infection?
   1. 3-year-old who has paroxysmal coughing and whose sibling has pertussis
   2. 5-year-old who has a new pruritic rash and a possible chickenpox infection
   3. 62-year-old who has a history of a methicillin-resistant *Staphylococcus aureus* (MRSA) abdominal wound infection
   4. 74-year-old who needs tuberculosis (TB) testing after being exposed to TB during a recent international airplane flight

6. You are caring for four clients who are receiving IV infusions of normal saline. Which client is at highest risk for bloodstream infection?
   1. Client with an implanted port in the right subclavian vein
   2. Client who has a midline IV catheter in the left antecubital fossa
   3. Client who has a nontunneled central line in the left internal jugular vein
   4. Client with a peripherally inserted central catheter (PICC) line in the right upper arm

7. You are caring for a client who has been admitted to the hospital with a leg ulcer that is infected with vancomycin-resistant *S. aureus* (VRSA). Which nursing action can you delegate to an LPN/LVN?
   1. Planning ways to improve the client's oral protein intake
   2. Teaching the client about home care of the leg ulcer
   3. Obtaining wound cultures during dressing changes
   4. Assessing the risk for further skin breakdown

8. A hospitalized 88-year-old client who has been receiving antibiotics for 10 days tells you that he is having frequent watery stools. Which action will you take first?
   1. Notify the physician about the loose stools.
   2. Obtain stool specimens for culture.
   3. Instruct the client about correct hand washing.
   4. Place the client on contact precautions.

PART 2 Common Health Scenarios

9. A client who states that he may have been contaminated by anthrax arrives at the ED. Which action included in the ED protocol for possible anthrax exposure will you take first?
   1. Notify hospital security personnel about the client.
   2. Escort the client to a decontamination room.
   3. Give ciprofloxacin (Cipro) 500 mg by mouth (PO).
   4. Assess the client for signs of infection.

10. A client with a vancomycin-resistant enterococcus (VRE) infection is admitted to the medical unit. Which action can be delegated to the UAP who is assisting with the client's care?
   1. Teaching the client and family members about means to prevent transmission of VRE
   2. Communicating with other departments when the client is transported for ordered tests
   3. Implementing contact precautions when providing care for the client
   4. Monitoring the results of ordered laboratory culture and sensitivity tests

11. A 23-year-old client comes to the outpatient clinic reporting increasing shortness of breath, diarrhea, abdominal pain, and epistaxis. Which action should you take first?
   1. Assist the client to pinch the anterior nares firmly for 5 minutes.
   2. Call an ambulance to take the client immediately to the hospital.
   3. Ask the client about any recent travel to Asia or the Middle East.
   4. Determine whether the client has had recommended immunizations.

12. You are the charge nurse on the medical unit. Which infection control activity should you delegate to an experienced UAP?
   1. Screening clients for upper respiratory tract symptoms
   2. Asking clients about the use of immunosuppressant medications
   3. Demonstrating correct hand washing to the clients' visitors
   4. Disinfecting blood pressure cuffs after clients are discharged

13. You are preparing to change the linens on the bed of a client who has a draining sacral wound infected by MRSA. Which PPE items will you plan to use? *(Select all that apply.)*
   1. Gown
   2. Gloves
   3. Goggles
   4. Surgical mask
   5. N95 respirator

14. A client who has frequent watery stools and a possible *Clostridium difficile* infection is hospitalized with dehydration. Which nursing action should the charge nurse delegate to an LPN/LVN?
   1. Performing ongoing assessments to determine the client's hydration status
   2. Explaining the purpose of ordered stool cultures to the client and family
   3. Administering the ordered metronidazole (Flagyl) 500 mg PO to the client
   4. Reviewing the client's medical history for any risk factors for diarrhea

15. As the infection control nurse in an acute care hospital, which action will you take to most effectively reduce the incidence of health care–associated infections?
   1. Require nursing staff to don gowns to change wound dressings for all clients.
   2. Ensure that dispensers for alcohol-based hand rubs are readily available in all client care areas of the hospital.
   3. Screen all newly admitted clients for colonization or infection with MRSA.
   4. Develop policies that automatically start antibiotic therapy for clients colonized by multidrug-resistant organisms.

16. In your role as the hospital infection control nurse, which policy will you implement to most effectively reduce the incidence of catheter-associated urinary tract infections (CAUTIs)?
   1. Limit the use of indwelling urinary catheters in all hospitalized clients.
   2. Ensure that clients with catheters have at least a 1500-mL fluid intake daily.
   3. Use urine dipstick testing to screen catheterized clients for asymptomatic bacteriuria.
   4. Require the use of antimicrobial/antiseptic impregnated catheters for catheterization.

17. You are admitting four clients with infections to the medical unit, but only one private room is available. Which client is it most appropriate to assign to the private room?
   1. Client with diarrhea caused by *C. difficile*
   2. Client with a wound infected with VRE
   3. Client with a cough who may have TB
   4. Client with toxic shock syndrome and fever

18. Which information about a client who has meningococcal meningitis is the best indicator that you can discontinue droplet precautions?
   1. Pupils are equal and reactive to light.
   2. Appropriate antibiotics have been given for 24 hours.
   3. Cough is productive of clear, nonpurulent mucus.
   4. Temperature is lower than 100° F (37.8° C).

19. You are administering vancomycin (Vancocin) 500 mg IV to a client with a MRSA wound infection when you notice that the client's neck and face are becoming flushed. Which action should you take next?
    1. Discontinue the vancomycin infusion.
    2. Slow the rate of the vancomycin infusion.
    3. Obtain an order for an antihistamine.
    4. Check the client's temperature.

20. A healthy 65-year-old woman who cares for a newborn grandchild has a clinic appointment in May. The client needs several immunizations, but tells you, "I hate shots! I will only take one today." Which immunization is most important to give?
    1. Influenza
    2. Herpes zoster
    3. Pneumococcal
    4. Tetanus, diphtheria, pertussis

21. You are caring for a client who is intubated and receiving mechanical ventilation. Which nursing actions are most essential in reducing the client's risk for ventilator-associated pneumonia (VAP)? *(Select all that apply.)*
    1. Keep the head of the client's bed elevated to at least 30 degrees.
    2. Assess the client's readiness for extubation at least daily.
    3. Ensure that the pneumococcal vaccine is administered.
    4. Use a kinetic bed to continuously change the client's position.
    5. Provide oral care with chlorhexidine solution at least daily.

22. You are preparing to insert a PICC line in a client's left forearm. Which solution will be best for cleaning the skin prior to the PICC insertion?
    1. 70% isopropyl alcohol
    2. Povidone-iodine (Betadine)
    3. 0.5% chlorhexidine in alcohol (Hibistat)
    4. Betadine followed by 70% isopropyl alcohol

23. You have received a needlestick injury after giving a client an intramuscular injection, but you have no information about the client's HIV status. What is the most appropriate method of obtaining this information about the client?
    1. You should personally ask the client to authorize HIV testing as soon as possible.
    2. The charge nurse should tell the client about the need for HIV testing.
    3. The occupational health nurse should discuss HIV status with the client.
    4. HIV testing should be performed the next time blood is drawn for other tests.

24. Which medication order for a client with a pulmonary embolism is most important to clarify with the prescribing physician before administration?
    1. Warfarin (Coumadin) 1.0 mg by mouth (PO)
    2. Morphine sulfate 2 to 4 mg IV
    3. Cephalexin (Keflex) 250 mg PO
    4. Heparin infusion at 900 units/hr

25. A client with atrial fibrillation is ambulating in the hallway on the coronary step-down unit and suddenly tells you, "I feel really dizzy." Which action should you take first?
    1. Help the client to sit down.
    2. Check the client's apical pulse.
    3. Take the client's blood pressure.
    4. Have the client breathe deeply.

26. The LPN/LVN whom you are supervising comes to you and says, "I gave the client with myasthenia gravis 90 mg of neostigmine (Prostigmin) instead of the ordered 45 mg!" In which order should you perform the following actions?
    1. Assess the client's heart rate.
    2. Complete a medication error report.
    3. Ask the LPN/LVN to explain how the error occurred.
    4. Notify the physician of the incorrect medication dose.
    _____, _____, _____, _____

27. You are caring for a confused and agitated client who has wrist restraints in place on both arms. Which action included in the client plan of care can you delegate to an LPN/LVN?
    1. Determining whether the client's mental status justifies the continued use of restraints
    2. Undoing and retying the restraints in order to improve client comfort
    3. Reporting the client's status and continued need for restraints to the health care provider
    4. Explaining the purpose of the restraints to the client's family members

28. You are checking medication orders that were received by telephone for a client with rheumatoid arthritis who was admitted with methotrexate toxicity. Which order is most important to clarify with the physician?
    1. Administer chlorambucil (Leukeran) 4 mg PO daily
    2. Infuse normal saline at 250 mL/hr for 4 hours
    3. Administer folic acid (Folacin) 2000 mcg PO daily
    4. Give cyanocobalamin (vitamin B_{12}) 10,000 mcg PO

Answer Key for this chapter begins on p. 174.

Common Health Scenarios   **PART 2**

CHAPTER 6

Respiratory Problems

1. An experienced LPN/LVN, under the supervision of the team leader RN, is providing nursing care for a patient with a respiratory problem. Which actions are appropriate to the scope of practice of an experienced LPN/LVN? *(Select all that apply.)*
   1. Auscultating breath sounds
   2. Administering medications via metered-dose inhaler (MDI)
   3. Completing in-depth admission assessment
   4. Checking oxygen saturation using pulse oximetry
   5. Developing the nursing care plan
   6. Evaluating the patient's technique for using MDIs

2. You are evaluating and assessing a patient with a diagnosis of chronic emphysema. The patient is receiving oxygen at a flow rate of 5 L/min by nasal cannula. Which finding concerns you immediately?
   1. Fine bibasilar crackles
   2. Respiratory rate of 8 breaths/min
   3. The patient sitting up and leaning over the nightstand
   4. A large barrel chest

3. The UAP tells you that a patient who is receiving oxygen at a flow rate of 6 L/min by nasal cannula is reporting nasal passage discomfort. What intervention should you suggest to improve the patient's comfort for this problem?
   1. Humidify the patient's oxygen.
   2. Use a simple face mask instead of a nasal cannula.
   3. Provide the patient with an extra pillow.
   4. Have the patient sit up in a chair at the bedside.

4. You are supervising a student nurse who is performing tracheostomy care for a patient. Which action by the student would cause you to intervene?
   1. Suctioning the tracheostomy tube before performing tracheostomy care
   2. Removing old dressings and cleaning off excess secretions
   3. Removing the inner cannula and cleaning using standard precautions
   4. Replacing the inner cannula and cleaning the stoma site

5. You are supervising an RN who floated from the medical-surgical unit to the emergency department. The nurse is providing care for a patient admitted with anterior epistaxis (nosebleed). Which directions would you clearly provide to the RN? *(Select all that apply.)*
   1. Position the patient supine and turned on his side.
   2. Apply direct lateral pressure to the nose for 5 minutes.
   3. Maintain standard body substance precautions.
   4. Apply ice or cool compresses to the nose.
   5. Instruct the patient not to blow the nose for several hours.

6. A patient with sleep apnea has a nursing diagnosis of Sleep Deprivation related to disrupted sleep cycle. Which action should you delegate to the UAP?
   1. Discussing weight-loss strategies such as diet and exercise with the patient
   2. Teaching the patient how to set up the bilevel positive airway pressure (BiPAP) machine before sleeping
   3. Reminding the patient to sleep on his side instead of his back
   4. Administering modafinil (Provigil) to promote daytime wakefulness

7. You are acting as preceptor for a newly-graduated RN during her second week of orientation. You would assign the new RN under your supervision to provide nursing care to which patients? *(Select all that apply.)*
   1. 38-year-old with moderate persistent asthma awaiting discharge
   2. 63-year-old with a tracheostomy needing tracheostomy care every shift
   3. 56-year-old with lung cancer who has just undergone left lower lobectomy
   4. 49-year-old just admitted with a new diagnosis of esophageal cancer
   5. 76-year-old newly diagnosed with type 2 diabetes

Common Health Scenarios   PART 2

8. You are providing care for a patient with recently diagnosed asthma. Which key points would you be sure to include in your teaching plan for this patient? *(Select all that apply.)*
   1. Avoid potential environmental asthma triggers such as smoke.
   2. Use the inhaler 30 minutes before exercising to prevent bronchospasm.
   3. Wash all bedding in cold water to reduce and destroy dust mites.
   4. Be sure to get at least 8 hours of rest and sleep every night.
   5. Avoid foods prepared with monosodium glutamate (MSG).

9. You are the team leader RN working with a student nurse. The student nurse is to teach a patient how to use an MDI without a spacer. Put in correct order the steps that the student nurse should teach the patient.
   1. Remove the inhaler cap and shake the inhaler.
   2. Open your mouth and place the mouthpiece 1 to 2 inches away.
   3. Breathe out completely.
   4. Hold your breath for at least 10 seconds.
   5. Press down firmly on the canister and breathe deeply through your mouth.
   6. Wait at least 1 minute between puffs.

   _____, _____, _____, _____, _____, _____

10. A patient has chronic obstructive pulmonary disease (COPD). Which intervention for airway management should you delegate to the UAP?
    1. Assisting the patient to sit up on the side of the bed
    2. Instructing the patient to cough effectively
    3. Teaching the patient to use incentive spirometry
    4. Auscultating breath sounds every 4 hours

11. The patient with COPD has a nursing diagnosis of Ineffective Breathing Pattern. Which is an appropriate action to delegate to the experienced LPN/LVN under your supervision?
    1. Observing how well the patient performs pursed-lip breathing
    2. Planning a nursing care regimen that gradually increases activity tolerance
    3. Assisting the patient with basic activities of daily living (ADLs)
    4. Consulting with the physical therapy department about reconditioning exercises

12. The patient with COPD tells the UAP that he did not get his annual flu shot this year and has not had a pneumonia vaccination. You would be sure to instruct the UAP to report which vital sign value?
    1. Blood pressure of 152/84 mm Hg
    2. Respiratory rate of 27 breaths/min
    3. Heart rate of 92 beats/min
    4. Oral temperature of 101.2° F (38.4° C)

13. You are responsible for the care of a postoperative patient with a thoracotomy. The patient has been given the nursing diagnosis of Activity Intolerance. Which action should you delegate to the UAP?
    1. Instructing the patient to alternate rest and activity periods
    2. Encouraging, monitoring, and recording nutritional intake
    3. Monitoring cardiorespiratory response to activity
    4. Planning activities for periods when the patient has the most energy

14. You are supervising a nursing student who is providing care for a thoracotomy patient with a chest tube. What finding would you clearly instruct the nursing student to notify you about immediately?
    1. Chest tube drainage of 10 to 15 mL/hr
    2. Continuous bubbling in the water-seal chamber
    3. Reports of pain at the chest tube site
    4. Chest tube dressing dated yesterday

15. After change of shift, you are assigned to care for the following patients. Which patient should you assess first?
    1. 68-year-old patient on a ventilator for whom a sterile sputum specimen must be sent to the laboratory
    2. 57-year-old with COPD and a pulse oximetry reading from the previous shift of 90% saturation
    3. 72-year-old with pneumonia who needs to be started on IV antibiotics
    4. 51-year-old with asthma who reports shortness of breath after using a bronchodilator inhaler

16. You are initiating a nursing care plan for a patient with pneumonia. Which intervention for cough enhancement should you delegate to the UAP?
    1. Teaching the patient about the importance of adequate fluid intake and hydration
    2. Assisting the patient to a sitting position with neck flexed, shoulders relaxed, and knees flexed
    3. Reminding the patient to use an incentive spirometer every 1 to 2 hours while awake
    4. Encouraging the patient to take a deep breath, hold it for 2 seconds, then cough two or three times in succession

17. The charge nurse is making assignments for the next shift. Which patient should be assigned to the fairly new nurse (6 months of experience) floated from the surgical unit to the medical unit?
    1. 58-year-old on airborne precautions for tuberculosis (TB)
    2. 65-year-old who just returned from bronchoscopy and biopsy
    3. 72-year-old who needs teaching about the use of incentive spirometry
    4. 69-year-old with COPD who is ventilator dependent

18. When a patient with TB is being prepared for discharge, which statement by the patient indicates a need for further teaching?
    1. "Everyone in my family needs to go and see the doctor for TB testing."
    2. "I will continue to take my isoniazid until I am feeling completely well."
    3. "I will cover my mouth and nose when I sneeze or cough and put my used tissues in a plastic bag."
    4. "I will change my diet to include more foods rich in iron, protein, and vitamin C."

19. You are admitting a patient for whom a diagnosis of pulmonary embolus must be ruled out. The patient's history and assessment reveal all of these findings. Which finding supports the diagnosis of pulmonary embolus?
    1. The patient was recently in a motor vehicle crash.
    2. The patient participated in an aerobic exercise program for 6 months.
    3. The patient gave birth to her youngest child 1 year ago.
    4. The patient was on bed rest for 6 hours after a diagnostic procedure.

20. Which intervention for a patient with a pulmonary embolus could be delegated to the LPN/LVN on your patient care team?
    1. Evaluating the patient's reports of chest pain
    2. Monitoring laboratory values for changes in oxygenation
    3. Assessing for symptoms of respiratory failure
    4. Auscultating the lungs for crackles

21. A patient with a pulmonary embolus is receiving anticoagulation with IV heparin. What instructions would you give the UAP who will help the patient with ADLs? *(Select all that apply.)*
    1. Use a lift sheet when moving and positioning the patient in bed.
    2. Use an electric razor when shaving the patient each day.
    3. Use a soft-bristled toothbrush or tooth sponge for oral care.
    4. Use a rectal thermometer to obtain a more accurate body temperature.
    5. Be sure the patient's footwear has a firm sole when the patient ambulates.

22. A patient with acute respiratory distress syndrome (ARDS) is receiving oxygen by nonrebreather mask, but arterial blood gas measurements still show poor oxygenation. As the nurse responsible for this patient's care, you would anticipate a physician order for what action?
    1. Perform endotracheal intubation and initiate mechanical ventilation.
    2. Immediately begin continuous positive airway pressure (CPAP) via the patient's nose and mouth.
    3. Administer furosemide (Lasix) 100 mg IV push immediately (STAT).
    4. Call a code for respiratory arrest.

23. You are the preceptor for an RN who is undergoing orientation to the intensive care unit. The RN is providing care for a patient with ARDS who has just been intubated in preparation for mechanical ventilation. You observe the nurse perform all of these actions. For which action must you intervene immediately?
    1. Assessing for bilateral breath sounds and symmetrical chest movement
    2. Auscultating over the stomach to rule out esophageal intubation
    3. Marking the tube 1 cm from where it touches the incisor tooth or nares
    4. Ordering a chest radiograph to verify that tube placement is correct

24. You are assigned to provide nursing care for a patient receiving mechanical ventilation. Which action should you delegate to an experienced UAP?
    1. Assessing the patient's respiratory status every 4 hours
    2. Taking vital signs and pulse oximetry readings every 4 hours
    3. Checking the ventilator settings to make sure they are as prescribed
    4. Observing whether the patient's tube needs suctioning every 2 hours

PART 2 Common Health Scenarios

25. After the respiratory therapist performs suctioning on a patient who is intubated, the UAP measures vital signs for the patient. Which vital sign value should the UAP report to the RN immediately?
    1. Heart rate of 98 beats/min
    2. Respiratory rate of 24 breaths/min
    3. Blood pressure of 168/90 mm Hg
    4. Tympanic temperature of 101.4° F (38.6° C)

26. You are making a home visit to a 50-year-old patient who was recently hospitalized with a right leg deep vein thrombosis and a pulmonary embolism. The patient's only medication is enoxaparin (Lovenox) subcutaneously. Which assessment information will you need to communicate to the physician?
    1. The patient says that her right leg aches all night.
    2. The right calf is warm to the touch and is larger than the left calf.
    3. The patient is unable to remember her husband's first name.
    4. There are multiple ecchymotic areas on the patient's arms.

27. The high-pressure alarm on a patient's ventilator goes off. When you enter the room to assess the patient, who has ARDS, the oxygen saturation monitor reads 87% and the patient is struggling to sit up. Which action should you take next?
    1. Reassure the patient that the ventilator will do the work of breathing for him.
    2. Manually ventilate the patient while assessing possible reasons for the high-pressure alarm.
    3. Increase the fraction of inspired oxygen (FIO_2) on the ventilator to 100% in preparation for endotracheal suctioning.
    4. Insert an oral airway to prevent the patient from biting on the endotracheal tube.

28. When assessing a 22-year-old patient who required emergency surgery and multiple transfusions 3 days ago, you find that the patient looks anxious and has labored respirations at a rate of 38 breaths/min. The oxygen saturation is 90% with the oxygen delivery at 6 L/min via nasal cannula. Which action is most appropriate?
    1. Increase the flow rate on the oxygen to 10 L/min and reassess the patient after about 10 minutes.
    2. Assist the patient in using the incentive spirometer and splint his chest with a pillow while he coughs.
    3. Administer the ordered morphine sulfate to the patient to decrease his anxiety and reduce the hyperventilation.
    4. Switch the patient to a nonrebreather mask at 95% to 100% FIO_2 and call the physician to discuss the patient's status.

29. You have just finished assisting the physician with a thoracentesis for a patient with recurrent left pleural effusion caused by lung cancer. The thoracentesis removed 1800 mL of fluid. Which patient assessment information is important to report to the physician?
    1. The patient starts crying and says she can't go on with treatment much longer.
    2. The patient reports sharp, stabbing chest pain with every deep breath.
    3. The blood pressure is 100/48 mm Hg and the heart rate is 102 beats/min.
    4. The dressing at the thoracentesis site has 1 cm of bloody drainage.

30. You are caring for a patient with emphysema and respiratory failure who is receiving mechanical ventilation through an endotracheal tube. To prevent ventilator-associated pneumonia (VAP), which action is most important to include in the plan of care?
    1. Administer ordered antibiotics as scheduled.
    2. Hyperoxygenate the patient before suctioning.
    3. Maintain the head of bed at a 30- to 45-degree angle.
    4. Suction the airway when coarse crackles are audible.

Answer Key for this chapter begins on p. 176.

CHAPTER 7

Cardiovascular Problems

1. You are working in the emergency department (ED) when a client arrives reporting substernal and left arm discomfort that has been going on for about 3 hours. Which laboratory test will be most useful in determining whether you should anticipate implementing the acute coronary syndrome (ACS) standard protocol?
   1. Creatine kinase MB level
   2. Troponin I level
   3. Myoglobin level
   4. C-reactive protein level

2. You are monitoring a 53-year-old client who is undergoing a treadmill stress test. Which client finding will require the most immediate action?
   1. Blood pressure of 152/88 mm Hg
   2. Heart rate of 134 beats/min
   3. Oxygen saturation of 91%
   4. Chest pain level of 3 (on a scale of 10)

3. The health care provider prescribes these actions for a client who was admitted with acute substernal chest pain. Which actions are appropriate to delegate to an experienced LPN/LVN who is working with you in the ED? *(Select all that apply.)*
   1. Attaching cardiac monitor leads
   2. Giving heparin 5000 units IV push
   3. Administering morphine sulfate 4 mg IV
   4. Obtaining a 12-lead electrocardiogram (ECG)
   5. Asking the client about pertinent medical history
   6. Having the client chew and swallow aspirin 162 mg

4. Based on this information in a client's medical record, which topic will you plan on including in the initial teaching plan for a client who has a new diagnosis of stage 1 hypertension?

Health History	Physical Exam	Social and Diet History
• Denies any chronic health problems • Takes no medications currently	• Height: 5 feet, 6 inches • Weight: 115 lb (52.3 kg) • BMI: 18.6	• Works as an accountant • 1 glass of wine once or twice weekly • Eats "fast food" frequently

   1. Benefits and adverse effects of beta-blockers
   2. Adverse effects of alcohol on blood pressure
   3. Methods for decreasing dietary caloric intake
   4. Low-sodium food choices when eating out

5. You make a home visit to evaluate a hypertensive client who has been taking enalapril (Vasotec). Which finding indicates that you need to contact the health care provider about a change in the drug therapy?
   1. Client reports frequent urination.
   2. Client's blood pressure is 138/86 mm Hg.
   3. Client coughs often during the visit.
   4. Client says, "I get dizzy sometimes."

6. While admitting a client, you obtain this information about her cardiovascular risk factors: Her mother and two siblings have had myocardial infarctions (MIs). The client smokes and has a 20 pack-year history of cigarette use. Her work as a mail carrier involves a lot of walking. She takes metoprolol (Lopressor) for hypertension, and her blood pressure has been in the range of 130/60 to 138/85 mm Hg. Which interventions will be important to include in the discharge plan for this client? *(Select all that apply.)*
   1. Referral to community programs that assist in smoking cessation
   2. Teaching about the impact of family history on cardiovascular risk
   3. Education about the need for a change in antihypertensive therapy
   4. Assistance in reducing the stress associated with her cardiovascular risk
   5. Discussion of the risks associated with having a sedentary lifestyle

7. You are the charge nurse for the coronary care step-down unit. Which client is best to assign to a float RN who has come for the day from the general medical-surgical unit?
   1. Client requiring discharge teaching about coronary artery stenting before going home today
   2. Client receiving IV furosemide (Lasix) to treat acute left ventricular failure
   3. Client who just transferred in from the radiology department after a coronary angioplasty
   4. Client just admitted with unstable angina who has orders for a heparin infusion and aspirin

8. At 9:00 PM, you admit a 63-year-old with a diagnosis of acute MI. Which finding is most important to communicate to the health care provider who is considering the use of fibrinolytic therapy with tissue plasminogen activator (alteplase [Activase]) for the client?
   1. The client was treated with alteplase about 8 months ago.
   2. The client takes famotidine (Pepcid) for esophageal reflux.
   3. The client has ST-segment elevations on the 12-lead ECG.
   4. The client has had continuous chest pain since 8:00 AM.

9. You are working with an experienced UAP and an LPN/LVN on the telemetry unit. A client who had an acute MI 3 days ago has a nursing diagnosis of Activity Intolerance related to fatigue and chest pain. Which nursing activity included in the care plan is best delegated to the LPN/LVN?
   1. Administering nitroglycerin (Nitrostat) if chest discomfort occurs during client activities
   2. Monitoring pulse, blood pressure, and oxygen saturation before and after client ambulation
   3. Teaching the client energy conservation techniques to decrease myocardial oxygen demand
   4. Explaining the rationale for alternating rest periods with exercise to the client and family

10. You are working in the ED caring for a client who was just admitted with left anterior chest pain, possible ACS. Which action will you take first?
    1. Insert an IV catheter.
    2. Auscultate heart sounds.
    3. Administer sublingual nitroglycerin.
    4. Draw blood for troponin I measurement.

11. An 80-year-old client on the coronary step-down unit tells you that he does not want to take the ordered docusate (Colace) because he does not have any problems with constipation. Which action is most appropriate?
    1. Document the medication on the client's chart as "refused."
    2. Mix the medication with food and administer it to the client.
    3. Explain that his decreased activity level may cause constipation.
    4. Reinforce that the docusate has been prescribed for a good reason.

12. You have given morphine sulfate 4 mg IV to a client who has an acute MI. When you evaluate the client's response 5 minutes after giving the medication, which finding indicates a need for immediate further action?
    1. Blood pressure decrease from 114/65 to 106/58 mm Hg
    2. Respiratory rate drop from 18 to 12 breaths/min
    3. Cardiac monitor indicating sinus rhythm at a rate of 96 beats/min
    4. Persisting chest pain at a level of 1 (on a scale of 0 to 10)

13. You are preparing to implement teaching about a heart-healthy diet and activity levels for a client who has had an MI and her husband. The client says, "I don't see why I need any teaching. I don't think I need to change anything right now." Which response is most appropriate?
    1. "Do you think your family may want you to make some lifestyle changes?"
    2. "Can you tell me why you don't feel that you need to make any changes?"
    3. "You are still in the stage of denial, but you will want this information later on."
    4. "Even though you don't want to change, it's important that you have this teaching."

14. You are caring for a hospitalized client with heart failure who is receiving captopril (Capoten) and spironolactone (Aldactone). Which laboratory value will be most important to monitor?
    1. Sodium level
    2. Blood urea nitrogen level
    3. Potassium level
    4. Alkaline phosphatase level

15. The health care provider telephones you with new prescriptions for a client with unstable angina who is already taking clopidogrel (Plavix). Which medication is most important to clarify further with the health care provider?
    1. Aspirin (Ecotrin) 162 mg daily
    2. Omeprazole (Prilosec) 20 mg daily
    3. Metoprolol (Lopressor) 50 mg daily
    4. Nitroglycerin patch (Nitrodur) 0.4 mg/hr

16. At 10:00 AM, a hospitalized client receives a new order for transesophageal echocardiography (TEE) as soon as possible. Which action will you take first?
    1. Put the client on "nothing by mouth" (NPO) status.
    2. Teach the client about the procedure.
    3. Insert an IV catheter in the client's forearm.
    4. Attach the client to a cardiac monitor.

17. You assess a client who has just returned to the recovery area after undergoing coronary arteriography. Which information is of most concern?
    1. Blood pressure is 144/78 mm Hg
    2. Pedal pulses are palpable at +1
    3. Left groin has a 3-cm bruised area
    4. Apical pulse is 122 beats/min and regular

18. You are working in an outpatient clinic where many vascular diagnostic tests are performed. Which task associated with vascular testing is most appropriate to delegate to an experienced UAP?
    1. Measuring ankle and brachial pressures in a client for whom the ankle-brachial index is to be calculated
    2. Checking blood pressure and pulse every 10 minutes in a client who is undergoing exercise testing
    3. Obtaining information about allergies from a client who is scheduled for left leg contrast venography
    4. Providing brief client teaching for a client who will undergo a right subclavian vein Doppler study

19. While working on the cardiac step-down unit, you are serving as preceptor to a newly graduated RN who has been in a 6-week orientation program. Which client will be best to assign to the new graduate?
    1. 19-year-old with rheumatic fever who needs discharge teaching before going home with a roommate today
    2. 33-year-old admitted a week ago with endocarditis who will be receiving ceftriaxone (Rocephin) 2 g IV
    3. 50-year-old with newly diagnosed stable angina who has many questions about medications and nursing care
    4. 75-year-old who has just been transferred to the unit after undergoing coronary artery bypass grafting yesterday

20. You are monitoring the cardiac rhythms of clients in the coronary care unit. Which client will need immediate intervention?
    1. Client admitted with heart failure who has atrial fibrillation with a rate of 88 beats/min while at rest
    2. Client with a newly implanted demand ventricular pacemaker who has occasional periods of sinus rhythm at a rate of 90 to 100 beats/min
    3. Client who has just arrived on the unit with an acute MI and has sinus rhythm at a rate of 76 beats/min with frequent premature ventricular contractions
    4. Client who recently started taking atenolol (Tenormin) and has a first-degree heart block, with a rate of 58 beats/min

21. Ventricular fibrillation is identified in an unresponsive 50-year-old client who has just arrived in the ED. Which action will you take first?
    1. Defibrillate at 200 J.
    2. Start cardiopulmonary resuscitation (CPR).
    3. Administer epinephrine (Adrenalin) 1 mg IV.
    4. Intubate and manually ventilate.

22. Two weeks ago, a 63-year-old client with heart failure received a new prescription for carvedilol (Coreg) 3.125 mg orally. When evaluating the client in the cardiology clinic, you obtain the following data. Which finding is of most concern?
    1. Reports of increased fatigue and activity intolerance
    2. Weight increase of 0.5 kg over a 1-week period
    3. Sinus bradycardia at a rate of 48 beats/min
    4. Traces of edema noted over both ankles

23. You have just received a change-of-shift report about these clients on the coronary step-down unit. Which one will you assess first?
    1. 26-year-old with heart failure caused by congenital mitral stenosis who is scheduled for balloon valvuloplasty later today
    2. 45-year-old with constrictive cardiomyopathy who developed acute dyspnea and agitation about 1 hour before the shift change
    3. 56-year-old who underwent coronary angioplasty and stent placement yesterday and has reported occasional chest pain since the procedure
    4. 77-year-old who was transferred from the intensive care unit 2 days ago after coronary artery bypass grafting and has a temperature of 100.6° F (38.1° C)

24. As the charge nurse in a long-term care facility that employs RNs, LPNs/LVNs, and UAPs, you have developed a plan for the ongoing assessment of all residents with a diagnosis of heart failure. Which activity included in the plan is most appropriate to delegate to an LPN/LVN team member?
    1. Weighing all residents with heart failure each morning
    2. Listening to lung sounds and checking for edema each week
    3. Reviewing all heart failure medications with residents every month
    4. Updating activity plans for residents with heart failure every quarter

25. During a home visit to an 88-year-old client who is taking digoxin (Lanoxin) 0.25 mg daily to treat heart failure and atrial fibrillation, you obtain this assessment information. Which finding is most important to communicate to the health care provider?
    1. Apical pulse of 68 beats/min and irregularly irregular
    2. Digoxin taken with meals
    3. Vision that is becoming "fuzzy"
    4. Lung crackles that clear after coughing

26. You are ambulating a cardiac surgery client who has a telemetry cardiac monitor when another staff member tells you that the client has developed supraventricular tachycardia at a rate of 146 beats/min. In which order will you take the following actions?
    1. Call the client's physician.
    2. Have the client sit down.
    3. Check the client's blood pressure.
    4. Administer PRN oxygen by nasal cannula.

    _____, _____, _____, _____

27. A client who has endocarditis with vegetation on the mitral valve suddenly reports severe left foot pain. You note that no pulse is palpable in the left foot and that it is cold and pale. Which action should you take next?
    1. Lower the client's left foot below heart level.
    2. Administer oxygen at 4 L/min to the client.
    3. Notify the client's physician about the change in status.
    4. Reassure the client that embolization is common in endocarditis.

28. A resident in a long-term care facility who has venous stasis ulcers is treated with an Unna boot. Which nursing activity included in the resident's care is best for you to delegate to the UAP?
    1. Teaching family members the signs of infection
    2. Monitoring capillary perfusion once every 8 hours
    3. Evaluating foot sensation and movement each shift
    4. Assisting the client in cleaning around the Unna boot

29. During the initial postoperative assessment of a client who has just been transferred to the postanesthesia care unit after repair of an abdominal aortic aneurysm, you obtain these data. Which finding has the most immediate implications for the client's care?
    1. Arterial line indicates a blood pressure of 190/112 mm Hg.
    2. Cardiac monitor shows frequent premature atrial contractions.
    3. There is no response to verbal stimulation.
    4. Urine output is 40 mL of amber urine.

30. You are developing a standardized care plan for the postoperative care of clients undergoing cardiac surgery. Which nursing activity included in the care plan will need to be performed by RN staff members?
    1. Removing chest and leg dressings on the second postoperative day and cleaning the incisions with antibacterial swabs
    2. Reinforcing client and family teaching about the need to deep breathe and cough at least every 2 hours while awake
    3. Developing an individual plan for discharge teaching based on discharge medications and needed lifestyle changes
    4. Administering oral analgesic medications as needed before helping the client out of bed on the first postoperative day

31. You are preparing to administer the following medications to a client with multiple health problems who has been hospitalized with deep vein thrombosis. Which medication is most important to double-check with another licensed nurse?
    1. Famotidine (Pepcid) 20 mg IV
    2. Furosemide (Lasix) 40 mg IV
    3. Digoxin (Lanoxin) 0.25 mg PO
    4. Warfarin (Coumadin) 2.5 mg PO

32. A client seen in the clinic with shortness of breath and fatigue is being evaluated for a possible diagnosis of heart failure. Which laboratory result will be most useful to monitor?
    1. Serum potassium
    2. B-type natriuretic peptide
    3. Blood urea nitrogen
    4. Hematocrit

Answer Key for this chapter begins on p. 178.

PART 2 Common Health Scenarios

CHAPTER 8

Hematologic Problems

1. You are reviewing the complete blood count for a patient who has been admitted for knee arthroscopy. Which value is most important to report to the physician before surgery?
   1. Hematocrit of 33%
   2. Hemoglobin level of 10.9 g/dL
   3. Platelet count of 426,000/mm³
   4. White blood cell count of 16,000/mm³

2. You are providing orientation for a new RN who is preparing to administer packed red blood cells (PRBCs) to a patient who had blood loss during surgery. Which action by the new RN requires that you intervene immediately?
   1. Waiting 20 minutes after obtaining the PRBCs before starting the infusion
   2. Starting an IV line for the transfusion using a 22-gauge catheter
   3. Priming the transfusion set using 5% dextrose in lactated Ringer's solution
   4. Telling the patient that the PRBCs may cause a serious transfusion reaction

3. A 32-year-old patient with sickle cell anemia is admitted to the hospital during a sickle cell crisis. Which action prescribed by the health care provider will you implement first?
   1. Give morphine sulfate 4 to 8 mg IV every hour as needed.
   2. Administer 100% oxygen using a nonrebreather mask.
   3. Start a 14-gauge IV line and infuse normal saline at 200 mL/hr.
   4. Give pneumococcal (Pneumovax) and *Haemophilus influenzae* (ActHIB) vaccines.

4. These activities are included in the care plan for a 78-year-old patient admitted to the hospital with anemia caused by possible gastrointestinal bleeding. Which activity can you delegate to an experienced UAP?
   1. Obtaining stool specimens for fecal blood test (Hemoccult) slides
   2. Having the patient sign a colonoscopy consent form
   3. Giving the prescribed polyethylene glycol electrolyte solution (GoLYTELY)
   4. Checking for allergies to contrast dye or shellfish

5. As charge nurse, you are making the daily assignments on the medical-surgical unit. Which patient is best assigned to a float nurse who has come from the post-anesthesia care unit (PACU)?
   1. 30-year-old patient with thalassemia major who has an order for subcutaneous infusion of deferoxamine (Desferal)
   2. 43-year-old patient with multiple myeloma who requires discharge teaching
   3. 52-year-old patient with chronic gastrointestinal bleeding who has returned to the unit after a colonoscopy
   4. 65-year-old patient with pernicious anemia who has just been admitted to the unit

6. You are making a room assignment for a newly arrived patient whose laboratory test results indicate pancytopenia. Which patient will be the best roommate for the new patient?
   1. Patient with digoxin toxicity
   2. Patient with viral pneumonia
   3. Patient with shingles
   4. Patient with cellulitis

7. A 67-year-old who is receiving chemotherapy for lung cancer is admitted to the hospital with thrombocytopenia. Which statement made by the patient when you are obtaining the admission history is of most concern?
   1. "I've noticed that I bruise more easily since the chemotherapy started."
   2. "My bowel movements are soft and dark brown."
   3. "I take one aspirin every morning because of my history of angina."
   4. "My appetite has decreased since the chemotherapy started."

8. After a car accident, a patient with a medical alert bracelet indicating hemophilia A is admitted to the emergency department (ED). Which action prescribed by the health care provider will you implement first?
   1. Transport to the radiology department for cervical spine radiography.
   2. Transfuse factor VII concentrate.
   3. Type and cross-match for 4 units of packed red blood cells (PRBCs).
   4. Infuse normal saline at 250 mL/hr.

9. As a home health nurse, you are obtaining an admission history for a patient who has deep vein thrombosis and is taking warfarin (Coumadin) 2 mg daily. Which statement by the patient is the best indicator that additional teaching about warfarin may be needed?
   1. "I have started to eat more healthy foods like green salads and fruit."
   2. "The doctor said that it is important to avoid becoming constipated."
   3. "Coumadin makes me feel a little nauseated unless I take it with food."
   4. "I will need to have some blood testing done once or twice a week."

10. A patient is admitted to the intensive care unit with disseminated intravascular coagulation associated with a gram-negative infection. Which assessment information has the most immediate implications for the patient's care?
    1. There is no palpable radial or pedal pulse.
    2. The patient reports chest pain.
    3. The patient's oxygen saturation is 87%.
    4. There is mottling of the hands and feet.

11. A 22-year-old with stage I Hodgkin disease is admitted to the oncology unit for radiation therapy. During the initial assessment, the patient tells you, "Sometimes I'm afraid of dying." Which response is most appropriate at this time?
    1. "Many individuals with this diagnosis have some fears."
    2. "Perhaps you should ask the doctor about medication."
    3. "Tell me a little bit more about your fear of dying."
    4. "Most people with stage I Hodgkin disease survive."

12. You receive a change-of-shift report about the following patients. Which one will you assess first?
    1. 26-year-old with thalassemia who has a hemoglobin level of 8 g/L and orders for a PRBC transfusion
    2. 44-year-old who was admitted 3 days previously in a sickle cell crisis and has orders for a computed tomographic scan
    3. 50-year-old with stage IV non-Hodgkin lymphoma who is crying and saying, "I'm not ready to die"
    4. 69-year-old with chemotherapy-induced neutropenia who has an oral temperature of 100.1° F (37.8° C)

13. A patient in a long-term care (LTC) facility who has chronic lymphocytic leukemia has a nursing diagnosis of Activity Intolerance related to weakness and anemia. Which nursing activity will you delegate to the UAP?
    1. Evaluating the patient's response to normal activities of daily living
    2. Checking the patient's blood pressure and pulse rate after ambulation
    3. Determining which self-care activities the patient can do independently
    4. Assisting the patient in choosing a diet that will improve strength

14. A transfusion of PRBCs has been infusing for 5 minutes when the patient becomes flushed and tachypneic and says, "I'm having chills. Please get me a blanket." Which action should you take first?
    1. Obtain a warm blanket for the patient.
    2. Check the patient's oral temperature.
    3. Stop the transfusion.
    4. Administer oxygen.

15. A group of patients is assigned to an RN-LPN/LVN team. The LPN/LVN should be assigned to provide patient care and administer medications to which patient?
    1. 36-year-old with chronic kidney failure who will need a subcutaneous injection of epoetin alfa (Procrit)
    2. 39-year-old with hemophilia B who has been admitted to receive a transfusion of PRBCs
    3. 50-year-old with newly diagnosed polycythemia vera who will require phlebotomy
    4. 55-year-old with a history of stem cell transplantation who has a bone marrow aspiration scheduled

16. You obtain the following data about a patient admitted with multiple myeloma. Which information has the most immediate implications for the patient's care?
    1. The patient reports chronic bone pain.
    2. The blood uric acid level is very elevated.
    3. The 24-hour urine test shows Bence Jones proteins.
    4. The patient reports new-onset leg numbness.

17. The nurse in the outpatient clinic is assessing a 22-year-old who required a splenectomy after a recent motor vehicle accident. Which information obtained during the assessment will be of most immediate concern to the nurse?
    1. The patient engages in unprotected sex.
    2. The oral temperature is 100° F (37.8° C).
    3. There is abdominal pain with light palpation.
    4. The patient admits to occasional marijuana use.

18. A patient with graft-versus-host disease (GVHD) after bone marrow transplantation is being cared for on the medical unit. Which nursing activity is best delegated to a travel RN?
    1. Administering oral cyclosporine (Sandimmune) to the patient
    2. Assessing the patient for signs of infection caused by GVHD
    3. Infusing 5% dextrose in 0.45% saline at 125 mL/hr into the patient
    4. Educating the patient about ways to prevent and detect infection

19. You are the charge nurse on an oncology unit when a patient with an absolute neutrophil count of 300/µL is admitted. Which staff member should you assign to provide care for this patient, under the supervision of an experienced oncology RN?
    1. LPN/LVN who has floated from the same-day surgery unit
    2. RN from a staffing agency who is being oriented to the oncology unit
    3. LPN/LVN with 2 years of experience on the oncology unit
    4. RN who recently transferred to the oncology unit from the ED

20. You are transferring a patient with newly-diagnosed chronic myeloid leukemia to an LTC facility. Which information is most important to communicate to the LTC charge nurse before transferring the patient?
    1. Philadelphia chromosome is present in the patient's blood smear.
    2. Glucose level is elevated as a result of prednisone (Deltasone) therapy.
    3. There has been a 20-lb weight loss over the last year.
    4. The patient's chemotherapy has resulted in neutropenia.

21. A patient with acute myelogenous leukemia is receiving induction-phase chemotherapy. Which assessment finding requires the most rapid action?
    1. Serum potassium level of 7.8 mEq/L
    2. Urine output less than intake by 400 mL
    3. Inflammation and redness of the oral mucosa
    4. Ecchymoses present on the anterior trunk

22. A patient who has been receiving cyclosporine (Sandimmune) following an organ transplantation is experiencing the following symptoms. Which one is of most concern?
    1. Bleeding of the gums while brushing the teeth
    2. Nontender lump in the right groin
    3. Occasional nausea after taking the medication
    4. Numbness and tingling of the feet

23. A patient with Hodgkin lymphoma who is receiving radiation therapy to the groin area has skin redness and tenderness in the area being irradiated. Which nursing activity should you delegate to the UAP caring for the patient?
    1. Checking the skin for signs of redness or peeling
    2. Assisting the patient in choosing appropriate clothing
    3. Explaining good skin care to the patient and family
    4. Cleaning the skin over the area daily with a mild soap

24. After you receive the change-of-shift report, which patient will you assess first?
    1. 20-year-old with possible acute myelogenous leukemia who has just arrived on the medical unit
    2. 38-year-old with aplastic anemia who needs teaching about decreasing infection risk before discharge
    3. 40-year-old with lymphedema who requests help in putting on compression stockings before getting out of bed
    4. 60-year-old with non-Hodgkin lymphoma who is refusing the prescribed chemotherapy regimen

Answer Key for this chapter begins on p. 181.

PART 2 Common Health Scenarios

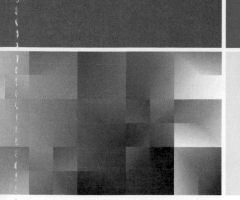

CHAPTER 9

Neurologic Problems

1. What is the priority nursing diagnosis for a client experiencing a migraine headache?
   1. Acute Pain related to biologic and chemical factors
   2. Anxiety related to change in or threat to health status
   3. Hopelessness related to deteriorating physiologic condition
   4. Risk for Injury related to side effects of medical therapy

2. You are creating a teaching plan for a client with newly-diagnosed migraine headaches. Which key items will you include in the teaching plan? *(Select all that apply.)*
   1. Foods that contain tyramine, such as alcohol and aged cheese, should be avoided.
   2. Drugs such as nitroglycerin (Nitrostat) and nifedipine (Procardia) should be avoided.
   3. Abortive therapy is aimed at eliminating the pain during the aura.
   4. A potential side effect of medications is rebound headache.
   5. Complementary therapies such as biofeedback and relaxation may be helpful.
   6. Estrogen therapy should be continued as prescribed by your physician.

3. After a client has a seizure, which action can you delegate to the UAP?
   1. Documenting the seizure
   2. Performing neurologic checks
   3. Taking the client's vital signs
   4. Restraining the client for protection

4. You are preparing to admit a client with a seizure disorder. Which actions can you delegate to an LPN/LVN?
   1. Completing the admission assessment
   2. Setting up oxygen and suction equipment
   3. Placing a padded tongue blade at the bedside
   4. Padding the side rails before the client arrives

5. A nursing student is teaching a client and family about epilepsy before the client's discharge. For which statement should you intervene?
   1. "You should avoid consumption of all forms of alcohol."
   2. "Wear your medical alert bracelet at all times."
   3. "Protect your loved one's airway during a seizure."
   4. "It's OK to take over-the-counter medications."

6. A client with Parkinson disease has received a nursing diagnosis of Impaired Physical Mobility related to neuromuscular impairment. You observe the UAP performing all of these actions. For which action must you intervene?
   1. Helping the client ambulate to the bathroom and back to bed
   2. Reminding the client not to look at his feet when he is walking
   3. Performing the client's complete bathing and oral care
   4. Setting up the client's tray and encouraging the client to feed himself

7. You are preparing to discharge a client with chronic low back pain. Which statement by the client indicates the need for additional teaching?
   1. "I will avoid exercise because the pain gets worse."
   2. "I will use heat or ice to help control the pain."
   3. "I will not wear high-heeled shoes at home or work."
   4. "I will purchase a firm mattress to replace my old one."

8. A client with a spinal cord injury (SCI) reports sudden severe throbbing headache that started a short time ago. Assessment of the client reveals increased blood pressure (168/94 mm Hg) and decreased heart rate (48 beats/min), diaphoresis, and flushing of the face and neck. What action should you take first?
   1. Administer the ordered acetaminophen (Tylenol).
   2. Check the Foley tubing for kinks or obstruction.
   3. Adjust the temperature in the client's room.
   4. Notify the physician about the change in status.

9. Which client should you, as charge nurse, assign to a new RN graduate who is on orientation to the neurologic unit?
   1. 28-year-old newly-admitted client with an SCI
   2. 67-year-old who had a stroke 3 days ago and has left-sided weakness
   3. 85-year-old with dementia who is to be transferred to long-term care today
   4. 54-year-old with Parkinson disease who needs assistance with bathing

10. A client with an SCI at level C3-C4 is being cared for in the emergency department (ED). What is the priority assessment?
    1. Determine the level at which the client has intact sensation.
    2. Assess the level at which the client has retained mobility.
    3. Check blood pressure and pulse for signs of spinal shock.
    4. Monitor respiratory effort and oxygen saturation level.

11. You are floated from the ED to the neurologic floor. Which action should you delegate to the UAP when providing nursing care for a client with an SCI?
    1. Assessing the client's respiratory status every 4 hours
    2. Taking the client's vital signs and recording every 4 hours
    3. Monitoring the client's nutritional status, including calorie counts
    4. Instructing the client how to turn, cough, and breathe deeply every 2 hours

12. You are helping a client with an SCI to establish a bladder retraining program. Which strategies may stimulate the client to void? *(Select all that apply.)*
    1. Stroking the client's inner thigh
    2. Pulling on the client's pubic hair
    3. Initiating intermittent straight catheterization
    4. Pouring warm water over the client's perineum
    5. Tapping the bladder to stimulate the detrusor muscle

13. A client with a cervical SCI has been placed in fixed skeletal traction with a halo fixation device. When caring for this client, the nurse may delegate which actions to an LPN/LVN? *(Select all that apply.)*
    1. Checking the client's skin for pressure from the device
    2. Assessing the client's neurologic status for changes
    3. Observing the halo insertion sites for signs of infection
    4. Cleaning the halo insertion sites with hydrogen peroxide
    5. Developing the nursing plan of care for the client

14. You are preparing a nursing care plan for a client with an SCI for whom the nursing diagnoses of Impaired Physical Mobility and Toileting Self-Care Deficit have been identified. The client tells you, "I don't know why we're doing all this. My life's over." Based on this statement, which additional nursing diagnosis takes priority?
    1. Risk for Injury related to altered mobility
    2. Imbalanced Nutrition: Less than Body Requirements
    3. Impaired Individual Resilience related to spinal cord injury
    4. Disturbed Body Image related to immobilization

15. Which client should be assigned to the traveling nurse, new to neurologic nursing care, who has been on the neurologic unit for 1 week?
    1. 34-year-old with newly diagnosed multiple sclerosis (MS)
    2. 68-year-old with chronic amyotrophic lateral sclerosis (ALS)
    3. 56-year-old with Guillain-Barré syndrome (GBS) in respiratory distress
    4. 25-year-old admitted with a C4-level SCI

16. A client with MS tells the UAP after physical therapy that she is too tired to take a bath. What is the priority nursing diagnosis at this time?
    1. Fatigue related to disease state
    2. Activity Intolerance due to generalized weakness
    3. Impaired Physical Mobility related to neuromuscular impairment
    4. Bathing Self-Care Deficit related to fatigue and neuromuscular weakness

17. An LPN/LVN, under your supervision, is providing nursing care for a client with GBS. What observation should you instruct the LPN/LVN to report immediately?
    1. Reports of numbness and tingling
    2. Facial weakness and difficulty speaking
    3. Rapid heart rate of 102 beats/min
    4. Shallow respirations and decreased breath sounds

18. The UAP reports to you, the RN, that a client with myasthenia gravis has an elevated temperature (102.2° F [39° C]), an increased heart rate (120 beats/min), and a rise in blood pressure (158/94 mm Hg) and was incontinent of urine and stool. What is your best first action at this time?
    1. Administer an acetaminophen suppository.
    2. Notify the physician immediately.
    3. Recheck vital signs in 1 hour.
    4. Reschedule the client's physical therapy.

19. You are providing care for a client with an acute hemorrhagic stroke. The client's spouse tells you that he has been reading a lot about strokes and asks why his wife has not received alteplase (Activase). What is your best response?
    1. "Your wife was not admitted within the time frame that alteplase is usually given."
    2. "This drug is used primarily for clients who experience an acute heart attack."
    3. "Alteplase dissolves clots and may cause more bleeding into your wife's brain."
    4. "Your wife had gallbladder surgery just 6 months ago, and this prevents the use of alteplase."

20. You are supervising a senior nursing student who is caring for a client with a right hemisphere stroke. Which action by the student nurse requires that you intervene?
    1. Instructing the client to sit up straight, and the client responding with a puzzled expression
    2. Moving the client's food tray to the right side of his over-bed table
    3. Assisting the client with passive range-of-motion (ROM) exercises
    4. Combing the hair on the left side of the client's head when the client always combs his hair on the right side

21. Which actions should you delegate to an experienced UAP when caring for a client with a thrombotic stroke who has residual left-sided weakness? *(Select all that apply.)*
    1. Assisting the client to reposition every 2 hours
    2. Reapplying pneumatic compression boots
    3. Reminding the client to perform active ROM exercises
    4. Assessing the extremities for redness and edema
    5. Setting up meal trays and assisting with feeding

22. A client who had a stroke needs to be fed. What instruction should you give to the UAP who will feed the client?
    1. Position the client sitting up in bed before you feed him.
    2. Check the client's gag and swallowing reflexes.
    3. Feed the client quickly, because there are three more you must feed.
    4. Suction the client's secretions between bites of food.

23. You have just admitted a client with bacterial meningitis who reports a severe headache with photophobia and has a temperature of 102.6° F (39.2° C) orally. Which prescribed intervention should be implemented first?
    1. Administer codeine 15 mg orally for the client's headache.
    2. Infuse ceftriaxone (Rocephin) 2000 mg IV to treat the infection.
    3. Give acetaminophen (Tylenol) 650 mg orally to reduce the fever.
    4. Give furosemide (Lasix) 40 mg IV to decrease intracranial pressure.

24. You are mentoring a student nurse in the intensive care unit (ICU) while caring for a client with meningococcal meningitis. Which action by the student requires that you intervene most rapidly?
    1. Entering the room without putting on a mask and gown
    2. Instructing the family that visits are restricted to 10 minutes
    3. Giving the client a warm blanket when he says he feels cold
    4. Checking the client's pupil response to light every 30 minutes

25. A 23-year-old with a recent history of encephalitis is admitted to the medical unit with new-onset generalized tonic-clonic seizures. Which nursing activities included in the client's care will be best to delegate to an LPN/LVN whom you are supervising? *(Select all that apply.)*
    1. Observing and documenting the onset and duration of any seizure activity
    2. Administering phenytoin (Dilantin) 200 mg by mouth (PO) three times a day
    3. Teaching the client about the need for frequent tooth brushing and flossing
    4. Developing a discharge plan that includes referral to the Epilepsy Foundation
    5. Assessing for adverse effects caused by new antiseizure medications

26. Which nursing action will be implemented first if a client has a generalized tonic-clonic seizure?
    1. Turn the client to one side.
    2. Give lorazepam (Ativan) 2 mg IV.
    3. Administer oxygen via nonrebreather mask.
    4. Assess the client's level of consciousness.

27. A client who recently started taking phenytoin to control simple partial seizures is seen in the outpatient clinic. Which information obtained during her chart review and assessment will be of greatest concern?
    1. The gums appear enlarged and inflamed.
    2. The white blood cell count is 2300/mm³.
    3. The client sometimes forgets to take the phenytoin until the afternoon.
    4. The client wants to renew her driver's license in the next month.

28. After you receive the change-of-shift report at 7:00 AM, which client will you assess first?
    1. 23-year-old with a migraine headache who reports severe nausea associated with retching
    2. 45-year-old who is scheduled for a craniotomy in 30 minutes and needs preoperative teaching
    3. 59-year-old with Parkinson disease who will need a swallowing assessment before breakfast
    4. 63-year-old with MS who has an oral temperature of 101.8° F (38.8° C) and flank pain

29. All of these nursing activities are included in the care plan for a 78-year-old man with Parkinson disease who has been referred to your home health agency. Which activities will you delegate to the UAP? *(Select all that apply.)*
    1. Checking for orthostatic changes in pulse and blood pressure
    2. Assessing for improvement in tremor after levodopa (L-dopa [Larodopa]) is given
    3. Reminding the client to allow adequate time for meals
    4. Monitoring for signs of toxic reactions to anti-Parkinson medications
    5. Assisting the client with prescribed strengthening exercises
    6. Adapting the client's preferred activities to his level of function

30. You are in charge of developing a standard plan of care in an Alzheimer disease care facility and are responsible for delegating and supervising resident care given by LPNs/LVNs and UAPs. Which activity is best to delegate to the LPN/LVN team leaders?
    1. Checking for improvement in resident memory after medication therapy is initiated
    2. Using the Mini-Mental State Examination to assess residents every 6 months
    3. Assisting residents in using the toilet every 2 hours to decrease risk for urinary incontinence
    4. Developing individualized activity plans after consulting with residents and family

31. A client who has Alzheimer disease is hospitalized with new-onset angina. Her husband tells you he does not sleep well because he needs to be sure she does not wander during the night. He insists on checking each of the medications you give the client to be sure they are "the same pills she takes at home." Based on this information, which nursing diagnosis is most appropriate for this client?
    1. Decreased Cardiac Output related to poor myocardial contractility
    2. Caregiver Role Strain related to continuous need for providing care
    3. Risk for Falls related to client wandering behavior during the night
    4. Ineffective Family Therapeutic Regimen Management related to poor client memory

32. You are caring for a client with a glioblastoma who is receiving dexamethasone (Decadron) 4 mg IV every 6 hours to relieve symptoms of right arm weakness and headache. Which assessment information will concern you the most?
    1. The client no longer recognizes family members.
    2. The blood glucose level is 234 mg/dL.
    3. The client reports a continuing headache.
    4. The daily weight has increased 1 kg.

33. A 70-year-old alcoholic client who has become lethargic, confused, and incontinent during the last week is admitted to the ED. His wife tells you that he fell down the stairs about a month ago, but that "he didn't have a scratch afterward." Which collaborative interventions will you implement first?
    1. Place the client on the hospital alcohol withdrawal protocol.
    2. Transport the client to the radiology department for a computed tomographic (CT) scan.
    3. Make a referral to the social services department.
    4. Give the client phenytoin 100 mg PO.

34. Which client in the neurologic ICU will be best to assign to an RN who has been floated from the medical unit?
    1. 26-year-old with a basilar skull fracture who has clear drainage coming out of the nose
    2. 42-year-old admitted several hours ago with a headache and a diagnosis of a ruptured berry aneurysm
    3. 46-year-old who was admitted 48 hours ago with bacterial meningitis and has an antibiotic dose due
    4. 65-year-old with an astrocytoma who has just returned to the unit after undergoing craniotomy

Answer Key for this chapter begins on p. 182.

CHAPTER 10

Visual and Auditory Problems

1. You are working in an ambulatory care clinic. A client calls to report redness of the sclera, itching of the eyes, and increased lacrimation for several hours. What should you direct the caller to do first?
   1. "Please call your physician" (i.e., refuse to advise).
   2. "Apply a cool compress to your eyes."
   3. "If you are wearing contact lenses, remove them."
   4. "Take an over-the-counter antihistamine."

2. At a community health clinic, you are teaching a community group about the prevention of accidental eye injuries. What is the most important thing to stress?
   1. Workplace policies for handling chemicals should be followed.
   2. Children and parents should be cautious about aggressive play.
   3. Protective eyewear should be worn during sports or hazardous work.
   4. Emergency eyewash stations should be established in the workplace.

3. Which clients would be best to assign to the most experienced nurse in an ambulatory care center that specializes in vision problems and eye surgery? *(Select all that apply.)*
   1. Client who requires postoperative instructions after cataract surgery
   2. Client who needs an eye pad and a metal shield applied
   3. Client who requests a home health referral for dressing changes and eyedrop instillation
   4. Client who needs teaching about self-administration of eyedrops
   5. Client who requires an assessment for recent and sudden loss of sight
   6. Client who requires preoperative teaching for laser trabeculoplasty

4. Place the following steps for eyedrop administration in the correct order.
   1. Gently press on the lacrimal duct for 1 minute.
   2. Gently pull the tissue underneath the eye downward to expose the lower conjunctival sac.
   3. Have the client gently close the eye and move it around.
   4. Have the client look up while you instill the number of prescribed drops.
   5. Hold the dropper and stabilize your hand on the client's forehead.
   6. Have the client sit down and tilt his or her head slightly backward.

   _____, _____, _____, _____, _____, _____

5. Which tasks are appropriate to delegate to an LPN/LVN who is functioning under the supervision of an RN? *(Select all that apply.)*
   1. Assessing the sexual implications for a client with oculogenital-type *Chlamydia trachomatis* infection
   2. Administering sulfacetamide sodium 10% (Sulf-10 Ophthalmic) to a child with conjunctivitis
   3. Reviewing hand-washing and hygiene practices with clients who have eye infections
   4. Showing clients how to gently cleanse eyelid margins to remove crusting
   5. Assessing nutritional factors for a client with age-related macular degeneration
   6. Reviewing the health history of a client to identify risk for ocular manifestations
   7. Performing a routine check of a client's visual acuity using the Snellen eye chart

6. You are interviewing an elderly woman and discover that she has been taking her glaucoma eyedrops by mouth for the past week. What should you do first?
   1. Call to obtain an order for tonometry so that her intraocular pressure can be checked.
   2. Try to determine how frequently and how much she has been ingesting.
   3. Ask her how she decided to take the drops orally instead of instilling them as eyedrops.
   4. Call the Poison Control Center and be prepared to describe untoward side effects.

7. You are working in a community health clinic and a client needs instructions for the care of a hordeolum (sty) on the right upper eyelid. What is the first treatment that the client should try?
   1. Apply warm compresses four times per day.
   2. Gently perform hygienic eyelid scrubs.
   3. Obtain a prescription for antibiotic drops.
   4. Contact the ophthalmologist.

8. Which finding should be immediately reported to the physician?
   1. A change in color vision
   2. Crusty yellow drainage on the eyelashes
   3. Increased lacrimation
   4. A curtainlike shadow across the visual field

9. In the care of a client who has sustained recent blindness, which tasks would be appropriate to delegate to a UAP? *(Select all that apply.)*
   1. Counseling the client to express grief or loss
   2. Assisting the client with ambulating in the hall
   3. Orienting the client to the surroundings
   4. Encouraging independence
   5. Obtaining supplies for hygienic care
   6. Storing personal items to reduce clutter
   7. Rearranging furniture to prevent falls

10. In discharge teaching after cataract surgery, the client and family should be told to immediately report which symptom to the physician?
    1. A scratchy sensation in the operative eye
    2. Loss of depth perception with the patch in place
    3. Poor vision 6-8 hours after patch removal
    4. Pain not relieved by prescribed medications

11. A client reports a sudden excruciating pain in the left eye with the visual change of colored halos around lights and blurred vision. Which interventions should you anticipate and perform for this emergency condition? *(Select all that apply.)*
    1. Prepare the client for photodynamic therapy.
    2. Instill a mydriatic agent, such as phenylephrine (Neo-Synephrine).
    3. Instill a miotic agent, such as pilocarpine (Isopto Carpine).
    4. Administer an oral hyperosmotic agent, such as isosorbide (Ismotic).
    5. Apply a cool compress to the forehead.
    6. Provide a darkened, quiet, and private space for the client.

12. Before giving a beta-adrenergic blocking glaucoma agent, you would make additional assessments and notify the physician if the client makes which statement?
    1. "My blood pressure runs a little high if I gain too much weight."
    2. "Occasionally I have palpitations, but they pass very quickly."
    3. "My joints feel stiff today, but that's just my arthritis."
    4. "My pulse rate is a little low today because I take digoxin."

13. You are supervising a new nurse who has just finished assessing a client who came to the clinic for redness and discomfort to the right eye. You review her documentation, which includes "visual acuity N/A." What should you do next?
    1. Do nothing; the documentation is minimal but acceptable.
    2. Ask her to explain her rationale for the documentation.
    3. Reassess the client yourself to validate her findings.
    4. Suggest that she contact the clinical educator for documentation tips.

14. Which tasks are appropriate to delegate to an LPN/LVN who is functioning under the supervision of a team leader or RN? *(Select all that apply.)*
    1. Irrigating the ear canal to loosen impacted cerumen
    2. Administering amoxicillin to a child with otitis media
    3. Reminding the client not to blow the nose after tympanoplasty
    4. Counseling a client with Ménière disease
    5. Suggesting communication techniques for the family of a hearing-impaired elder
    6. Assessing a client with labyrinthitis for headache and level of consciousness

15. You are interviewing an elderly client who reports that "lately there has been a roaring sound in my ears." What additional assessments should you include? *(Select all that apply.)*
    1. Obtain a medication history.
    2. Ask about exposure to loud noises.
    3. Observe the canal for earwax or foreign body.
    4. Assess for signs and symptoms of ear infection.
    5. Ask about frequency of ear hygiene.

16. A cheerful elderly widow comes to the community clinic for her annual checkup. She is in reasonably good health, but she has a hearing loss of 40 dB. She confides, "I don't get out much. I used to be really active, but the older I get, the more trouble I have hearing. It can be really embarrassing." What is the priority nursing diagnosis?
    1. Risk for Situational Low Self-Esteem related to perceived inability to interact
    2. Impaired Social Interaction related to progressive hearing loss
    3. Deficient Knowledge related to pathophysiologic processes
    4. Ineffective Coping related to change in sensory abilities

17. Which physical assessment findings should be reported to the physician?
    1. Pearly gray or pink tympanic membrane
    2. Dense whitish ring at the circumference of the tympanum
    3. Bulging red or blue tympanic membrane
    4. Cone of light at the innermost part of the tympanum

18. Which description by a client reporting vertigo would concern you the most?
    1. Dizziness with hearing loss
    2. Episodic vertigo
    3. Vertigo without hearing loss
    4. "Merry-go-round" vertigo

19. In assisting clients with vertigo and balance problems, which team member (RN, LPN/LVN, MD, physical therapist, UAP), working under appropriate supervision, should be assigned to complete each task?
    1. Assess and identify the cause of the vertigo. _____
    2. Assist the client in routine position change and ambulation. _____
    3. Administer antivertigo agents such as meclizine (Antivert). _____
    4. Obtain informed consent for a labyrinthectomy. _____
    5. Assess situations that lead to or exacerbate vertigo. _____
    6. Review the need for adaptive aids such as a walker or cane. _____

20. You performed postoperative stapedectomy teaching several days ago for a client. Which comment by the client concerns you the most?
    1. "I'm going to take swimming lessons in a couple of months."
    2. "I have to take a long overseas flight in several weeks."
    3. "I can't wait to get back to my regular weightlifting class."
    4. "I have been coughing a lot with my mouth open."

21. Place the following steps for ear irrigation in the correct order.
    1. Use an otoscope to ascertain that the eardrum is intact and that there is no evidence of infection.
    2. Place the tip of the syringe at an angle in the external canal.
    3. Watch for fluid return and signs of cerumen.
    4. If cerumen does not appear, wait 10 minutes and repeat the irrigation.
    5. Fill a syringe with warm irrigating solution.
    6. After completion of the irrigation, have the client turn the head to the side to facilitate drainage.
    7. Apply gentle but continuous pressure to the syringe plunger.

    _____, _____, _____, _____, _____, _____, _____

PART 2 Common Health Scenarios

Answer Key for this chapter begins on p. 185.

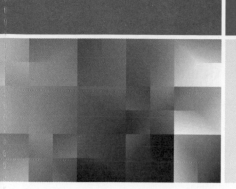

CHAPTER 11

Musculoskeletal Problems

1. You are initiating a nursing care plan for a patient with osteoporosis. All of these nursing interventions apply to the nursing diagnosis Risk for Falls. Which intervention should you delegate to the UAP?
   1. Identifying environmental factors that increase risk for falls
   2. Monitoring gait, balance, and fatigue level with ambulation
   3. Collaborating with the physical therapist (PT) to provide the patient with a walker
   4. Assisting the patient with ambulation to the bathroom and in the halls

2. You are preparing to teach a patient with a new diagnosis of osteoporosis about strategies to prevent falls. Which teaching points will you be sure to include? *(Select all that apply.)*
   1. Wear a hip protector when ambulating.
   2. Remove throw rugs and other obstacles at home.
   3. Exercise to help build your strength.
   4. Expect a few bumps and bruises when you go home.
   5. Rest when you are tired.

3. Your assessment reveals all of these data when you are admitting a patient with Paget disease. Which finding should you notify the physician about first?
   1. There is a bowing of both legs and the knees are asymmetrical.
   2. The base of the skull is invaginated (platybasia).
   3. The patient is only 5 feet tall and weighs 120 lb.
   4. The skull is soft, thick, and larger than normal.

4. The charge nurse observes an LPN/LVN providing all of these interventions for a patient with Paget disease. Which action requires that the charge nurse intervene?
   1. Administering 600 mg of ibuprofen (Advil) to the patient
   2. Encouraging the patient to perform PT-recommended exercises
   3. Applying ice and gentle massage to the patient's lower extremities
   4. Reminding the patient to drink milk and eat cottage cheese

5. As charge nurse, you are making assignments for the day shift. Which patient would you assign to the nurse who was floated from the postanesthesia care unit (PACU) for the day?
   1. 35-year-old with osteomyelitis who needs teaching before hyperbaric oxygen therapy
   2. 62-year-old with osteomalacia who is being discharged to a long-term care facility
   3. 68-year-old with osteoporosis given a new orthotic device whose knowledge of its use must be assessed
   4. 72-year-old with Paget disease who has just returned from surgery for total knee replacement

6. You delegate the measurement of vital signs to an experienced UAP. Osteomyelitis has been diagnosed in a patient. Which vital sign value would you instruct the UAP to report immediately?
   1. Temperature of 101° F (38.3° C)
   2. Blood pressure of 136/80 mm Hg
   3. Heart rate of 96 beats/min
   4. Respiratory rate of 24 breaths/min

7. You are working with a UAP to provide care for six patients. At the beginning of the shift, you carefully tell the UAP what patient interventions and tasks she is expected to perform. To be sure that your communication is appropriate, you refer to the "Four Cs." List the Four Cs below.

   _____

   _____

   _____

   _____

8. You are caring for a patient with carpal tunnel syndrome (CTS) who has been admitted for surgery. Which intervention should you delegate to the UAP?
   1. Initiating placement of a splint for immobilization during the day
   2. Assessing the patient's wrist and hand for discoloration and brittle nails
   3. Assisting the patient with daily self-care measures such as bathing and eating
   4. Testing the patient for painful tingling in the four digits of the hand

Common Health Scenarios   **PART 2**

9. You observe a UAP performing all of these interventions for a patient with CTS. Which action requires that you intervene immediately?
   1. Arranging the patient's lunch tray and cutting his meat
   2. Providing warm water and assisting the patient with his bath
   3. Replacing the patient's splint in hyperextension position
   4. Reminding the patient not to lift very heavy objects

10. A patient is scheduled for endoscopic carpal tunnel release surgery in the morning. What would you be sure to teach the patient?
    1. Pain and numbness will be experienced for several days to weeks.
    2. Immediately after surgery, the patient will no longer need assistance.
    3. After surgery, the dressing will be large and there will be lots of drainage.
    4. The patient's pain and paresthesia will no longer be present.

11. As charge nurse, you assign the nursing care of a patient who has just returned from open carpal tunnel release surgery to an experienced LPN/LVN, who will perform under the supervision of an RN. Which instructions would you provide for the LPN/LVN? *(Select all that apply.)*
    1. Check the patient's vital signs every 15 minutes in the first hour.
    2. Check the dressing for drainage and tightness.
    3. Elevate the patient's hand above the heart.
    4. The patient will no longer need pain medication.
    5. Check the neurovascular status of the fingers every hour.

12. You are preparing the patient who had carpal tunnel release surgery for discharge. Which information is important to provide to this patient?
    1. The surgical procedure is a cure for CTS.
    2. Hand movements will be restricted for 4 to 6 weeks after surgery.
    3. Frequent doses of pain medication will no longer be necessary.
    4. The health care provider should be notified immediately if there is any pain or discomfort.

13. When receiving discharge instructions, a patient with osteoporosis makes all of these statements. Which statement indicates to you that the patient needs additional teaching?
    1. "I take my ibuprofen every morning as soon as I get up."
    2. "My daughter removed all of the throw rugs in my home."
    3. "My husband helps me every afternoon with range-of-motion exercises."
    4. "I rest in my reclining chair every day for at least an hour."

14. A patient has a fractured femur. Which finding would you instruct the UAP to report immediately?
    1. The patient reports pain.
    2. The patient appears confused.
    3. The patient's blood pressure is 136/88 mm Hg.
    4. The patient voided using the bedpan.

15. After you receive the change-of-shift report, which patient should you assess first?
    1. 42-year-old with CTS who reports pain
    2. 64-year-old with osteoporosis awaiting discharge
    3. 28-year-old with a fracture who reports that the cast is tight
    4. 56-year-old with a left leg amputation who reports phantom pain

16. A patient with a fractured fibula is receiving skeletal traction and has skeletal pins in place. What would you instruct the UAP to report immediately?
    1. The patient wants to change position in bed.
    2. There is a small amount of clear fluid at the pin sites.
    3. The traction weights are resting on the floor.
    4. The patient reports pain and muscle spasm.

17. The nursing diagnosis for a patient with a fracture of the right ankle is Impaired Physical Mobility. As charge nurse, you observe a newly-graduated RN perform all of these interventions. For which action should you intervene?
    1. Encouraging the patient to go from a lying to a standing position
    2. Administering pain medication before the patient begins exercises
    3. Explaining to the patient and family the purpose of the exercise program
    4. Reminding the patient about the correct use of crutches

18. The charge nurse is assigning the nursing care of a patient who had a left below-the-knee amputation 1 day ago to an experienced LPN/LVN, who will function under your supervision. What will you tell the LPN/LVN is the major focus for the patient's care today?
    1. To attain pain control over phantom pain
    2. To monitor for signs of sufficient tissue perfusion
    3. To assist the patient to ambulate as soon as possible
    4. To elevate the residual limb when the patient is supine

19. A patient with a right above-the-knee amputation asks you why he has phantom limb pain. What is your best response?
    1. "Phantom limb pain is not explained or predicted by any one theory."
    2. "Phantom limb pain occurs because your body thinks your leg is still present."
    3. "Phantom limb pain will not interfere with your activities of daily living."
    4. "Phantom limb pain is not real pain but is remembered pain."

20. During morning care, a patient with a below-the-knee amputation asks the UAP about prostheses. How will you instruct the UAP to respond?
    1. "You should get a prosthesis so that you can walk again."
    2. "Wait and ask your doctor that question the next time he comes in."
    3. "It's too soon to be worrying about getting a prosthesis."
    4. "I'll ask the nurse to come in and discuss this with you."

21. During assessment of a patient with fractures of the medial ulna and radius, you find all of these data. Which assessment finding should you report to the health care provider immediately?
    1. The patient reports pressure and pain.
    2. The cast is in place and is dry and intact.
    3. The skin is pink and warm to the touch.
    4. The patient can move all the fingers and the thumb.

22. A patient who underwent a right above-the-knee amputation 4 days ago also has a diagnosis of depression. Which order would you clarify with the health care provider?
    1. Give fluoxetine (Prozac) 40 mg once a day.
    2. Administer acetaminophen with codeine (Tylenol-Codeine) 1 or 2 tablets every 4 hours as needed.
    3. Assist the patient to the bedside chair every shift.
    4. Reinforce the dressing to the right residual limb as needed.

Answer Key for this chapter begins on p. 186.

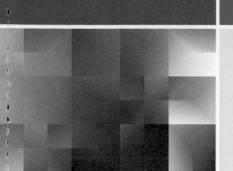

CHAPTER 12

Gastrointestinal and Nutritional Problems

1. When a client is being prepared for a colonoscopy procedure, which task is most suitable to delegate to the UAP?
   1. Explaining the need for a clear liquid diet 1 to 3 days before the procedure
   2. Reinforcing "nothing by mouth" status 8 hours before the procedure
   3. Administering laxatives 1 to 3 days before the procedure
   4. Administering an enema the night before the procedure

2. You would be most concerned about an order for a total parenteral nutrition (TPN) fat emulsion for a client with which condition?
   1. Gastrointestinal (GI) obstruction
   2. Severe anorexia nervosa
   3. Chronic diarrhea and vomiting
   4. Fractured femur

3. You are preparing to administer TPN through a central line. Place the following steps for administration in the correct order.
   1. Use aseptic technique when handling the injection cap.
   2. Thread the IV tubing through an infusion pump.
   3. Check the solution for cloudiness or turbidity.
   4. Connect the tubing to the central line.
   5. Select and flush the correct tubing and filter.
   6. Set the infusion pump at the prescribed rate.
   7. Confirm the order for TPN prior to administration.

   _____, _____, _____, _____, _____, _____, _____

4. You are caring for a client with peptic ulcer disease. Which assessment finding is the most serious?
   1. Projectile vomiting
   2. Burning sensation 2 hours after eating
   3. Coffee-ground emesis
   4. Boardlike abdomen with shoulder pain

5. You are taking an initial history for a client seeking surgical treatment for obesity. Which finding should be called to the attention of the surgeon before proceeding with additional history taking or physical assessment?
   1. Obesity for approximately 5 years
   2. History of counseling for body dysmorphic disorder
   3. Failure to reduce weight with other forms of therapy
   4. Body weight 100% above the ideal for age, gender, and height

6. You are taking report on an elderly client who was admitted with abdominal pain and nausea, vomiting, and diarrhea. The client also has a history of chronic dementia. Which comment by the night shift nurse concerns you the most?
   1. The client has a flat affect and rambling and repetitive speech.
   2. The client has memory impairments and thinks the year is 1948.
   3. The client lacks motivation and demonstrates early morning awakening.
   4. The client has a fluctuating level of consciousness and mood swings.

7. In the care of a client with gastroesophageal reflux disease, which task would be appropriate to assign to a UAP?
   1. Sharing successful strategies for weight reduction
   2. Encouraging the client to express concerns about lifestyle modification
   3. Reminding the client not to lie down for 2 to 3 hours after eating
   4. Explaining the rationale for eating small frequent meals

8. You are providing immediate postoperative care for a client who had fundoplication to reinforce the lower esophageal sphincter for the purpose of a hiatal hernia repair. What is the priority action for the care of this client?
   1. Elevate the head of the bed at least 30 degrees.
   2. Assess the nasogastric tube for yellowish-green drainage.
   3. Assist the client to start taking a clear liquid diet.
   4. Assess the client for gas bloat syndrome.

9. Which client is the most appropriate to assign to an LPN/LVN, under the supervision of an RN?
   1. Client with oral cancer who is scheduled in the morning for glossectomy
   2. Obese client returned from surgery after a vertical banded gastroplasty
   3. Client with anorexia nervosa who has muscle weakness and decreased urine output
   4. Client with intermittent nausea and vomiting related to chemotherapy

10. The postoperative care of a morbidly obese client is being planned. Which task best utilizes the expertise of the LPN/LVN?
    1. Obtaining an oversized blood pressure cuff and a large-size bed
    2. Setting up a reinforced trapeze bar
    3. Assisting in the planning of toileting, turning, and ambulation
    4. Assigning tasks to UAPs and other ancillary staff

11. A client with proctitis needs a rectal suppository. A senior nursing student assigned to care for this client tells you that she is afraid to insert a suppository because she has never done it before. What is the most appropriate action in supervising this student?
    1. Give the medication yourself and tell the student to talk to the instructor.
    2. Ask the student to leave the clinical area because she is unprepared.
    3. Reassign the client to an LPN/LVN and send the student to observe.
    4. Show the student how to insert the suppository and talk to the instructor.

12. You are teaching the client and family how to perform colostomy irrigation. Place the following information in the correct order.
    1. Hang the container at about shoulder height.
    2. Allow the solution to flow slowly and steadily for 5 to 10 minutes.
    3. Put 500 to 1000 mL of lukewarm water in the container.
    4. Clip the irrigation sleeve and have the client walk for 30 to 45 minutes for secondary evacuation.
    5. Lubricate the stoma cone and gently insert the tubing tip into the stoma.
    6. Clean, rinse, and dry the skin, and apply a new drainage pouch.
    7. Put on a pair of clean gloves.
    8. Allow 15 to 20 minutes for the initial evacuation.
    ____, ____, ____, ____, ____, ____, ____, ____

13. You are caring for a client with a nasogastric (NG) tube. Which task can be delegated to an experienced UAP?
    1. Removing the NG tube per physician order
    2. Securing the tape if the client accidentally dislodges the tube
    3. Disconnecting the suction to allow ambulation to the toilet
    4. Reconnecting the suction after the client has ambulated

14. You are planning a treatment and prevention program for chronic fecal incontinence for an elderly client. Which intervention should you try first?
    1. Administer a glycerin suppository 15 minutes before evacuation time.
    2. Insert a rectal tube at specified intervals each day.
    3. Assist the client to the bedpan or toilet 30 minutes after meals.
    4. Use incontinence briefs or adult-sized diapers.

15. A client hospitalized with ulcerative colitis reports 10 to 20 small diarrhea stools per day, with abdominal pain before defecation. The client appears depressed and underweight and is uninterested in self-care or suggested therapies. What is the priority nursing diagnosis?
    1. Diarrhea related to irritated bowel
    2. Imbalanced Nutrition: Less than Body Requirements related to nutrient loss
    3. Acute Pain related to increased GI motility
    4. Ineffective Self-Health Management related to treatment plan

16. While transferring a dirty laundry bag, a UAP sustains a puncture wound to the finger from a contaminated needle. The unit has several clients with hepatitis and acquired immunodeficiency syndrome (AIDS); the needle source is unknown. Place in order of priority the instructions that should be given to the UAP.
    1. Have blood test(s) performed per protocol.
    2. Complete and file an incident report.
    3. Perform a thorough aseptic hand washing.
    4. Report to the occupational health nurse.
    5. Follow up for results and counseling.
    6. Begin prophylactic drug therapy.
    ____, ____, ____, ____, ____, ____

17. You are caring for an obese postoperative client who underwent surgery for bowel resection. As the client is moving in bed, he comments, "Something popped open." Upon examination you note wound evisceration. Place in order the steps for handling this complication.
    1. Cover the intestine with sterile moistened gauze.
    2. Stay calm and stay with the client.
    3. Check the vital signs, especially blood pressure and pulse.
    4. Have a colleague gather sterile supplies and contact the physician.
    5. Put the client into semi-Fowler position with knees slightly flexed.
    6. Prepare the client for surgery as ordered.
    ____, ____, ____, ____, ____, ____

18. You are providing postoperative care for a client who underwent laparoscopic cholecystectomy. What should be reported immediately to the physician?
    1. The client cannot void 5 hours postoperatively.
    2. The client reports shoulder pain.
    3. The client reports right upper quadrant pain.
    4. Output does not equal input for the first few hours.

19. In the care of a client with acute viral hepatitis, which task should be delegated to the UAP?
    1. Emptying the bedpan while wearing gloves
    2. Playing games or engaging the client in diversional activities
    3. Monitoring dietary preferences
    4. Reporting signs and symptoms of jaundice

20. You are caring for a client with cirrhosis and portal hypertension. Which statement by the client concerns you the most?
    1. "I'm very constipated and have been straining during bowel movements."
    2. "I can't button my pants anymore because my belly is so swollen."
    3. "I have a tight sensation in my lower legs when I forget to put my feet up."
    4. "When I sleep, I have to sit in a recliner so that I can breathe more easily."

21. For clients coming to the ambulatory care GI clinic, which task would be most appropriate to assign to an LPN/LVN?
    1. Teaching a client self-care measures for an ulcer
    2. Assisting the physician in incision and drainage of a pilonidal cyst
    3. Evaluating a client's response to sitz baths for an anorectal abscess
    4. Describing the basic pathophysiology of an anal fistula to a client

22. A client underwent an exploratory laparotomy 2 days ago. The physician should be called immediately for which physical assessment finding?
    1. Abdominal distention and rigidity
    2. Displacement of the NG tube by the client
    3. Absent or hypoactive bowel sounds
    4. Nausea and occasional vomiting

23. You must rearrange the room assignments for several clients. Which two clients would be best to put in the same room?
    1. 35-year-old woman with copious intractable diarrhea and vomiting
    2. 43-year-old woman who underwent cholecystectomy 2 days ago
    3. 53-year-old woman with pain related to alcohol-associated pancreatitis
    4. 62-year-old woman with colon cancer receiving chemotherapy and radiation
    _____, _____

24. You are caring for a client who was recently admitted for severe diverticulitis. Which task is appropriate to delegate for the care of this client?
    1. Tell the unit secretary to call radiology and schedule a barium enema.
    2. Instruct the LPN/LVN to give PRN laxatives when the client reports constipation.
    3. Advise the nursing student to help the client ambulate up and down the hall.
    4. Tell the UAP that a stool specimen must be saved to test for occult blood.

25. You are caring for a client who was admitted to your medical-surgical unit for observation after being evaluated in the emergency department for blunt trauma to the abdomen. Which instructions are appropriate to give to the UAP?
    1. Check the client's skin temperature and report if the skin feels cool.
    2. Check the urine in the urometer every hour and observe for red- or pink-tinged urine.
    3. Check vital signs every hour and report all of the values.
    4. Check the client's pain and report worsening of pain or discomfort.

26. Place the steps for performing colostomy care in the correct order.
    1. Fit the pouch snugly around the stoma.
    2. Assess the color and appearance of the stoma.
    3. Wash the skin with mild soap and rinse with warm water.
    4. Apply a skin barrier to protect the peristomal skin.
    5. Dry the skin carefully.
    6. Don a pair of clean gloves and remove the old pouch.
    _____, _____, _____, _____, _____, _____

PART 2 Common Health Scenarios

27. Clients who are undernourished or starved for prolonged periods are at risk for refeeding syndrome when nourishment is first given. What is the priority nursing assessment to prevent complications associated with this syndrome?
    1. Monitor for peripheral edema, crackles in the lungs, and jugular vein distention.
    2. Monitor for decreased bowel sounds, nausea, bloating, and abdominal distention.
    3. Observe for signs of secret purging and ingestion of water to increase weight.
    4. Assess for alternating constipation and diarrhea and pale clay-colored stools.

28. You are caring for a client who was admitted for advanced cirrhosis. The client has massive ascites, peripheral dependent edema in the lower extremities, nausea and vomiting, and dyspnea related to pressure on the diaphragm. For the nursing diagnosis of Excess Fluid Volume, which indicator is the most reliable for tracking fluid retention?
    1. Auscultating the lung fields for crackles every day
    2. Measuring the abdominal girth every morning
    3. Performing daily weights with the same amount of clothing
    4. Checking the extremities for pitting edema and comparing to baseline

29. A client with end-stage liver disease is talking to you about being on the transplant list. Which statement by the client concerns you the most?
    1. "I have a family history of diabetes."
    2. "I had symptoms of asthma when I was a kid."
    3. "I am going to cut down on my drinking very soon."
    4. "I am not very good about taking prescribed medication."

30. You are supervising a nursing student who is caring for a client who had a cholecystectomy. There is a T-tube in place. You would intervene if the student performs which action?
    1. Maintains the client in a semi-Fowler position
    2. Checks the amount, color, and consistency of the drainage
    3. Gently aspirates the drainage from the tube
    4. Inspects the skin around the tube for redness or irritation

Answer Key for this chapter begins on p. 188.

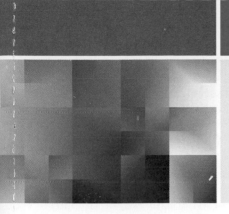

CHAPTER 13

Diabetes Mellitus

1. You are preparing to review a teaching plan for a patient with type 2 diabetes mellitus. To determine the patient's level of compliance with his prescribed diabetic regimen, which value would you be sure to review?
   1. Fasting glucose level
   2. Oral glucose tolerance test results
   3. Glycosylated hemoglobin (HgbA$_{1c}$) level
   4. Fingerstick glucose findings for 24 hours

2. A patient has newly-diagnosed type 2 diabetes. Which task should you delegate to a UAP?
   1. Arranging a consult with the dietitian
   2. Assessing the patient's insulin injection technique
   3. Teaching the patient to use a glucometer to monitor glucose at home
   4. Reminding the patient to check glucose level before each meal

3. A nursing diagnosis for a patient with newly-diagnosed diabetes is Risk for Injury related to sensory alterations. Which key points should you include in the teaching plan for this patient? *(Select all that apply.)*
   1. "Clean and inspect your feet every day."
   2. "Be sure that your shoes fit properly."
   3. "Nylon socks are best to prevent friction on your toes from shoes."
   4. "Only a podiatrist should trim your toenails."
   5. "Report any nonhealing skin breaks to your health care provider."

4. An LPN/LVN's assessment of two diabetic patients reveals all of these findings. Which would you instruct the LPN/LVN to report immediately?
   1. Fingerstick glucose reading of 185 mg/dL
   2. Numbness and tingling in both feet
   3. Profuse perspiration
   4. Bunion on the left great toe

5. The plan of care for a diabetic patient includes all of these interventions. Which intervention should you delegate to a UAP?
   1. Checking to make sure that the patient's bath water is not too hot
   2. Discussing community resources for diabetic outpatient care
   3. Teaching the patient to perform daily foot inspection
   4. Assessing the patient's technique for drawing insulin into a syringe

6. A 58-year-old with type 2 diabetes was admitted to your unit with a diagnosis of chronic obstructive pulmonary disease (COPD) exacerbation. When you prepare a care plan for this patient, what would you be sure to include? *(Select all that apply.)*
   1. Fingerstick blood glucose checks before meals and at bedtime
   2. Sliding-scale insulin dosing as ordered
   3. Bed rest until the COPD exacerbation is resolved
   4. Teaching about the Atkins diet for weight loss
   5. Demonstration of the components of foot care

7. A UAP tells you that, while assisting with the morning care of a postoperative patient with type 2 diabetes who has been given insulin, the patient asked if she will always need to take insulin now. What is your priority for teaching the patient?
   1. Explain to the patient that she is now considered to have type 1 diabetes.
   2. Tell the patient to monitor fingerstick glucose level every 4 hours after discharge.
   3. Teach the patient that a person with type 2 diabetes does not always need insulin.
   4. Talk with the patient about the relationship between illness and increased glucose levels.

8. An LPN/LVN is to administer rapid-acting insulin (Lispro) to a patient with type 1 diabetes. What essential information would you be sure to tell the LPN/LVN?
   1. Give this insulin after the patient's food tray has been delivered and the patient is ready to eat.
   2. Only give this insulin if the patient's fingerstick glucose reading is above 200 mg/dL.
   3. This insulin mimics the basal glucose control of the pancreas.
   4. Rapid-acting insulin is the only insulin that can be given subcutaneously or IV.

9. In the care of a patient with type 2 diabetes, which actions can you delegate to a UAP? *(Select all that apply.)*
   1. Providing the patient with extra packets of artificial sweetener for coffee
   2. Assessing how well the patient's shoes fit
   3. Recording the liquid intake from the patient's breakfast tray
   4. Teaching the patient what to do if dizziness or lightheadedness occurs
   5. Checking and recording the patient's blood pressure

10. In the emergency department during initial assessment of a newly-admitted patient with diabetes, the nurse discovers all of these findings. Which finding should be reported to the health care provider immediately?
    1. Hammer toe of the left second metatarsophalangeal joint
    2. Rapid respiratory rate with deep inspirations
    3. Numbness and tingling bilaterally in the feet and hands
    4. Decreased sensitivity and swelling of the abdomen

11. You are caring for a diabetic patient who is developing diabetic ketoacidosis (DKA). Which task delegation is most appropriate?
    1. Ask the unit clerk to page the physician to come to the unit.
    2. Ask the LPN/LVN to administer IV push insulin according to a sliding scale.
    3. Ask the UAP to hang a new bag of normal saline.
    4. Ask the UAP to get the patient a cup of orange juice.

12. You are serving as preceptor to a nurse who has recently graduated and passed the RN licensure examination. The new nurse has only been on the unit for 2 days. Which patient should you assign to the new nurse?
    1. 68-year-old with diabetes who is showing signs of hyperglycemia
    2. 58-year-old with diabetes who has cellulitis of the left ankle
    3. 49-year-old with diabetes who has just returned from the postanesthesia care unit after a below-knee amputation
    4. 72-year-old with diabetes with DKA who is receiving IV insulin

13. A patient with diabetes has hot, dry skin; rapid and deep respirations; and a fruity odor to his breath. As charge nurse, you observe a newly-graduated RN performing all the following patient tasks. Which one requires that you intervene immediately?
    1. Checking the patient's fingerstick glucose level
    2. Encouraging the patient to drink orange juice
    3. Checking the patient's order for sliding-scale insulin dosing
    4. Assessing the patient's vital signs every 15 minutes

14. A patient has newly-diagnosed type 2 diabetes. Which action should you assign to an LPN/LVN instead of a UAP?
    1. Measuring the patient's vital signs every shift
    2. Checking the patient's glucose level before each meal
    3. Administering subcutaneous insulin on a sliding scale as needed
    4. Assisting the patient with morning care

15. A patient with type 1 diabetes reports feeling dizzy. What should the nurse do first?
    1. Check the patient's blood pressure.
    2. Give the patient some orange juice.
    3. Give the patient's morning dose of insulin.
    4. Use a glucometer to check the patient's glucose level.

16. While working in the diabetes clinic, you obtain this information about an 8-year-old with type 1 diabetes. Which finding is most important to address when planning child and parent education?
    1. Most recent hemoglobin A_{1c} level of 7.8%
    2. Many questions about diet choices from the parents
    3. Child's participation in soccer practice after school 2 days a week
    4. Morning preprandial glucose range of 55 to 70 mg/dL

17. Which actions can the school nurse delegate to UAPs who are working with a 7-year-old child with type 1 diabetes in an elementary school? *(Select all that apply.)*
    1. Obtaining information about the child's usual insulin use from the parents
    2. Administering oral glucose tablets when blood glucose level falls below 60 mg/dL
    3. Teaching the child about what foods have high carbohydrate levels
    4. Obtaining blood glucose readings using the child's blood glucose monitor
    5. Reminding the child to have a snack after the physical education class

18. While you are performing an admission assessment on a patient with type 2 diabetes, he tells you that he routinely drinks 3 beers a day. What is your priority follow-up question at this time?
    1. "Do you have any days when you do not drink?"
    2. "When during the day do you drink your beers?"
    3. "Do you drink any other forms of alcohol?"
    4. "Have you ever had a lipid profile completed?"

19. The UAP reports to you that a patient with type 1 diabetes has a question about exercise. What important points would you be sure to teach this patient? *(Select all that apply.)*
    1. Exercise guidelines are based on blood glucose and urine ketone levels.
    2. Be sure to test your blood glucose only after exercising.
    3. You can exercise vigorously if your blood glucose is between 100 and 250 mg/dL.
    4. Exercise will help resolve the presence of ketones in your urine.
    5. A 5- to 10-minute warm-up and cool-down period should be included in your exercise.

20. The experienced UAP has been delegated to take vital signs and check fingerstick glucose on a diabetic patient who is postoperative. Which vital sign change would you instruct the UAP to report immediately?
    1. Blood pressure increase from 132/80 mm Hg to 138/84 mm Hg
    2. Temperature increase from 98.4° F (36.8° C) to 99° F (37.2° C)
    3. Respiratory rate increase from 18 breaths/min to 22 breaths/min
    4. Glucose increase from 190 mg/dL to 236 mg/dL

21. You are the preceptor for a senior nursing student who will teach a diabetic patient about self-care during sick days. For which statement by the student must you intervene?
    1. "When you are sick, be sure to monitor your blood glucose at least every 4 hours."
    2. "Test your urine for ketones whenever your blood glucose level is less than 240 mg/dL."
    3. "To prevent dehydration, drink 8 ounces of sugar-free liquid every hour while you are awake."
    4. "Continue to eat your meals and snacks at the usual times."

22. You are caring for an 81-year-old adult with type 2 diabetes, hypertension, and peripheral vascular disease. Which admission assessment findings increase the patient's risk for development of hyperglycemic-hyperosmolar syndrome (HHS)? *(Select all that apply.)*
    1. Hydrochlorothiazide (HCTZ) prescribed to control her diabetes
    2. Weight gain of 6 pounds over the past month
    3. Avoids consuming liquids in the evening
    4. Blood pressure of 168/94 mm Hg
    5. Urine output of 50 to 75 mL/hr

23. You are orienting a new graduate nurse who is providing diabetes education for a patient about insulin injection. For which teaching statement by the new nurse must you intervene?
    1. "To prevent lipohypertrophy, be sure to rotate injection sites from the abdomen to the thighs."
    2. "To correctly inject the insulin, lightly grasp a fold of skin and inject at a 90-degree angle."
    3. "Always draw your regular insulin into the syringe first before your NPH insulin."
    4. "Avoid injecting the insulin into scarred sites because those areas slow the absorption rate of insulin."

24. The patient with type 2 diabetes is "nothing by mouth" (NPO) for a cardiac catheterization. An LPN/LVN who is administering medications to this patient asks you (the supervising RN) whether the patient should receive his ordered repaglinide (Prandin). What is your best response?
    1. "Yes, because this drug will increase the patient's insulin secretion and prevent hyperglycemia."
    2. "No, because this drug may cause the patient to experience gastrointestinal symptoms such as nausea."
    3. "No, because this drug should be given 1 to 30 minutes before meals and the patient is NPO."
    4. "Yes, because this drug should be taken 3 times a day whether the patient eats or not."

25. You are caring for a diabetic patient admitted with hypoglycemia that occurred at home. Which teaching points for treatment of hypoglycemia at home would you include in a teaching plan for the patient and family before discharge? *(Select all that apply.)*
    1. Signs and symptoms of hypoglycemia include hunger, irritability, weakness, headache, and blood glucose less than 60 mg/dL.
    2. Treat hypoglycemia with 4 to 8 g of carbohydrate such as glucose tablets or ¼ cup of fruit juice.
    3. Retest blood glucose in 30 minutes.
    4. Repeat the carbohydrate treatment if the symptoms do not resolve.
    5. Eat a small snack of carbohydrate and protein if the next meal is more than an hour away.

Answer Key for this chapter begins on p. 190.

CHAPTER 14

Other Endocrine Problems

1. A patient is admitted to the medical unit with possible Graves disease (hyperthyroidism). Which assessment finding supports this diagnosis?
   1. Periorbital edema
   2. Bradycardia
   3. Exophthalmos
   4. Hoarse voice

2. Which change in vital signs would you instruct the UAP to report immediately for a patient with hyperthyroidism?
   1. Rapid heart rate
   2. Decreased systolic blood pressure
   3. Increased respiratory rate
   4. Decreased oral temperature

3. For a patient with hyperthyroidism, which task will you delegate to an experienced UAP?
   1. Instructing the patient to report any occurrence of palpitations, dyspnea, vertigo, or chest pain
   2. Monitoring the apical pulse, blood pressure, and temperature every 4 hours
   3. Drawing blood to measure levels of thyroid-stimulating hormone, triiodothyronine, and thyroxine
   4. Teaching the patient about side effects of the drug propylthiouracil

4. As the shift begins, you are assigned to care for the following patients. Which patient should you assess first?
   1. 38-year-old with Graves disease and a heart rate of 94 beats/min
   2. 63-year-old with type 2 diabetes and fingerstick glucose level of 137 mg/dL
   3. 58-year-old with hypothyroidism and a heart rate of 48 beats/min
   4. 49-year-old with Cushing disease and dependent edema rated as 1+

5. A patient is hospitalized with adrenocortical insufficiency. Which nursing activity should you delegate to a UAP?
   1. Reminding the patient to change positions slowly
   2. Assessing the patient for muscle weakness
   3. Teaching the patient how to collect a 24-hour urine sample
   4. Revising the patient's nursing plan of care

6. Assessment findings for a patient with Cushing disease include all of the following. For which finding would you notify the physician immediately?
   1. Purple striae present on the abdomen and thighs
   2. Weight gain of 1 lb since the previous day
   3. Dependent edema rated as 1+ in the ankles and calves
   4. Crackles bilaterally in the lower lobes of the lungs

7. A patient with pheochromocytoma underwent surgery to remove his adrenal glands. Which nursing intervention should you delegate to a UAP?
   1. Revising the nursing care plan to include strategies to provide a calm and restful environment postoperatively
   2. Instructing the patient to avoid smoking and drinking caffeine-containing beverages
   3. Assessing the patient's skin and mucous membranes for signs of adequate hydration
   4. Monitoring lying and standing blood pressure every 4 hours with a cuff placed on the same arm

8. For the patient with pheochromocytoma, which physical assessment technique should you instruct an LPN/LVN to avoid?
   1. Listening for abdominal bowel sounds in all four quadrants
   2. Palpating the abdomen in all four quadrants
   3. Checking the blood pressure every hour
   4. Assessing the mucous membranes for hydration status

9. A patient with adrenal insufficiency is to be discharged and will take prednisone (Deltasone) 10 mg orally each day. Which instruction would you be sure to teach the patient?
   1. Excessive weight gain or swelling should be reported to the physician.
   2. Changing positions rapidly may cause hypotension.
   3. A diet with foods low in sodium may be beneficial.
   4. Signs of hypoglycemia may occur while taking this drug.

10. You are caring for a patient who has just undergone hypophysectomy for hyperpituitarism. Which post-operative finding requires immediate intervention?
    1. Presence of glucose in the nasal drainage
    2. Presence of nasal packing in the nares
    3. Urine output of 40 to 50 mL/hr
    4. Patient reports of thirst

11. Which patients should you, as the charge nurse, assign to the care of an LPN/LVN, under the supervision of the RN team leader?
    1. 51-year-old who has just undergone bilateral adrenalectomy
    2. 83-year-old with type 2 diabetes and chronic obstructive pulmonary disease
    3. 38-year-old with myocardial infarction preparing for discharge
    4. 72-year-old with mental status changes admitted from a long-term care facility

12. You are providing care for a patient who underwent thyroidectomy 2 days ago. Which laboratory value requires close monitoring by a nurse?
    1. Calcium level
    2. Sodium level
    3. Potassium level
    4. White blood cell count

13. A 24-year-old patient with diabetes insipidus makes all of these statements when you are preparing the patient for discharge from the hospital. Which statement indicates to you that the patient needs additional teaching?
    1. "I will drink fluids equal to the amount of my urine output."
    2. "I will weigh myself every day using the same scale."
    3. "I will wear my medical alert bracelet at all times."
    4. "I will gradually wean myself off the vasopressin."

14. You are preparing a care plan for a patient with Cushing disease. Which nursing diagnoses would you be sure to include? *(Select all that apply.)*
    1. Risk for Injury related to the potential for bruising
    2. Disturbed Body Image
    3. Imbalanced Nutrition: Less than Body Requirements
    4. Risk for Injury related to the potential for hypertension
    5. Risk for Infection

15. When providing care for a patient with Addison disease, you should be alert for which laboratory value change?
    1. Decreased hematocrit
    2. Increased sodium level
    3. Decreased potassium level
    4. Decreased calcium level

16. A female patient is admitted with a diagnosis of primary hypofunction of the adrenal glands. Which assessment finding supports this diagnosis?
    1. Patchy areas of pigment loss over the face
    2. Decreased muscle strength
    3. Greatly increased urine output
    4. Scalp alopecia

17. You are instructing a senior nursing student on the techniques for palpation of the thyroid gland. What precaution would you be sure to include when instructing the student about thyroid palpation?
    1. Always stand to the side of the patient.
    2. Instruct the patient not to swallow.
    3. Palpate using one hand and then the other.
    4. Always palpate the thyroid gland gently.

18. Two UAPs are assisting a patient with Cushing disease to move up in bed. Which action by the UAPs requires your immediate intervention?
    1. Positioning themselves on opposite sides of the patient's bed
    2. Grasping under the patient's arms to pull him up in bed
    3. Lowering the side rails of the patient's bed before moving him
    4. Removing the pillow before moving the patient up in bed

19. You are caring for the following patients with endocrine disorders. Which one must you assess first?
    1. 21-year-old with diabetes insipidus whose urine output overnight was 2000 mL
    2. 55-year-old with syndrome of inappropriate antidiuretic hormone secretion (SIADH) who is demanding that the UAP refill his water pitcher
    3. 65-year-old with Addison disease whose morning potassium level is 6.2 mEq/L
    4. 48-year-old with Cushing disease with a weight gain of 1.5 lb over the past 4 days

20. Which health care provider orders for the patient with Addison disease should you delegate to the experienced UAP? *(Select all that apply.)*
    1. Weigh the patient every morning.
    2. Obtain fingerstick glucose before each meal and at bedtime.
    3. Check vital signs every 2 hours.
    4. Monitor for cardiac dysrhythmias.
    5. Administer oral prednisone 10 mg every morning.
    6. Record intake and output.

21. The LPN/LVN asks you why the patient with Cushing disease has bruising and petechiae across her abdomen. What is your best response?
    1. "Patients with Cushing disease often have bleeding disorders."
    2. "Patients with Cushing disease have very fragile capillaries."
    3. "Please ask the patient if she slipped or fell during the night."
    4. "Thin and delicate skin can result in development of bruising."

22. The patient with hyperparathyroidism who is not a candidate for surgery asks you why she is receiving IV normal saline and IV furosemide. What is your best response?
    1. "This therapy is to protect your kidney function."
    2. "You are receiving these therapies to prevent edema formation."
    3. "Diuretic and hydration therapies are used to reduce your serum calcium."
    4. "These therapies may help to improve your candidacy for surgery."

23. Which actions should you delegate to the LPN/LVN for the care of a patient with hypothyroidism? *(Select all that apply.)*
    1. Assessing and recording the rate and depth of respirations
    2. Auscultating lung sounds every 4 hours
    3. Creating an individualized nursing care plan for the patient
    4. Administering sedation medications every 6 hours
    5. Checking blood pressure, heart rate, and respirations every 4 hours
    6. Reminding the patient to report any episodes of chest pain or discomfort

24. You are caring for a patient with hyperthyroidism who had a partial thyroidectomy yesterday. Which change in assessment would you report to the health care provider immediately?
    1. Temperature elevation to 100.2° F
    2. Heart rate increase from 64 beats/min to 76 beats/min
    3. Respiratory rate decrease from 26 breaths/min to 16 breaths/min
    4. Pulse oximetry reading of 92%

25. You admit a patient whose assessment reveals prominent brow ridge, large hands and feet, and large lips and nose. Which pituitary hormone do you suspect is elevated?
    1. Thyroid-stimulating hormone
    2. Growth hormone
    3. Adrenocorticotropic hormone
    4. Vasopressin antidiuretic hormone

PART 2   Common Health Scenarios

Answer Key for this chapter begins on p. 192.

CHAPTER 15

Integumentary Problems

1. You are caring for a client who has just had a squamous cell carcinoma removed from the face. Which activity can you delegate to an experienced LPN/LVN?
   1. Teaching the client about risk factors for squamous cell carcinoma
   2. Showing the client how to care for the surgical site at home
   3. Monitoring the surgical site for swelling, bleeding, or pain
   4. Discussing the reasons for avoiding aspirin use for a week after surgery

2. You are employed as the charge nurse in a long-term care (LTC) facility that employs RNs, LPNs/LVNs, and UAPs. When you are planning care for a resident with a stage III sacral pressure ulcer, which nursing intervention is best to delegate to an LPN/LVN?
   1. Choosing the type of dressing to be used on the ulcer
   2. Using the Norton scale to assess for pressure ulcer risk factors
   3. Assisting the client in changing position at frequent intervals
   4. Cleaning and changing the dressing on the ulcer every morning

3. You have just received a change-of-shift report for the burn unit. Which client should you assess first?
   1. Client with deep partial-thickness burns on both legs who reports severe and continuous leg pain
   2. Client who has just arrived from the emergency department with facial burns sustained in a house fire
   3. Client who has just been transferred from the post-anesthesia care unit after having skin grafts applied to the anterior chest
   4. Client admitted 3 weeks ago with full-thickness leg and buttock burns who has been waiting for 3 hours to receive discharge teaching

4. You are performing a sterile dressing change for a client with infected deep partial-thickness burns of the chest and abdomen. List the steps of the care plan in the order in which each should be accomplished.
   1. Apply silver sulfadiazine (Silvadene) ointment.
   2. Obtain specimens for aerobic and anaerobic wound cultures.
   3. Administer morphine sulfate 10 mg IV.
   4. Débride the wound of eschar using gauze sponges.
   5. Cover the wound with a sterile gauze dressing.
   _____, _____, _____, _____, _____

5. You are the nurse manager in the burn unit. Which client is best to assign to an RN who has floated from the oncology unit?
   1. 23-year-old who has just been admitted with burns over 30% of the body after a warehouse fire
   2. 36-year-old who requires discharge teaching about nutrition and wound care after having skin grafts
   3. 45-year-old with infected partial-thickness back and chest burns who has a dressing change scheduled
   4. 57-year-old with full-thickness burns on both arms who needs assistance in positioning hand splints

6. You perform a skin assessment on a 70-year-old new resident in an LTC facility. Which finding is of most concern?
   1. Numerous striae are noted across the abdomen and buttocks.
   2. All the toenails are thickened and yellow.
   3. Silver scaling is present on the elbows and knees.
   4. An irregular border is seen on a black mole on the scalp.

7. Which assessment finding calls for the most immediate further assessment or intervention?
   1. Bluish color around the lips and earlobes
   2. Yellow color of the skin and sclera
   3. Bilateral erythema of the face and neck
   4. Dark brown spotting on the chest and back

8. A 22-year-old woman who has been taking isotretinoin (Claravis) to treat severe cystic acne makes all these statements while being seen for a follow-up examination. Which statement is of most concern?
   1. "My husband and I are thinking of starting a family soon."
   2. "I don't think there has been much improvement in my skin."
   3. "Sometimes I get nauseated after taking the medication."
   4. "I have been having problems driving when it gets dark."

9. A client is scheduled for patch testing to determine allergies to several substances. Which action associated with this test should you delegate to a medical assistant working in the allergy clinic?
   1. Explaining the purpose of the testing to the client
   2. Examining the patch area for evidence of a reaction
   3. Scheduling a follow-up appointment for the client in 2 days
   4. Monitoring the client for anaphylactic reactions to the testing

10. You are preparing to discharge four clients from the hospital and are planning their discharge teaching. Which client will it be most important to instruct about the need to use sunscreen?
    1. 32-year-old with a urinary tract infection who is being discharged with a prescription for tetracycline (Sumycin)
    2. Fair-skinned 55-year-old who has just had neck surgery and who plans to walk in the yard for 15 minutes twice daily
    3. Dark-skinned 62-year-old who has had keloids injected with hydrocortisone (Solu-Cortef)
    4. 78-year-old with a red, pruritic rash caused by an allergic reaction to penicillin (Bicillin)

11. As a home health nurse, you are caring for a 72-year-old client who has a nursing diagnosis of Impaired Skin Integrity related to poor nutrition, bladder incontinence, and immobility. Which nursing actions should you delegate to the UAP?
    1. Telling the client and family to apply the skin barrier cream in a smooth, even layer
    2. Completing a diet assessment and suggesting changes in diet to improve the client's nutrition
    3. Reminding the family to help the client to the commode every 2 hours during the day
    4. Evaluating the client for improvement in documented areas of skin breakdown or damage

12. You are the charge nurse in an LTC facility that employs RNs, LPNs/LVNs, and UAPs as staff members. An 80-year-old client has candidiasis in the skinfolds of the abdomen and groin. Which intervention is best to delegate to an LPN/LVN?
    1. Applying nystatin (Mycostatin) powder to the area three times daily
    2. Cleaning the skinfolds every 8 hours with mild soap and drying thoroughly
    3. Evaluating the need for further antifungal treatment at least weekly
    4. Assessing for ongoing risk factors for skin breakdown and infection

13. After reviewing the medical record for a client who has an oral herpes simplex infection following chemotherapy, which nursing diagnosis will you address as the priority?

Physical Assessment	Nutritional Assessment	Social/Emotional Assessment
• Vesicular lesions throughout mouth and lips	• Taking only a few bites of each meal	• States "I feel like a monster with these herpes sores all over my face!"
• Reports level 9 (0 to 10 scale) oral pain	• 2-lb (1-kg) weight loss in last 3 days	• Refuses to see visitors

1. Social Isolation related to anxiety about herpes infection
2. Acute Pain related to the presence of extensive herpes simplex lesions
3. Imbalanced Nutrition: Less than Body Requirements related to decreased oral intake
4. Disturbed Body Image related to the appearance of oral lesions

14. A client admitted to the emergency department (ED) reports itching of the trunk and groin. You note multiple reddened wheals on the chest, back, and groin. Which question is most appropriate to ask next?
    1. "Do you have a family history of eczema?"
    2. "Have you been using sunscreen regularly?"
    3. "How do you usually manage stress?"
    4. "Are you taking any new medications?"

15. A client who has extensive blister injuries to the back and both legs caused by exposure to toxic chemicals at work is admitted to the ED. Which ordered intervention will you implement first?
    1. Infuse lactated Ringer's solution at 250 mL/hr.
    2. Rinse the back and legs with 4 L of sterile normal saline.
    3. Obtain blood for a complete blood count and electrolyte levels.
    4. Document the percentage of total body surface area burned.

16. You have just received the change-of-shift report in the burn unit. Which client requires the most immediate assessment or intervention?
    1. 22-year-old admitted 4 days previously with facial burns due to a house fire who has been crying since recent visitors left
    2. 34-year-old who returned from skin-graft surgery 3 hours ago and is reporting level 8 pain (on a scale of 0 to 10)
    3. 45-year-old with partial-thickness leg burns who has a temperature of 102.6° F (39.2° C) and a blood pressure of 98/46 mm Hg
    4. 57-year-old who was admitted with electrical burns 24 hours ago and has a blood potassium level of 5.1 mEq/L

17. You take the health history of a 60-year-old client who has been admitted to the same-day surgery unit for elective facial dermabrasion. Which information is most important to convey to the plastic surgeon?
    1. The client does not routinely use sunscreen.
    2. The client has a family history of melanoma.
    3. The client has not eaten anything for 8 hours.
    4. The client takes 325 mg of aspirin daily.

18. You are the charge nurse on a medical-surgical unit and are working with a newly-graduated RN who has been on orientation to the unit for 3 weeks. Which client is best to assign to the new graduate?
    1. 34-year-old who was just admitted to the unit with periorbital cellulitis
    2. 40-year-old who needs discharge instructions after having skin grafts to the thigh
    3. 67-year-old who requires a dressing change after hydrotherapy for a pressure ulcer
    4. 78-year-old who needs teaching before a punch biopsy of a facial lesion

19. When you are evaluating a client who has been taking prednisone (Deltasone) 30 mg daily to treat contact dermatitis, which finding is most important to report to the health care provider?
    1. The blood glucose level is 136 mg/dL.
    2. The client states, "I am eating all the time."
    3. The client reports epigastric pain.
    4. The blood pressure is 148/84 mm Hg.

20. As charge nurse, you are providing orientation for a newly-hired RN. Which action by the new RN requires the most immediate action?
    1. Obtaining an anaerobic culture specimen from a superficial burn wound
    2. Giving doxycycline (Vibramycin) with a glass of milk to a client with cellulitis
    3. Discussing the use of herpes zoster vaccine with a 25-year-old client
    4. Teaching a newly admitted burn client about the use of pressure garments

PART 2 Common Health Scenarios

Answer Key for this chapter begins on p. 193.

CHAPTER 16

Renal and Urinary Problems

1. You are providing nursing care for a 24-year-old female patient admitted to the unit with a diagnosis of cystitis. Which intervention should you delegate to the UAP?
   1. Teaching the patient how to secure a clean-catch urine sample
   2. Assessing the patient's urine for color, odor, and sediment
   3. Reviewing the nursing care plan and add nursing interventions
   4. Providing the patient with a clean-catch urine sample container

2. Which laboratory result is of most concern to you for an adult patient with cystitis?
   1. Serum white blood cell (WBC) count of 9000/mm^3
   2. Urinalysis results showing 1 or 2 WBCs present
   3. Urine bacteria count of 100,000 colonies per milliliter
   4. Serum hematocrit of 36%

3. As charge nurse, you would assign the nursing care of which patient to an LPN/LVN, working under the supervision of an RN?
   1. 48-year-old with cystitis who is taking oral antibiotics
   2. 64-year-old with kidney stones who has a new order for lithotripsy
   3. 72-year-old with urinary incontinence who needs bladder training
   4. 52-year-old with pyelonephritis who has severe acute flank pain

4. You are admitting a 66-year-old male patient suspected of having a urinary tract infection (UTI). Which piece of the patient's medical history supports this diagnosis?
   1. Patient's wife had a UTI 1 month ago
   2. Followed for prostate disease for 2 years
   3. Intermittent catheterization 6 months ago
   4. Kidney stone removal 1 year ago

5. A patient is being admitted to rule out interstitial cystitis. What should your plan of care for this patient include?
   1. Take daily urine samples for urinalysis.
   2. Maintain accurate intake and output records.
   3. Obtain an admission urine sample to determine electrolyte levels.
   4. Teach the patient about the cystoscopy procedure.

6. You are supervising a new RN graduate who is on orientation to the unit. The new RN asks you why the patient with uncomplicated cystitis is being discharged with orders for ciprofloxacin (Cipro) 250 mg twice a day for only 3 days. What is your best response?
   1. "We should check with the physician, because the patient should take this drug for 10 to 14 days."
   2. "A 3-day course of ciprofloxacin is not the appropriate treatment for a patient with uncomplicated cystitis."
   3. "Research has shown that, with a 3-day course of ciprofloxacin, there is increased patient adherence to the plan of care."
   4. "Longer courses of antibiotic therapy are required for hospitalized patients to prevent nosocomial infections."

7. A 28-year-old married female patient with cystitis requires instruction about how to prevent future UTIs, and you have delegated this teaching to a newly-graduated RN. Which statement by the new nurse requires that you intervene?
   1. "You should always drink 1 to 3 L of fluid every day."
   2. "Empty your bladder regularly even if you do not feel the urge to urinate."
   3. "Drinking cranberry juice daily will decrease the number of bacteria in your bladder."
   4. "It's okay to soak in the tub with bubble bath because it will keep you clean."

8. You are creating a nursing care plan for older adult patients with incontinence. For which patient will a bladder-training program be an appropriate intervention?
   1. Patient with functional incontinence caused by mental status changes
   2. Patient with stress incontinence due to weakened bladder neck support
   3. Patient with urge incontinence and abnormal detrusor muscle contractions
   4. Patient with transient incontinence related to loss of cognitive function

9. A patient with incontinence will be taking oxybutynin chloride (Ditropan) 5 mg by mouth three times a day after discharge. Which information would you be sure to teach this patient before discharge?
   1. "Drink fluids or use hard candy when you experience a dry mouth."
   2. "Be sure to notify your physician if you experience a dry mouth."
   3. "If necessary, your physician can increase your dose up to 40 mg/day."
   4. "You should take this medication with meals to avoid stomach ulcers."

10. You are providing care for a patient with reflex urinary incontinence. Which action could be appropriately delegated to a new LPN/LVN?
    1. Teaching the patient bladder emptying by the Credé method
    2. Demonstrating how to perform intermittent self-catheterization
    3. Discussing the side effects of bethanechol chloride (Urecholine)
    4. Reinforcing the importance of proper hand washing to prevent infection

11. A patient has urolithiasis and is passing the stones into the lower urinary tract. What is the priority nursing diagnosis for the patient at this time?
    1. Acute Pain
    2. Risk for Infection
    3. Risk for Injury
    4. Anxiety related to the risk for recurrent stones

12. You are supervising a nurse on orientation to the unit who is discharging a patient admitted with kidney stones who underwent lithotripsy. Which statement by the nurse to the patient requires that you intervene?
    1. "You should finish all of your antibiotics to make sure that you don't get a UTI."
    2. "Remember to drink at least 3 L of fluids every day to prevent another stone from forming."
    3. "Report any signs of bruising to your physician immediately, since this indicates bleeding."
    4. "You can return to work in 2 days to 6 weeks, depending on what your physician prescribes."

13. As charge nurse, you must rearrange room assignments to admit a new patient. Which two patients would be best suited to be roommates?
    1. 58-year-old with urothelial cancer receiving multiagent chemotherapy
    2. 63-year-old with kidney stones who has just undergone open ureterolithotomy
    3. 24-year-old with acute pyelonephritis and severe flank pain
    4. 76-year-old with urge incontinence and a UTI
    _____, _____

14. The nursing diagnosis of Constipation related to compression of the intestinal tract has been identified in a patient with polycystic kidney disease. Which nursing care action should you delegate to a newly-trained LPN/LVN?
    1. Instructing the patient about foods that are high in fiber
    2. Teaching the patient about foods that assist in promoting bowel regularity
    3. Assessing the patient for previous bowel problems and bowel routine
    4. Administering docusate sodium (Colace) 100 mg by mouth twice a day

15. In a male patient who must undergo intermittent catheterization, you are preparing to insert a catheter to assess the patient for postvoid residual. Place the steps for catheterization in the correct order.
    1. Assist the patient to the bathroom and ask the patient to attempt to void.
    2. Retract the foreskin and hold the penis at a 60- to 90-degree angle.
    3. Open the catheterization kit and put on sterile gloves.
    4. Lubricate the catheter and insert it through the meatus of the penis.
    5. Position the patient supine in bed or with the head slightly elevated.
    6. Drain all the urine present in the bladder into a container.
    7. Cleanse the glans penis starting at the meatus and working outward.
    8. Remove the catheter, clean the penis, and measure the amount of urine returned.
    _____, _____, _____, _____, _____, _____, _____, _____

16. You are the admitting nurse for a patient with nephrotic syndrome. Which assessment finding supports this diagnosis?
    1. Edema formation
    2. Hypotension
    3. Increased urine output
    4. Flank pain

17. A patient has renal cell carcinoma (adenocarcinoma of the kidney). You are providing orientation to a new nurse on the unit, who asks you why this patient is not receiving chemotherapy. What is your best response?
    1. "The prognosis for this form of cancer is very poor, and we will be providing only comfort measures."
    2. "Nephrectomy is the preferred treatment as chemotherapy has been shown to have only limited effectiveness against this type of cancer."
    3. "Research has shown that the most effective means of treating this form of cancer is with radiation therapy."
    4. "Radiofrequency ablation is a minimally invasive procedure that is the best way to treat renal cell carcinoma."

18. You are teaching a patient how best to prevent renal trauma after an injury that required a left nephrectomy. Which points would you include in your teaching plan? *(Select all that apply.)*
    1. Always wear a seat belt.
    2. Avoid all contact sports.
    3. Practice safe walking habits.
    4. Wear protective clothing to participate in contact sports.
    5. Use caution when riding a bicycle.

19. You are providing nursing care for a patient with acute kidney failure for whom a nursing diagnosis of Excess Fluid Volume related to compromised regulatory mechanisms has been identified. Which actions should you delegate to an experienced UAP? *(Select all that apply.)*
    1. Measuring and recording vital sign values every 4 hours
    2. Weighing the patient every morning using a standing scale
    3. Administering furosemide (Lasix) 40 mg orally twice a day
    4. Reminding the patient to save all urine for intake and output measurement
    5. Assessing breath sounds every 4 hours
    6. Ensuring that the patient's urinal is within reach

20. A UAP reports to you that a patient with acute kidney failure has had a urine output of 350 mL over the past 24 hours after receiving furosemide 40 mg IV push. The UAP asks you how this can happen. What is your best response?
    1. "During the oliguric phase of acute kidney failure, patients often do not respond well to either fluid challenges or diuretics."
    2. "There must be some sort of error. Someone must have failed to record the urine output."
    3. "A patient with acute kidney failure retains sodium and water, which counteracts the action of the furosemide."
    4. "The gradual accumulation of nitrogenous waste products results in the retention of water and sodium."

21. You are the charge nurse. Which patient will you assign to a nurse floated to your unit from the surgical intensive care unit (ICU)?
    1. Patient with kidney stones scheduled for lithotripsy this morning
    2. Patient who has just undergone surgery for renal stent placement
    3. Newly-admitted patient with an acute UTI
    4. Patient with chronic kidney failure who needs teaching on peritoneal dialysis

22. Your patient is receiving IV piggyback doses of gentamicin (Garamycin) every 12 hours. Which would be your priority for monitoring during the period that the patient is receiving this drug?
    1. Serum creatinine and blood urea nitrogen levels
    2. Patient weight every morning
    3. Intake and output every shift
    4. Temperature

23. A patient in whom acute kidney failure has been diagnosed has had a urine output of 1560 mL for the past 8 hours. The LPN/LVN who is caring for this patient, under your supervision, asks you how a patient with kidney failure can have such a large urine output. What is your best response?
    1. "The patient's kidney failure was due to hypovolemia and we have given him IV fluids to correct the problem."
    2. "Acute kidney failure patients go through a diuretic phase when their kidneys begin to recover and may put out as much as 10 L of urine per day."
    3. "With that much urine output, there must have been a mistake in the patient's diagnosis."
    4. "An increase in urine output like this is an indicator that the patient is entering the recovery phase of acute kidney failure."

24. A patient on the medical-surgical unit with acute kidney failure is to begin continuous arteriovenous hemofiltration (CAVH) as soon as possible. What is the priority action at this time?
    1. Call the charge nurse and transfer the patient to the ICU.
    2. Develop a teaching plan for the patient that focuses on CAVH.
    3. Assist the patient with morning bath and mouth care before transfer.
    4. Notify the physician that the patient's mean arterial pressure is 68 mm Hg.

25. You are caring for a patient admitted with dehydration secondary to deficient antidiuretic hormone (ADH). Which specific gravity value supports this diagnosis?
    1. 1.010
    2. 1.035
    3. 1.020
    4. 1.002

26. You are supervising a senior nursing student who is caring for a 78-year-old scheduled for an intravenous pyelography. What information would you be sure to stress about this procedure to the nursing student?
    1. "After the procedure, monitor urine output because the contrast dye increases the risk for kidney failure in older adults."
    2. "The purpose of this procedure is to measure kidney size."
    3. "Because this procedure assesses kidney function, there is no need for a bowel prep."
    4. "Keep the patient NPO after the procedure because during the procedure the patient will receive drugs that affect the gag reflex."

Answer Key for this chapter begins on p. 195.

1. You are assessing a long-term-care client with a history of benign prostatic hyperplasia (BPH). Which information will require the most immediate action?
   1. The client states that he always has trouble starting his urinary stream.
   2. The chart shows an elevated level of prostate-specific antigen.
   3. The bladder is palpable above the symphysis pubis and the client is restless.
   4. The client says he has not voided since having a glass of juice 4 hours ago.

2. While performing a breast examination on a 22-year-old client, you obtain the following data. Which finding is of most concern?
   1. Both breasts have many nodules in the upper outer quadrants.
   2. The client reports bilateral breast tenderness with palpation.
   3. The breast on the right side is slightly larger than the left breast.
   4. An irregularly shaped, nontender lump is palpable in the left breast.

3. After undergoing a modified radical mastectomy, a client is transferred to the postanesthesia care unit (PACU). Which nursing action is best to delegate to an experienced LPN/LVN?
   1. Monitoring the client's dressing for any signs of bleeding
   2. Documenting the initial assessment on the client's chart
   3. Communicating the client's status report to the charge nurse on the surgical unit
   4. Teaching the client about the importance of using pain medication as needed

4. You are working with a UAP to care for a client who has had a right breast lumpectomy and axillary lymph node dissection. Which nursing action can you delegate to the UAP?
   1. Teaching the client why blood pressure measurements are taken on the left arm
   2. Elevating the client's arm on two pillows to promote lymphatic drainage
   3. Assessing the client's right arm for lymphedema
   4. Reinforcing the dressing if it becomes saturated

5. You obtain the following assessment data about your client who has had a transurethral resection of the prostate (TURP) and has continuous bladder irrigation. Which finding indicates the most immediate need for nursing intervention?
   1. The client states that he feels a continuous urge to void.
   2. The catheter drainage is light pink with occasional clots.
   3. The catheter is taped to the client's thigh.
   4. The client reports painful bladder spasms.

6. A 67-year-old client with BPH has a new prescription for tamsulosin (Flomax). Which statement about tamsulosin is most important to include when teaching this client?
   1. "This medication will improve your symptoms by shrinking the prostate."
   2. "The force of your urinary stream will probably increase."
   3. "Your blood pressure will decrease as a result of taking this medication."
   4. "You should avoid sitting up or standing up too quickly."

7. You are caring for a client who has just returned to the surgical unit after a TURP. Which assessment finding will require the most immediate action?
   1. Blood pressure reading of 153/88 mm Hg
   2. Catheter that is draining deep red blood
   3. Client not wearing antiembolism hose
   4. Client reports of abdominal cramping

8. After a radical prostatectomy, a client is ready to be discharged. Which nursing action included in the discharge plan should be delegated to an experienced LPN/LVN?
   1. Reinforcing the client's need to check his temperature daily
   2. Teaching the client how to care for his retention catheter
   3. Documenting a discharge assessment in the client's chart
   4. Instructing the client about the prescribed narcotic analgesic

9. The day after a radical prostatectomy, your client has blood clots in the urinary catheter and reports bladder spasms. The client says that his right calf is sore and that he feels short of breath. Which action will you take first?
   1. Irrigate the catheter with 50 mL of sterile saline.
   2. Administer oxybutynin (Ditropan) 5 mg orally.
   3. Apply warm packs to the client's right calf.
   4. Measure oxygen saturation using pulse oximetry.

10. After arriving for your shift in the emergency department (ED), you receive a change-of-shift report about all of these clients. Which one do you need to assess first?
    1. 19-year-old with scrotal swelling and severe pain that has not decreased with elevation of the scrotum
    2. 25-year-old who has a painless indurated lesion on the glans penis
    3. 44-year-old with an elevated temperature, chills, and back pain associated with recurrent prostatitis
    4. 77-year-old with abdominal pain and acute bladder distention

11. A 79-year-old who has just returned to the surgical unit following a TURP reports acute bladder spasms. In which order will you perform the following prescribed actions?
    1. Administer acetaminophen/oxycodone 325 mg/5 mg (Percocet) 2 tablets.
    2. Irrigate the retention catheter with 30 to 50 mL of sterile normal saline.
    3. Infuse 500 mL of 5% dextrose in lactated Ringer's solution over 2 hours.
    4. Offer the client oral fluids to at least 2500 to 3000 mL daily. _____, _____, _____, _____

12. A 68-year-old client who is ready for discharge from the ED has a new prescription for nitroglycerin (Nitrostat) 0.4 mg sublingual as needed for angina. Which client information has the most immediate implications for teaching?
    1. The client has BPH and some urinary hesitancy.
    2. The client's father and two brothers all have had myocardial infarctions.
    3. The client uses sildenafil (Viagra) several times weekly for erectile dysfunction.
    4. The client is unable to remember when he first experienced chest pain.

13. You are caring for a 21-year-old client who had a left orchiectomy for testicular cancer on the previous day. Which nursing activity will you delegate to an LPN/LVN?
    1. Educating the client about post-orchiectomy chemotherapy and radiation
    2. Administering the prescribed "as needed" (PRN) oxycodone (Roxicodone) to the client
    3. Teaching the client how to perform testicular self-examination on the remaining testicle
    4. Assessing the client's knowledge level about post-orchiectomy fertility

14. You are the charge nurse on the oncology unit. Which client is best to assign to an RN who has floated from the ED?
    1. Client who needs doxorubicin (Adriamycin) to treat metastatic breast cancer
    2. Client who needs discharge teaching after surgery for stage II ovarian cancer
    3. Client with metastatic prostate cancer who requires frequent assessment and treatment for breakthrough pain
    4. Client with testicular cancer who requires preoperative teaching about orchiectomy and lymph node resection

15. After you receive the change-of-shift report, in which order will you assess these clients assigned to your care?
    1. 22-year-old who has questions about how to care for the drains placed in her breast reconstruction incision
    2. Anxious 44-year-old who is scheduled to be discharged today after undergoing a total vaginal hysterectomy
    3. 69-year-old who reports level 5 pain (on a scale of 0 to 10) after undergoing perineal prostatectomy 2 days ago
    4. Usually oriented 78-year-old who has new-onset confusion after having a bilateral orchiectomy the previous day _____, _____, _____, _____

16. A client has had a needle biopsy of the prostate gland using the transrectal approach. Which statement is most important to include in the client teaching plan?
    1. "The doctor will call you about the test results in a day or two."
    2. "Serious infections may occur as a complication of this test."
    3. "You will need to call the doctor if you develop a fever or chills."
    4. "It is normal to have a small amount of rectal bleeding after the test."

17. You are working on the PACU caring for a 32-year-old client who has just arrived after undergoing dilation and curettage to evaluate infertility. Which assessment finding should be immediately communicated to the surgeon?
    1. Blood pressure of 162/90 mm Hg
    2. Saturation of the perineal pad after the first 30 minutes
    3. Oxygen saturation of 91% to 95%
    4. Sharp, continuous, level 8 (out of 10) abdominal pain

18. When you are developing the plan of care for a home health client who has been discharged after a radical prostatectomy, which activities will you delegate to the home health aide? *(Select all that apply.)*
    1. Monitoring the client for symptoms of urinary tract infection
    2. Helping the client to connect the catheter to the leg bag
    3. Checking the client's incision for appropriate wound healing
    4. Assisting the client in ambulating for increasing distances
    5. Helping the client shower at least every other day

19. You are working in the ED when a client with possible toxic shock syndrome is admitted. Which prescribed intervention will you implement first?
    1. Remove the client's tampon.
    2. Obtain blood specimens for culture.
    3. Give acetaminophen (Tylenol) 650 mg.
    4. Infuse nafcillin (Unipen) 1000 mg IV.

20. When assessing a client with cervical cancer who had a total abdominal hysterectomy yesterday, you obtain the following data. Which information has the most immediate implications for planning of the client's care?
    1. Fine crackles are audible at the lung bases.
    2. The client's right calf is swollen, and she reports calf tenderness.
    3. The client uses the patient-controlled analgesia device every 30 minutes.
    4. Urine in the collection bag is amber and clear.

21. You observe a student nurse who is caring for a client who has an intracavitary radioactive implant in place to treat cervical cancer. Which action by the student requires that you intervene immediately?
    1. Standing next to the client for 5 minutes while assisting with her bath
    2. Asking the client how she feels about losing her childbearing ability
    3. Assisting the client to the bedside commode for a bowel movement
    4. Offering to get the client whatever she would like to eat or drink

22. A client who underwent an abdominal hysterectomy 3 days ago reports burning with urination. Her urine output during the previous shift was 210 mL, and her temperature is 101.3° F (38.5° C). Which of these actions prescribed by the health care provider will you implement first?
    1. Insert a straight catheter PRN for output of less than 300 mL/8 hr.
    2. Administer acetaminophen (Tylenol) 650 mg orally.
    3. Send a urine specimen to the laboratory for culture and sensitivity testing.
    4. Administer ceftizoxime (Cefizox) 1 g IV every 12 hours.

23. An 86-year-old woman had an anterior and posterior colporrhaphy (A & P repair) several days ago. Her retention catheter was removed 8 hours ago. Which assessment finding requires that you act most rapidly?
    1. The oral temperature is 100.7° F (38.2° C).
    2. The abdomen is firm and tender to palpation above the symphysis pubis.
    3. Breath sounds are decreased, with fine crackles audible at both bases.
    4. The apical pulse is 86 beats/min and slightly irregular.

24. You are providing orientation for a new RN on the medical-surgical unit. The new RN takes the following actions while caring for a client with severe pelvic inflammatory disease (PID). Which action by the new RN is most important to correct quickly?
    1. Telling the client that she should avoid using tampons in the future
    2. Offering the client an ice pack to decrease her abdominal pain
    3. Positioning the client flat in bed while helping her take a bath
    4. Teaching the client that she should not have intercourse for 2 months

PART 2 Common Health Scenarios

25. Which information obtained when taking a client's health history will be most important in determining whether the client should receive the human papillomavirus (HPV) immunization?
    1. Client is 19 years old
    2. Client is sexually active
    3. Client has a positive pregnancy test
    4. Client has tested positive for HPV previously

26. Three days after undergoing a pelvic exenteration procedure, a client reports dizziness after experiencing a sudden "giving" sensation along her abdominal incision. You find that the wound edges are open and loops of intestine are protruding. Which action should you take first?
    1. Notify the surgeon that wound evisceration has occurred.
    2. Cover the wound with saline-soaked dressings.
    3. Use swabs to obtain aerobic and anaerobic wound cultures.
    4. Call for assistance from the Rapid Response Team.

27. You are working on a medical unit staffed with LPNs/LVNs and UAPs when a client with stage IV ovarian cancer and recurrent ascites is admitted for paracentesis. Which activity is best to delegate to an experienced LPN/LVN?
    1. Obtaining a paracentesis tray from the central supply area
    2. Completing the short-stay client admission form
    3. Measuring vital signs every 15 minutes after the procedure
    4. Providing discharge instructions after the procedure

28. While you are working in the clinic, a healthy 32-year-old woman whose sister is a carrier of the *BRCA* gene asks you which form of breast cancer screening is the most effective for her. Which response is best?
    1. "An annual mammogram is usually sufficient screening for women your age."
    2. "Monthly self-breast examination is recommended because of your higher risk."
    3. "A yearly breast examination by a health care provider should be scheduled."
    4. "Magnetic resonance imaging is recommended in addition to annual mammography."

Answer Key for this chapter begins on p. 196.

CHAPTER 18

Problems in Pregnancy and Childbearing

1. A 30-year-old woman with type 1 diabetes mellitus comes to the clinic for preconception care. What is the priority education for her at this time?
   1. Her insulin requirements will likely increase during the second and third trimesters of pregnancy.
   2. Infants of diabetic mothers can be macrosomic, which can result in more difficult delivery and higher likelihood of cesarean section.
   3. Breast feeding is highly recommended, and insulin use is not a contraindication.
   4. Achievement of optimal glycemic control at this time is of utmost importance in preventing congenital anomalies.

2. Which task could be appropriately assigned to the UAP working with you at the obstetric clinic?
   1. Checking the blood pressure of a patient who is 36 weeks pregnant and reports a headache
   2. Removing the adhesive skin closure strips of a patient who had a cesarean section 2 weeks ago
   3. Giving community resource information and emergency numbers to a prenatal patient whom you suspect is experiencing domestic violence
   4. Dispensing a breast pump with instruction to a lactating patient having trouble with milk supply 4 weeks postpartum

3. You are working in the obstetric triage area, and several patients have just come in. Which patient should you assess first?
   1. A 17-year-old gravida 1, para 0 (G1P0) woman at 40 weeks' gestation with contractions every 6 minutes who is crying loudly and is surrounded by anxious family members
   2. A 22-year-old G3P2 woman at 38 weeks' gestation with contractions every 3 minutes who is requesting to go to the bathroom to have a bowel movement
   3. A 32-year-old G4P3 woman at 27 weeks' gestation who noted vaginal bleeding today following intercourse
   4. A 27-year-old G2P1 woman at 37 weeks' gestation who experienced spontaneous rupture of membranes 30 minutes ago but feels no contractions

4. A 19-year-old G1P0 patient at 40 weeks' gestation who is in labor is being treated with magnesium sulfate for seizure prophylaxis in preeclampsia. Which are priority assessments with this medication? *(Select all that apply.)*
   1. Check deep tendon reflexes.
   2. Observe for vaginal bleeding.
   3. Check the respiratory rate.
   4. Note the urine output.
   5. Monitor for calf pain.

5. Which action would best demonstrate evidence-based nursing practice in the care of a patient who is 1 day postpartum and reporting nipple soreness while breast-feeding?
   1. Give the baby a bottle after 5 minutes of nursing to allow soreness to resolve.
   2. Assess the mother-baby couplet for nursing position and latch, and correct as indicated.
   3. Advise the use of a breast pump until nipple soreness resolves.
   4. Advise alternating breast and bottle feedings to avoid excess sucking at the nipple.

6. A 24-year-old G2P1 woman is being admitted in active labor at 39 weeks' gestation. What prenatal data would be most important to know in your care of this patient at this time?
   1. Hemoglobin level of 11 g/dL at 28 weeks' gestation
   2. Positive result on test for group B streptococci at 36 weeks' gestation
   3. Urinary tract infection with *Escherichia coli* treated at 20 weeks' gestation
   4. Elevated level on glucose screening test at 28 weeks' gestation followed by normal 3-hour glucose tolerance test results at 29 weeks' gestation

7. You are working as a telephone triage nurse in the prenatal clinic. Which telephone call would require immediate notification of the provider?
   1. Patient reports leaking vaginal fluid at 34 weeks' gestation
   2. Patient reports nausea and vomiting at 8 weeks' gestation
   3. Patient reports pedal edema at 39 weeks' gestation
   4. Patient reports vaginal itching at 20 weeks' gestation

8. You are the RN in the labor and delivery unit caring for a 25-year-old G3P2 patient in active labor. You have identified late fetal heart decelerations and decreased variability in the fetal heart rate. You have notified the provider on call, who feels that the pattern is acceptable. What would be your priority action at this time?
   1. Advise the patient that a different provider will be called because you do not agree with the advice of the first provider.
   2. Discuss your concerns with another labor and delivery nurse.
   3. Document your conversation with the provider accurately, including the provider's interpretation and recommendation, and continue close observation of the fetal heart rate.
   4. Go up the chain of command and communicate your assessment of the fetal heart rate findings clearly to the next appropriate provider.

9. What would be the appropriate first nursing action when caring for a 20-year-old G1P0 woman at 39 weeks' gestation who is in active labor and for whom an assessment reveals mild variable fetal heart rate decelerations?
   1. Change the maternal position.
   2. Notify the provider.
   3. Prepare for delivery.
   4. Readjust the fetal monitor.

10. A 24-year-old G1P0 patient, who is receiving oxytocin (Pitocin), is in labor at 41 weeks' gestation. Which are appropriate nursing actions in the presence of late fetal heart rate decelerations? *(Select all that apply.)*
    1. Discontinue the oxytocin.
    2. Decrease the maintenance IV fluid rate.
    3. Administer oxygen to the mother by mask.
    4. Place the woman in high Fowler position.
    5. Notify the provider.

11. A pregnant woman at 12 weeks' gestation tells you that she is a vegetarian. What would be the first appropriate nursing action?
    1. Recommend vitamin B_{12} and iron supplementation.
    2. Recommend consumption of protein drinks daily.
    3. Obtain a 24-hour diet recall history.
    4. Determine the reason for her vegetarian diet.

12. A 26-year-old G1P1 patient who underwent cesarean section 24 hours ago tells the nurse that she is having some trouble breast-feeding. Which tasks could be appropriately delegated to the UAP on the postpartum floor? *(Select all that apply.)*
    1. Providing the mother with an ordered abdominal binder
    2. Assisting the mother with breast-feeding
    3. Taking the mother's vital signs
    4. Checking the amount of lochia present
    5. Assisting the mother with ambulation

13. You are the charge nurse in the labor and delivery unit. Which action by a newly graduated RN during a delivery complicated by shoulder dystocia would require your immediate intervention?
    1. Applying fundal pressure
    2. Applying suprapubic pressure
    3. Requesting immediate presence of the neonatologist
    4. Flexing the maternal legs back across the maternal abdomen

14. Which statements by a new father indicate that additional discharge teaching is needed for this family, who had their first baby 24 hours ago? *(Select all that apply.)*
    1. "We have a crib ready for our baby with lots of stuffed animals and two quilts that my mother made."
    2. "My wife wants to receive the flu shot before she goes home."
    3. "We will bring our baby to the pediatrician in 3 weeks."
    4. "I will give the baby formula at night so my wife can rest. She will breast-feed in the daytime."
    5. "We will always put our baby to sleep in a face-up position."

15. As the charge nurse in the labor and delivery unit, you need to assign two patients to one of the RNs because of a staffing shortage. Normally on your unit the nurse-patient ratio is 1:1. Which two patients would you assign to the RN?
    1. 30-year-old G1P0 woman, 40 weeks, 2 cm/90% effaced/−1 station
    2. 25-year-old G3P2 woman, 38 weeks, 8 cm/100% effaced/0 station
    3. 26-year-old G1P1 woman who delivered via normal vaginal delivery 15 minutes ago
    4. 17-year-old G1P0 woman with premature rupture of membranes, no labor at 35 weeks
    5. 40-year-old G6P5 woman with contractions at 28 weeks who has not yet been evaluated by the provider _____, _____

16. While assessing a 29-year-old G2P2 patient who had a normal spontaneous vaginal delivery 30 minutes ago, you note a large amount of red vaginal bleeding. What would be your first priority nursing action?
    1. Check vital signs.
    2. Notify the provider.
    3. Firmly massage the uterine fundus.
    4. Put the baby to breast.

17. A 30-year-old G1P0 woman at 39 weeks experienced a fetal demise and has just delivered a female infant. Her husband is at the bedside. Which are appropriate nursing actions at this time? *(Select all that apply.)*
    1. Offer the option of autopsy to the parents.
    2. Stay with the parents and offer supportive care.
    3. Place the infant on the maternal abdomen.
    4. Clean and wrap the baby and offer the infant to the parents to view or hold when desired.
    5. Ask the parents if there are any special rituals in their religion or culture for a baby who has died that they would like to have done.

18. A 27-year-old patient underwent a primary cesarean section because of breech presentation 24 hours ago. Which assessment finding would be of the most concern?
    1. Small amount of lochia rubra
    2. Temperature of 99° F (37.2° C)
    3. Slight redness of the left calf
    4. Pain rated as 3 of 10 in the incisional area

19. A 22-year-old G1P0 woman is being given an epidural anesthetic for pain control during labor and birth. Which are appropriate nursing actions when epidural anesthesia is used during labor? *(Select all that apply.)*
    1. Request the anesthesiologist to discontinue the epidural anesthetic when the patient's cervix is completely dilated to allow the patient to sense the urge to push.
    2. Insert a Foley catheter, because the woman is likely to be unable to void.
    3. Encourage pushing efforts when the cervix is completely dilated in the absence of an urge to push.
    4. Encourage the patient to turn from side to side during the course of labor.
    5. Teach the patient that pain relief can be expected to last 1 to 2 hours.

20. A 36-year-old G1P0 patient has received an epidural anesthetic. Her cervix is 6 cm dilated. Her blood pressure is currently 60/38 mm Hg. Which would be appropriate priority nursing actions? *(Select all that apply.)*
    1. Place the patient in high Fowler position.
    2. Turn the patient to a lateral position.
    3. Notify the anesthesiologist.
    4. Prepare for emergency cesarean section.
    5. Decrease the IV fluid rate.

21. A 17-year-old G1P0 woman at 40 weeks is in labor. She has chosen natural childbirth with assistance from a doula. Her mother and her boyfriend are at the bedside. What nursing action can help the patient achieve her goal of an unmedicated labor and birth?
    1. Encourage the patient to stay in bed.
    2. Allow the patient's support people to provide labor support and minimize nursing presence.
    3. Assess the effectiveness of the labor support team and offer suggestions as indicated.
    4. Offer pain medication on a regular basis so the patient knows it is available if desired.

22. A 25-year-old G2P1 patient has come to the obstetric triage room at 32 weeks reporting painless vaginal bleeding. You are providing orientation for a new RN on the unit. Which statement by the new RN to the patient would require your prompt intervention?
    1. "I'm going to check your vital signs."
    2. "I'm going to apply a fetal monitor to check the baby's heart rate and to see if you are having contractions."
    3. "I'm going to perform a vaginal examination to see if your cervix is dilated."
    4. "I'm going to feel your abdomen to check the position of the baby."

23. A 30-year-old G6P5 woman at 12 weeks has just begun prenatal care, and her initial laboratory work reveals that she has tested positive for human immunodeficiency virus (HIV) infection. What would be priority evidence-based nursing education for this patient today?
    1. Medication for HIV infection is safe and can greatly reduce transmission of HIV to the infant.
    2. Breast feeding is still recommended due to the great benefits to the infant.
    3. Pregnancy is known to accelerate the course of HIV disease in the mother.
    4. Cesarean section is not recommended because of the increased risk of HIV transmission with the bleeding at surgery.

24. A 22-year-old woman is 6 weeks postpartum. In the clinic she admits to crying every day, feeling overwhelmed, and sometimes thinking that she may hurt the baby. What would be the priority nursing action at this time?
    1. Advise the patient of community resources, parent groups, and depression hotlines.
    2. Counsel the mother that the "baby blues" are common at this time and assess her nutrition, rest, and availability of help at home.
    3. Contact the provider to evaluate the patient before allowing her to leave the clinic.
    4. Advise the woman that she cannot use medication for depression because she is breast feeding.

PART 2 Common Health Scenarios

25. A 23-year-old G1P0 patient at 10 weeks states that she exercises 5 days a week. You have discussed exercise in pregnancy with her. Which statement by the patient indicates that more teaching of evidence-based principles is needed?
    1. "I will continue to exercise 5 days a week."
    2. "I will reduce my exercise at this time in my pregnancy to reduce the risk of miscarriage but will increase it in the second trimester."
    3. "I will drink more fluid before and after exercising."
    4. "I will stop playing football while I am pregnant."

26. A 3-day-old breast-fed infant is brought to the clinic by his parents for routine assessment following a normal full-term delivery without complications. Which statement by the parents suggests an abnormal finding on a newborn of this age?
    1. "The baby urinated only 3 times yesterday."
    2. "The bowel movement of the baby was dark at first, but yesterday it was greenish yellow."
    3. "The baby cried for 2 hours last night."
    4. "The baby ate four times in the past 24 hours."

27. A full-term newborn is at the clinic with his parents. He is 4 days old. His birth weight was 7 pounds. Which assessment made by the RN is most significant?
    1. The infant's weight today is 6 pounds 9 ounces.
    2. The infant's skin is peeling.
    3. The infant's breast tissue is swollen.
    4. There is a yellow discharge from the infant's right eye.

28. You have received orders to initiate phototherapy on a 36-hour-old newborn with an elevated bilirubin level. What instructions will you give the student nurse who is assisting in the care of the infant? *(Select all that apply.)*
    1. Cover the infant's eyes with a mask.
    2. Monitor the infant's temperature closely.
    3. Keep the infant "nothing by mouth" (NPO) during the treatment.
    4. Apply ointment to the infant's skin prior to light exposure.
    5. Offer the infant sterile water feedings during the treatment.

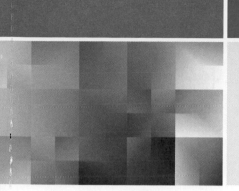

CHAPTER 19

Pediatric Problems

1. In caring for a 3-year-old with pain, which assessment question would be the most useful?
   1. "Can you point to the pain with one finger and tell me what that pain feels like inside of you?"
   2. "If number 1 were a little pain and number 10 were a big pain, what number would your pain be?"
   3. "The smiling face has 'no hurting'; the crying face has a 'really big hurting.' Which face is most like your hurting?"
   4. "One chip is 'a little bit of hurt' and four chips are 'the most hurt.' How many chips would you take for your hurt?"

2. Which pediatric pain patient should be assigned to a newly-graduated RN?
   1. Adolescent who has sickle cell disease and was recently weaned from morphine delivered via a patient-controlled analgesia device to an oral analgesic; he has been continually asking for an increased dose
   2. Child who needs premedication before reduction of a fracture; the child has been crying and is resistant to any touch to the arm or other procedures
   3. Child who is receiving palliative end-of-life care; the child is receiving narcotics around the clock to relieve suffering, but there is a progressive decrease in alertness and responsiveness
   4. Child who has chronic pain and whose medication and nonpharmacologic regimen has recently been changed; the mother is anxious to see if the new regimen is successful

3. You are caring for several children with cancer and are reviewing morning laboratory results for all of your patients. Which of these patient conditions combined with the indicated laboratory result causes you the greatest immediate concern?
   1. Nausea and vomiting with a potassium level of 3.3 mEq/L
   2. A nosebleed with a platelet count of 100,000/mm^3
   3. Fever with an absolute neutrophil count of 450/mm^3
   4. Fatigue with a hemoglobin level of 8 g/dL

4. A 6-year-old who received chemotherapy and had anorexia is now cheerfully eating peanut butter, yogurt, and applesauce. When the mother arrives, the child refuses to eat and throws the dish on the floor. What is your best response to this behavior?
   1. Remind the child that foods tasted good today and will help the body to get strong.
   2. Allow the mother and child time alone to review and control the behavior.
   3. Ask the mother to leave until the child can finish eating and then invite her back.
   4. Explain to the mother that the behavior could be a normal expression of anger.

5. An 8-year-old child has stomatitis secondary to chemotherapy. Which task would be best to delegate to the UAP?
   1. Reporting evidence of severe mucosal ulceration
   2. Assisting the child in swishing and spitting an anesthetic mouthwash
   3. Assessing the child's ability and willingness to drink through a straw
   4. Helping the patient to eat a bland, moist, soft diet

6. As the pediatric unit charge nurse, you are making patient assignments for the evening shift. Which patient is most appropriate to assign to an experienced LPN/LVN?
   1. 1-year-old with severe combined immunodeficiency disease who is scheduled to receive chemotherapy in preparation for a stem cell transplant
   2. 2-year-old with Wiskott-Aldrich syndrome who has orders for a platelet transfusion
   3. 3-year-old who has chronic graft-versus-host disease and is incontinent of loose stools
   4. 6-year-old who received chemotherapy a week ago and is admitted with increasing lethargy and a temperature of 101° F (38.3° C)

7. You are the pediatric unit charge nurse working with a new RN. Which action by the new RN requires the most immediate action on your part?
   1. Placing a child who has chemotherapy-induced neutropenia into a negative-pressure room
   2. Wearing goggles to change the linens of a patient who has diarrhea caused by *Clostridium difficile*
   3. Instructing UAPs to use an N95 respirator mask when caring for a child who has pertussis
   4. Admitting a new patient with respiratory syncytial virus (RSV) infection to a room with another child who has RSV

8. You are preparing to care for a 6-year-old who has just undergone allogeneic stem cell transplantation and will need protective environmental isolation. Which nursing tasks will you delegate to the UAP? *(Select all that apply.)*
   1. Stocking the patient's room with the needed personal protective equipment items
   2. Teaching the patient to perform thorough hand washing after using the bathroom
   3. Reminding visitors to wear a respirator mask, gloves, and gown
   4. Posting the precautions for protective isolation on the door of the patient's room
   5. Talking to the family members about the reasons for the isolation

9. You are a public school nurse. Which action will you take to have the most impact on the incidence of infectious diseases in the school?
   1. Make soap and water readily available in the classrooms.
   2. Ensure that students are immunized according to national recommendations.
   3. Provide written information about infection control to all parents.
   4. Teach students how to cover their mouths when they cough or sneeze.

10. While working in the pediatric clinic, you receive a telephone call from the parent of a 13-year-old who is receiving chemotherapy for leukemia. The patient's sibling has chickenpox (varicella). Which action will you anticipate taking next?
    1. Administer varicella-zoster immune globulin to the patient.
    2. Teach the parent about the correct use of acyclovir (Zovirax).
    3. Educate the parent about contact and airborne precautions.
    4. Prepare to admit the patient to a private room in the hospital.

11. You are the charge nurse on the pediatric unit when a pediatrician calls wanting to admit a child with rubeola (measles). Which factor is of most concern in determining whether to admit the child to your unit?
    1. The unit is staffed with fewer RNs than usual.
    2. No negative-airflow rooms are available.
    3. The infection control nurse liaison is not present today.
    4. There are several children receiving chemotherapy.

12. A 16-year-old with cystic fibrosis is admitted with increased shortness of breath and possible pneumonia. Which nursing activity is most important to include in the patient's care?
    1. Allowing the patient to decide whether she needs aerosolized medications
    2. Placing the patient in a private room to decrease the risk of further infection
    3. Scheduling postural drainage and chest physio-therapy (CPT) every 4 hours
    4. Planning activities to allow for at least 8 hours of uninterrupted sleep

13. You have obtained this assessment information about a 3-year-old who has just returned to the pediatric unit after having a tonsillectomy. Which finding requires the most immediate follow-up?
    1. Frequent swallowing
    2. Hypotonic bowel sounds
    3. Reports of a sore throat
    4. Heart rate of 112 beats/min

14. You are providing nursing care for a newborn infant with respiratory distress syndrome (RDS) who is receiving nasal continuous positive airway pressure ventilation. Which assessment finding is most important to report to the health care provider?
    1. Apical pulse rate of 156 beats/min
    2. Crackles audible in both lungs
    3. Tracheal deviation to the right
    4. Oxygen saturation of 93%

15. You are assisting with the delivery of a 31-week gestational age premature newborn who requires intubation for RDS. Which medication will you anticipate will be needed first for this infant?
    1. Theophylline (Theolair, Theochron)
    2. Surfactant (Exosurf)
    3. Dexamethasone (Decadron)
    4. Albuterol (Proventil)

16. You obtain this information when assessing a 3-year-old with uncorrected tetralogy of Fallot who is crying. Which finding requires immediate action?
    1. The apical pulse rate is 118 beats/min.
    2. A loud systolic murmur is heard in the pulmonic area.
    3. There is marked clubbing of all of the child's nail beds.
    4. The lips and oral mucosa are dusky in color.

17. After receiving the change-of-shift report, which patient should you assess first?
    1. 18-month-old with coarctation of the aorta who has decreased pedal pulses
    2. 3-year-old with rheumatic fever who reports severe knee pain
    3. 5-year-old with endocarditis who has crackles audible throughout both lungs
    4. 8-year-old with Kawasaki disease who has a temperature of 102.2° F (39° C)

18. As the pediatric unit charge nurse, you are working with a newly-graduated RN who has been on orientation in the unit for 2 months. Which patient should you assign to the new RN?
    1. 2-year-old with a ventricular septal defect for whom digoxin (Lanoxin) 90 mcg by mouth has been prescribed
    2. 4-year-old who had a pulmonary artery banding and has just been transferred in from the intensive care unit
    3. 9-year-old with mitral valve endocarditis whose parents need teaching about IV antibiotic administration
    4. 16-year-old with a heart transplant who was admitted with a low-grade fever and tachycardia

19. You are obtaining the history and physical information for a child who is recovering from Kawasaki disease and receives aspirin therapy. Which information about this patient will concern you most?
    1. The child attends a day-care center 5 days a week.
    2. The child's fingers have areas of peeling skin.
    3. The child is very irritable and cries frequently.
    4. The child has not received any immunizations.

20. You are working with an LPN/LVN who is caring for a 10-year-old who has severe abdominal, hip, and knee pain caused by a sickle cell crisis. Which action taken by the LPN/LVN requires that you intervene immediately?
    1. Suggesting genetic counseling to the patient
    2. Positioning cold packs on the patient's knees
    3. Placing a "No Visitors" sign on the patient's door
    4. Checking the patient's temperature every 2 hours

21. You have just received a change-of-shift report about these pediatric patients. Which patient will you assess first?
    1. 1-year-old with hemophilia B who was admitted because of decreased responsiveness
    2. 3-year-old with von Willebrand disease who has a dose of desmopressin (DDAVP) scheduled
    3. 7-year-old with acute lymphocytic leukemia who has chemotherapy-induced thrombocytopenia
    4. 16-year-old with sickle cell disease who reports acute right lower quadrant abdominal pain

22. You are reviewing the complete blood count for a 3-year-old who has been diagnosed with idiopathic thrombocytopenic purpura. Which information should you report immediately to the health care provider?
    1. Increased eosinophil level
    2. Hemoglobin level of 6.1 g/dL
    3. Platelet count of 40,000/mm^3
    4. Elevated reticulocyte count

23. A 4-year-old with acute lymphocytic leukemia has these medications ordered. Which one is most important to double-check with another licensed nurse?
    1. Prednisone (Deltasone) 1 mg by mouth (PO)
    2. Amoxicillin (Amoxil) 250 mg PO
    3. Methotrexate (Rheumatrex) 10 mg PO
    4. Filgrastim (Neupogen) 5 mcg subcutaneously

24. You are the charge nurse on the pediatric neurologic unit when the health care provider calls with new medication prescriptions for several patients with seizure disorders. Which prescription is most important to verify with the provider?
    1. Ibuprofen (Motrin) 10 mg/kg for a 2-year-old having a febrile seizure
    2. Phenytoin (Dilantin) 300 mg/day for a 6-year-old with tonic-clonic seizures
    3. Valproic acid (Depakote) 15 mg/kg/day for an 11-year-old with absence seizures
    4. Carbamazepine (Tegretol) 100 mg every 8 hours for a 70-kg 17-year-old with complex seizures

25. You are caring for a 3-year-old who has returned to the pediatric intensive care unit after insertion of a ventriculoperitoneal shunt to correct hydrocephalus. Which assessment finding is most important to communicate to the surgeon?
    1. The child is crying and says, "It hurts!"
    2. The right pupil is 1 mm larger than the left pupil.
    3. The cardiac monitor shows a heart rate of 130 beats/min.
    4. The head dressing has a 2-cm area of bloody drainage.

PART 2 Common Health Scenarios

26. You are caring for a newborn with a myelomeningocele who is awaiting surgical closure of the defect. Which assessment finding is of most concern?
    1. Bulging of the sac when the infant cries
    2. Oozing of stool from the anal sphincter
    3. Flaccid paralysis of both legs
    4. Temperature of 101.8° F (38.8° C)

27. An excited mother calls you for advice. "My child got cleaning solution in her eyes and I rinsed her eyes with water for a few minutes. What should I do? She is still screaming!" What do you instruct the caller to do first?
    1. Comfort the child and check her vision.
    2. Continue to irrigate the eyes with water.
    3. Call the Poison Control Center.
    4. Call 911 to request an ambulance.

28. A new nurse is caring for a child with a foreign body in the ear canal who has not yet been evaluated by the health care provider. You would intervene if the new nurse performs which action?
    1. Inspects the pinna for trauma
    2. Obtains history for type of object
    3. Prepares to irrigate the canal with warm water
    4. Uses an otoscope to check for perforation

29. You receive the following shift report on an adolescent with anorexia: The patient is 5 kg under her target weight. Her self-esteem has improved, but she continues to refer to herself as "fatty." She is able to appropriately verbalize a diet and exercise plan. What is the priority nursing diagnosis?
    1. Imbalanced Nutrition: Less than Body Requirements
    2. Disturbed Body Image
    3. Risk for Situational Low Self-Esteem
    4. Ineffective Health Maintenance

30. A 2-year-old child who has abdominal pain is diagnosed with intussusception. A hydrostatic reduction has been performed, and the health care provider has informed the parents that surgery is the next step. Which finding should be reported immediately before surgery proceeds?
    1. Palpable sausage-shaped abdominal mass
    2. Passage of normal brown stool
    3. Passage of currant jelly–like stools
    4. Frequent nausea and vomiting

31. A parent calls the emergency department (ED), saying "I think my toddler might have swallowed a little toy. He is breathing okay, but I don't know what to do." What is the most essential question to ask the caller?
    1. "Has he vomited?"
    2. "Have you been checking his stools?"
    3. "What do you think he swallowed?"
    4. "Has he been coughing?"

32. You are teaching a group of day-care workers about how to avoid transmission of hepatitis A in day-care settings. What is the single most effective measure to emphasize?
    1. Hand hygiene should be performed often to prevent and control the spread of infection.
    2. Children in whom hepatitis has been diagnosed should not share toys with others.
    3. Children with episodes of fecal incontinence should be isolated from others.
    4. Immunizations are recommended before children are admitted into day-care settings.

33. These medications have been prescribed for a 9-year-old with deep partial- and full-thickness burns. Which medication is most important to double-check with another licensed nurse before administration?
    1. Silver sulfadiazine (Silvadene) ointment
    2. Famotidine (Pepcid) 20 mg IV
    3. Lorazepam (Ativan) 0.5 mg PO
    4. Multivitamin (Centrum Kids) 1 tablet PO

34. You are caring for a 5-year-old whose mother asks why he still wets the bed. What is your best response?
    1. "He is old enough that he should no longer be wetting the bed."
    2. "Most children outgrow bed-wetting by the time they start school."
    3. "His bed-wetting may be due to an immature bladder or deep sleep pattern."
    4. "He will probably stop once he realizes how embarrassing it is to wet the bed."

35. Which intervention for the 5-year-old child who still wets the bed would be best assigned to the UAP?
    1. Reminding the child to use the bathroom before going to bed
    2. Teaching the mother about moisture alarm devices
    3. Administering the prescribed dose of imipramine (Tofranil)
    4. Discussing research related to the use of hypnosis with the mother

36. A 16-year-old in the adolescent health clinic tells you that she has been sexually active for 6 months, "but only with my boyfriend." Screening for which sexually transmitted disease (STD) will be most important for this patient?
    1. Syphilis
    2. Genital herpes simplex
    3. Human papillomavirus
    4. Chlamydia

37. The health care provider has ordered cooling measures for a child with fever who is likely to be discharged when the temperature comes down. Which task will you delegate to the UAP?
    1. Providing explanations of nursing actions to the family
    2. Assisting the child in removing outer clothing
    3. Advising the parent to use acetaminophen (Tylenol) instead of aspirin
    4. Monitoring the child's level of consciousness and orientation level

38. A tearful parent brings a child to the ED after the child takes an unknown amount of children's chewable vitamins at an unknown time. The child is currently alert and asymptomatic. What information should be immediately reported to the physician?
    1. The ingested children's chewable vitamins contain iron.
    2. The child has been treated previously for ingestion of toxic substances.
    3. The child has been treated several times before for accidental injuries.
    4. The child was nauseated and vomited once at home.

39. You are preparing a child for IV conscious sedation before repair of a facial laceration. What information should you immediately report to the health care provider?
    1. The parent is unsure about the child's tetanus immunization status.
    2. The child is upset and pulls out the IV.
    3. The parent declines the IV conscious sedation.
    4. The parent wants information about the IV conscious sedation.

40. A teenager arrives in the triage area alert and ambulatory, but his clothes are covered with blood. His friends are yelling, "We were goofing around and he got poked in the abdomen with a stick!" Which comment would be of most concern?
    1. "There was a lot of blood and we used three bandages."
    2. "He pulled the stick out, just now, because it was hurting him."
    3. "The stick was really dirty and covered with mud."
    4. "He's a diabetic, so he needs attention right away."

41. The ED receives multiple individuals, mostly children, who were injured when the roof of a day-care center collapsed because of a heavy snowfall. Based on physiologic differences in children compared with adults, for which injuries and complications will the nurse assess first? *(Select all that apply.)*
    1. Head injuries
    2. Bradycardia or junctional arrhythmias
    3. Hypoxemia
    4. Liver and spleen contusions
    5. Hypothermia
    6. Fractures of the long bones
    7. Lumbar spines injuries

Answer Key for this chapter begins on p. 201.

PART 2 Common Health Scenarios

CHAPTER 20

Emergencies and Disasters

1. You are the charge nurse in an emergency department (ED) and must assign two staff members to cover the triage area. Which team is the most appropriate for this assignment?
   1. An advanced practice nurse and an experienced LPN/LVN
   2. An experienced LPN/LVN and an inexperienced RN
   3. An experienced RN and an inexperienced RN
   4. An experienced RN and an experienced UAP

2. You are working in the triage area of an ED, and the following four clients approach the triage desk at the same time. List the order in which you will assess these clients.
   1. Ambulatory, dazed 25-year-old man with a bandaged head wound
   2. Irritable infant with a fever, petechiae, and nuchal rigidity
   3. 35-year-old jogger with a twisted ankle who has a pedal pulse and no deformity
   4. 50-year-old woman with moderate abdominal pain and occasional vomiting _____, _____, _____, _____

3. When a primary survey of a trauma client is conducted, what is considered one of the priority actions?
   1. Obtain a complete set of vital sign measurements.
   2. Palpate and auscultate the abdomen.
   3. Perform a brief neurologic assessment.
   4. Check the pulse oximetry reading.

4. A 56-year-old client comes to the triage area with left-sided chest pain, diaphoresis, and dizziness. What is the priority action?
   1. Initiate continuous electrocardiographic monitoring.
   2. Notify the ED physician.
   3. Administer oxygen via nasal cannula.
   4. Establish IV access.

5. A client is admitted through the ED for treatment of a strangulated intestinal obstruction with perforation. What interventions do you anticipate for this emergency condition? *(Select all that apply.)*
   1. Preparation for surgery
   2. Barium enema examination
   3. Nasogastric (NG) tube insertion
   4. Abdominal radiography
   5. IV fluid administration
   6. IV administration of broad-spectrum antibiotics
   7. Morphine via a client-controlled analgesia device

6. It is the summer season, and clients with signs and symptoms of heat-related illness come to the ED. Which client needs attention first?
   1. Elderly person with reports of dizziness and syncope after standing in the sun for several hours to view a parade
   2. Marathon runner who reports severe leg cramps and nausea, and shows tachycardia, diaphoresis, pallor, and weakness
   3. Relatively healthy homemaker who reports that the air conditioner has been broken for days and who manifests tachypnea, hypotension, fatigue, and profuse diaphoresis
   4. Homeless person with altered mental status, poor muscle coordination, and hot, dry, ashen skin; and whose duration of heat exposure is unknown

7. You respond to a call for help from the ED waiting room. An elderly client is lying on the floor. List the order in which you must carry out the following actions.
   1. Perform the chin lift or jaw thrust maneuver.
   2. Establish unresponsiveness.
   3. Initiate cardiopulmonary resuscitation (CPR).
   4. Call for help and activate the code team.
   5. Instruct a UAP to get the crash cart. _____, _____, _____, _____, _____

Common Health Scenarios

PART 2

8. The emergency medical service team has transported a client with severe chest pain. As the client is being transferred to the emergency stretcher, you note unresponsiveness, cessation of breathing, and no palpable pulse. Which task is appropriate to delegate to the UAP?
   1. Performing chest compressions
   2. Initiating bag-valve mask ventilation
   3. Assisting with oral intubation
   4. Placing the defibrillator pads

9. An anxious 24-year-old college student reports tingling sensations, palpitations, and sore chest muscles. Deep, rapid breathing and carpal spasms are noted. What priority nursing action should you take?
   1. Notify the physician immediately.
   2. Administer supplemental oxygen.
   3. Have the student breathe into a paper bag.
   4. Obtain an order for an anxiolytic medication.

10. An experienced traveling nurse has been assigned to work in the ED; however, this is the nurse's first week on the job. Which area of the ED is the most appropriate assignment for this nurse?
    1. Trauma team
    2. Triage
    3. Ambulatory or fast-track clinic
    4. Pediatric medicine team

11. In the care of a client who has experienced sexual assault, which task is most appropriate for an LPN/LVN to perform?
    1. Assessing immediate emotional state and physical injuries
    2. Collecting hair samples, saliva specimens, and scrapings beneath fingernails
    3. Providing emotional support and supportive communication
    4. Ensuring that the chain of custody of evidence is maintained

12. You are caring for a client with frostbite to the feet. Place the following interventions in the correct order.
    1. Apply a loose, sterile, bulky dressing.
    2. Give pain medication.
    3. Remove the client from the cold environment.
    4. Immerse the feet in warm water of 105° F to 115° F (40.6° C to 46.1° C).
    5. Monitor for compartment syndrome. _____, _____, _____, _____, _____

13. The LPN/LVN is performing care for a client who sustained an amputation of the first and second digits in a chainsaw accident. Which actions would require immediate intervention by the supervising RN? *(Select all that apply.)*
    1. Gently cleansing the amputated digits and the hand with a povidone-iodine (Betadine)/normal saline solution
    2. Cleansing the amputated digits and placing them directly into an ice slurry
    3. Wrapping the cleansed digits in saline-moistened gauze, sealing them in a plastic bag, and placing them in an ice slurry
    4. Cleansing the digits with sterile normal saline and placing them in a sterile cup with sterile normal saline
    5. Placing the amputated digits in the correct anatomic position and then wrapping the hand and digits with sterile gauze.

14. You are giving discharge instructions to a woman who has been treated for contusions and bruises sustained during an episode of domestic violence. What is your priority intervention for this client?
    1. Arrange transportation to a safe house.
    2. Make a referral to a counselor.
    3. Advise the client about contacting the police.
    4. Make an appointment to follow up on the injuries.

15. You notify the ED physician about a client who reports abdominal pain, nausea and vomiting, and fever. The abdomen is distended, rigid, and boardlike, and there is rebound tenderness. Later you see an order for discharge and a follow-up appointment in the morning. You reexamine the client and the symptoms seem worse. What should you do first?
    1. Contact the nursing supervisor and express your concerns.
    2. Express your findings and concerns to the physician.
    3. Discharge the client, but stress the importance of follow-up.
    4. Follow the physician's orders and write an incident report.

16. An intoxicated client comes in with slurred speech, mild confusion, and uncooperative behavior. The client cannot provide a good history but admits to "drinking a few on the weekend." What is the priority nursing action for this client?
    1. Obtain an order for determining blood alcohol level.
    2. Contact the family to obtain additional history and baseline information.
    3. Administer naloxone (Narcan) 2 to 4 mg as ordered.
    4. Administer IV fluid with supplemental thiamine as ordered.

17. When an unexpected death occurs in the ED, which task is most appropriate to delegate to the UAP?
    1. Escorting the family to a place of privacy
    2. Going with the organ donor specialist to talk to the family
    3. Assisting with postmortem care
    4. Helping the family to collect belongings

18. After emergency endotracheal intubation, you must verify tube placement and secure the tube. List in order the steps that are required to perform this function.
    1. Obtain an order for a chest radiograph to document tube placement.
    2. Secure the tube in place.
    3. Auscultate the chest during assisted ventilation.
    4. Confirm that the breath sounds are equal and bilateral.
    5. Check exhaled carbon dioxide levels. _____, _____, _____, _____, _____

19. A man, with a known history of alcohol abuse, has been in police custody for 48 hours. Initially, anxiety, sweating, and tremors were noted. Now, disorientation, hallucination, and hyperreactivity are observed. The medical diagnosis is delirium tremens. What is the priority nursing diagnosis?
    1. Risk for Injury related to seizures
    2. Risk for Other-Directed Violence related to hallucinations
    3. Risk for Situational Low Self-Esteem related to police custody
    4. Risk for Imbalanced Nutrition: Less than Body Requirements related to chronic alcohol abuse

20. You are assigned to telephone triage. A client who was just stung by a common honeybee calls for advice. The client reports pain and localized swelling but has no respiratory distress or other systemic signs of anaphylaxis. What is the first action that you should direct the caller to perform?
    1. Call 911.
    2. Remove the stinger by scraping.
    3. Apply a cool compress.
    4. Take an oral antihistamine.

21. You are assessing a client who has sustained a cat bite to the left hand. The cat's immunizations are up to date. The date of the client's last tetanus shot is unknown. Which is the priority nursing diagnosis?
    1. Risk for Infection related to organisms specific to cat bites
    2. Impaired Skin Integrity related to puncture wounds
    3. Ineffective Health Maintenance related to immunization status
    4. Risk for Impaired Physical Mobility related to potential tendon damage

22. The following clients come to the ED reporting acute abdominal pain. Prioritize them for care in order of the severity of their conditions.
    1. 35-year-old man reporting severe intermittent cramps with three episodes of watery diarrhea 2 hours after eating
    2. 11-year-old boy with a low-grade fever, right lower quadrant tenderness, nausea, and anorexia for the past 2 days
    3. 40-year-old woman with moderate right upper quadrant pain who has vomited small amounts of yellow bile and whose symptoms have worsened over the past week
    4. 65-year-old man with a pulsating abdominal mass and sudden onset of "tearing" pain in the abdomen and flank within the past hour
    5. 23-year-old woman reporting dizziness and severe left lower quadrant pain who states she is possibly pregnant
    6. 50-year-old woman who reports gnawing midepigastric pain that is worse between meals and during the night _____, _____, _____, _____, _____, _____

23. The nursing manager decides to form a committee to address the issue of violence against ED personnel. Which combination of employees would be best suited to fulfill this assignment?
    1. ED physicians and charge nurses
    2. Experienced RNs and experienced paramedics
    3. RNs, LPNs/LVNs, and UAPs
    4. At least one representative from each group of ED personnel

24. You are caring for a client with multiple injuries sustained during a head-on car collision. Which assessment finding takes priority?
    1. A deviated trachea
    2. Unequal pupils
    3. Ecchymosis in the flank area
    4. Irregular apical pulse

25. A client involved in a one-car rollover comes in with multiple injuries. List in order of priority the interventions that must be initiated for this client.
    1. Secure two large-bore IV lines and infuse normal saline.
    2. Use the chin lift or jaw thrust maneuver to open the airway.
    3. Assess for spontaneous respirations.
    4. Give supplemental oxygen via mask.
    5. Obtain a full set of vital sign measurements.
    6. Remove the client's clothing.
    7. Insert a Foley catheter if not contraindicated. _____, _____, _____, _____, _____, _____, _____

26. A group of people arrive at the ED by private car reporting extreme periorbital swelling, cough, and tightness in the throat. There is a strong odor emanating from their clothes. They report exposure to a "gas bomb" that was set off in their house. What is the priority action?
    1. Measure vital signs and listen to lung sounds.
    2. Direct the clients to the decontamination area.
    3. Instruct clients to don personal protective equipment.
    4. Direct the clients to the cold or clean zone for immediate treatment.

27. In the work setting, what is your primary responsibility in preparing for management of disasters, including natural disasters and bioterrorism incidents?
    1. Knowing the agency's emergency response plan
    2. Being aware of the signs and symptoms of potential agents of bioterrorism
    3. Knowing how and what to report to the Centers for Disease Control and Prevention (CDC)
    4. Making ethical decisions about exposing self to potentially lethal substances

28. Emergency and ambulatory care nurses are among the first health care workers to encounter victims of a bioterrorist attack. List in order of priority the actions that should be taken by ED staff in the event of a biochemical incident.
    1. Report to the public health department or CDC per protocol.
    2. Decontaminate the affected individuals in a separate area.
    3. Protect the environment for the safety of personnel and nonaffected clients.
    4. Don personal protective equipment.
    5. Perform triage according to protocol. _____, _____, _____, _____, _____

29. You are talking to a group of people about an industrial explosion in which many people were killed or injured. Which individual has the greatest risk for psychiatric difficulties, such as post-traumatic stress disorder, related to the incident?
    1. Individual who repeatedly watched television coverage of the event
    2. Person who recently learned that her son was killed in the incident
    3. Individual who witnessed the death of a co-worker during the explosion
    4. Person who was injured and trapped for several hours before rescue

30. Identify the five most critical elements in performing disaster triage for multiple victims.
    1. Obtain past medical and surgical histories.
    2. Check airway, breathing, and circulation.
    3. Assess the level of consciousness.
    4. Visually inspect for gross deformities, bleeding, and obvious injuries.
    5. Note color, presence of moisture, and temperature of the skin.
    6. Obtain a history of allergies to food or medicine.
    7. Check vital signs, including pulse and respirations.
    8. Obtain a list of current medications.
    9. Inquire about the last tetanus shot. _____, _____, _____, _____, _____

31. You are working in a small rural community hospital. There is a fire in a local church, and six injured clients have arrived at the hospital. Many others are expected to arrive soon, and other hospitals are 5 hours away. Using disaster triage principles, place the following six clients in the order in which they should receive medical attention.
    1. 52-year-old man in full cardiac arrest who has been receiving CPR continuously for the past 60 minutes
    2. Firefighter who is showing combative behavior and has respiratory stridor
    3. 60-year-old woman with full-thickness burns to the hands and forearms
    4. Teenager with a crushed leg that is very swollen who is anxious and has tachycardia
    5. 3-year-old child with respiratory distress and burns over more than 70% of the anterior body
    6. 12-year-old with wheezing and very labored respirations unrelieved by an asthma inhaler _____, _____, _____, _____, _____, _____

Answer Key for this chapter begins on p. 204.

CHAPTER 21

Psychiatric–Mental Health Problems

Note: In this chapter, the term "mental health assistant" is used, rather than the more familiar "UAP." Different facilities and localities will use different titles for assistive personnel. The key point to remember in assigning tasks or making patient assignments is that UAPs who routinely work on a medical-surgical unit will have different skill sets than mental health assistants, who usually work on a psychiatric unit.

1. A patient with a diagnosis of hypochondriasis has made multiple clinic visits and undergone diagnostic tests for "cancer," with no evidence of organic disease. Today he declares, "I have a brain tumor. I can feel it growing. My appointment is tomorrow, but I can't wait!" What is the most therapeutic response?
   1. Present reality: "Sir, you have been seen many times in this clinic and had many diagnostic tests. The results have always been negative."
   2. Encourage expression of feelings: "Let me spend some time with you. Tell me about what you are feeling and why you think you have a brain tumor."
   3. Set boundaries: "Sir, I will take your vital signs, but then I am going to call your case manager so that you can discuss the scheduled appointment."
   4. Respect the patient's wishes: "Sir, sit down and I will make sure that you see the physician right away. Don't worry; we will take care of you."

2. You are caring for a patient in whom a conversion disorder was recently diagnosed. She is experiencing a sudden loss of vision after witnessing a violent fight between her husband and adult-age son. What is the priority therapeutic approach to use with this patient?
   1. Reassure her that her blindness is temporary and will resolve with time
   2. Gently point out that she seems to be able to see well enough to function independently
   3. Encourage expression of feelings and link emotional trauma to the blindness
   4. Teach ways to cope with blindness, such as methodically arranging personal items

3. As the charge nurse, you are reviewing the assignment sheet for an acute psychiatric unit. Which experienced team member should be reassigned?
   1. Male LVN assigned to a male patient with chronic depression and excessive rumination
   2. Young male mental health assistant assigned to a female adolescent with anorexia nervosa
   3. Female RN assigned to a newly admitted female patient who has command hallucinations and delusions of persecution
   4. Older female RN with medical-surgical experience assigned to a male patient with Alzheimer disease

4. You arrive home and find that the house of your neighbor (Jane) is on fire. A fireman is physically restraining her from running back into the house. What is the best response?
   1. "Jane, come and sit in my house until this is over with."
   2. "Jane, calm down and let the fireman do his job."
   3. "Jane, look at me and hold my hand."
   4. "Jane, tell me why you are struggling so hard."

5. There is a patient on the medical-surgical unit who has been there for several months. He is hostile, rude, and belligerent, and no one likes to interact with him. How should you handle the assignment?
   1. Rotate the assignment schedule so that no one has to care for him more than once or twice a week.
   2. Pair a float nurse and a nursing student and assign the patient to that team because they will have a fresh perspective toward the patient.
   3. Identify two or three experienced nurses as primary caregivers and develop a plan that includes psychosocial interventions.
   4. Assign yourself as primary caregiver so that you can role-model how patients should be treated.

6. A patient diagnosed with paranoid schizophrenia tells you that, "Dr. Smith has killed several other patients and now he is trying to kill me." What is the best response?
   1. "I have worked here a long time. No one has died. You are safe here."
   2. "What has Dr. Smith done to make you think he would like to kill you?"
   3. "All of the staff, including Dr. Smith, are here to ensure your safety."
   4. "Whenever you are concerned or nervous, talk to me or any of the nurses."

7. A nursing student reports to you that he has observed several types of behavior among the patients. Which patient needs priority assessment?
   1. A patient who is having command hallucinations
   2. A patient who is demonstrating clang associations
   3. A patient who is verbalizing ideas of reference
   4. A patient who is using neologisms

8. Mr. J. has a panic disorder and it appears that he is having some problems controlling his anxiety. Which symptoms concern you the most?
   1. His heart rate is increased and he reports chest tightness.
   2. He demonstrates tachypnea and carpopedal spasms.
   3. He is pacing to and fro and pounding his fists together.
   4. He is muttering to himself and is easily startled.

9. You are interviewing a patient with suicidal ideations and a history of major depression. Which comment concerns you the most?
   1. "I have had problems with depression most of my adult life."
   2. "My father and my brother both committed suicide."
   3. "My wife is having health problems and she relies on me."
   4. "I am afraid to kill myself, and I wished I had more courage."

10. A patient comes into the walk-in clinic and tells you that he wants to be admitted to an alcohol rehabilitation program. Which question is the most important to ask?
    1. "What made you decide to enter a program at this time?"
    2. "How much alcohol do you usually consume in a day?"
    3. "When was the last time you had a drink?"
    4. "Have you been in a rehabilitation program before?"

11. A patient on the acute psychiatric unit develops neuroleptic malignant syndrome. Which task should be delegated to the mental health assistant?
    1. Wiping the patient's body with cool moist towels
    2. Monitoring vital signs every 15 minutes
    3. Attaching the patient to the electrocardiogram (ECG) monitor
    4. Assisting the RN to transfer the patient to the medical intensive care unit (ICU)

12. Which patient should be assigned to a newly-graduated nurse who has just started on the acute psychiatric unit?
    1. Patient who is frequently admitted for borderline personality disorder and suicidal gesture
    2. Patient admitted yesterday for disorganized schizophrenia and psychosis
    3. Patient newly admitted to determine differential diagnosis of depression, dementia, or delirium
    4. Patient newly diagnosed with major depression and rumination about loss and suicide

13. Which task can be assigned to a medical-surgical UAP who has been temporarily floated to the acute psychiatric unit to help out?
    1. Performing one-to-one observation of a patient who is suicidal
    2. Assisting the occupational therapist to conduct a craft class
    3. Accompanying an elderly patient who wanders on a walk outside
    4. Assisting the medication nurse who is having problems with a patient

14. The team has to apply restraints to a combative patient in order to prevent harm to others or to self. Which action requires your intervention?
    1. Mental health assistant uses a quick-release knot to secure the restraint
    2. Physician secures the restraint to the side rail
    3. RN checks the pulses distal to the restraints
    4. LPN/LVN explains to the patient why he is being restrained

15. A well-known celebrity is admitted to your psychiatric unit. Several RNs from other units drop by and express an interest in seeing the patient. What is the best response?
    1. "Please be discreet and do not interrupt the work flow."
    2. "How did you find out that the patient was admitted to this unit?"
    3. "Please wait. I need to call the nursing supervisor about this request."
    4. "I'm sorry; the patient has asked that only family be allowed to visit."

16. An LPN/LVN complains to you (charge nurse) that she is always assigned to the same patient with chronic depression. What should you do?
    1. Look at the assignment sheet and see if there is any way to switch assignments with another LPN/LVN.
    2. Tell her to care for the patient today, but that you will remember the request for future assignments.
    3. Remind her that continuity of care and patient-centered care are the primary goals.
    4. Explain that patients with chronic conditions are more likely to fall under the LPN/LVN scope of practice.

17. The emergency department (ED) is calling to report on a patient who will be admitted to your acute psychiatric unit. He has a history of bipolar disorder and was in an altercation that resulted in the death of another. He has contusions, abrasions and minor lacerations. What is the priority question that you should ask?
    1. "When will the patient be transferred?"
    2. "Will a police officer be with him while he is on the unit?"
    3. "Why isn't the patient being admitted to the trauma unit?"
    4. "What is the patient's current mood and behavior?"

18. A patient needs Klonopin 1 mg by mouth. The pharmacy delivers clonidine 0.1-mg tablets. A nursing student asks you if Klonopin and clonidine are two different names for the same drug. Place the following steps in the correct sequence so that you can teach the nursing student how to prevent medication errors.
    1. Advise the pharmacy of any corrections as appropriate.
    2. Recognize that "look-alike, sound-alike" drugs increase the chances of error.
    3. Consult a medication book to verify the purpose of the drugs and generic and brand names.
    4. Check the original medication order to verify what was prescribed.
    5. Write an incident report, as appropriate, if you believe that a system error is occurring.
    6. Call the physician for clarification of the order as appropriate. _____, _____, _____, _____, _____, _____

19. A patient is displaying muscle spasms of the tongue, face, and neck, and his eyes are locked in an upward gaze. He has been prescribed haloperidol (Haldol). What is the priority action?
    1. Encourage him to look at you and stay with him until the spasms pass.
    2. Place the patient on aspiration precautions until the spasms subside.
    3. Obtain an order for intramuscular or IV diphenhydramine (Benadryl).
    4. Obtain an order for and administer an antiseizure medication.

20. Several patients are taking antipsychotic medications and are having medication side effects. Place the following patients in priority order for additional assessment and appropriate interventions.
    1. A patient who is taking trifluoperazine (Stelazine) and has a temperature of 103.6° F (39.8° C) with tachycardia, muscular rigidity, and dysphagia
    2. A patient who is taking fluphenazine (Prolixin) and has dry mouth and dry eyes, urinary hesitancy, constipation, and photosensitivity
    3. A patient who is taking loxapine (Loxitane) and has a protruding tongue with lip smacking and spastic facial distortions
    4. A patient who is taking clozapine (Clozaril) and reports a sore throat, fever, malaise, and flulike symptoms that began about 6 weeks ago after starting the new antipsychotic medication; white blood cell count is 2000/mm^3 _____, _____, _____, _____

21. You are reviewing the principle of "least restrictive" interventions with the staff. Place the following interventions in the correct ascending order from the least restrictive to the most restrictive.
    1. Escort the patient to a quiet room for a time out.
    2. Restrain the patient's arms and legs with soft cloth restraints.
    3. Verbally instruct the patient to stop the unacceptable behavior (i.e., yelling, arguing) and move to another part of the day room.
    4. Accompany the patient out into the garden courtyard.
    5. Restrain the patient's upper extremities with wrist restraints.
    6. Place the patient in an isolation room with a mental health assistant observing. _____, _____, _____, _____, _____, _____

22. Which behavior would be the most problematic and require vigilance to prevent danger to self or others?
    1. Avolition
    2. Echolalia
    3. Motor agitation
    4. Stupor

23. A patient comes in to the clinic with nausea, constipation, and "excruciating stomach pain." Over a period of several years, this patient has come in two or three times a month with the same report, but multiple diagnostic tests have consistently yielded negative results for physical disorders. What is the priority nursing intervention for this patient?
    1. Advocate for the patient to have a psychiatric consultation.
    2. Ensure that the patient sees the same health care provider for continuity.
    3. Perform a physical assessment to identify any physical abnormalities.
    4. Assess for concurrent symptoms of depression or anxiety.

24. An elderly man was admitted for palliative care of terminal pancreatic cancer. The wife stated, "We don't want hospice; he wants treatment." The patient requested discharge and home health visits. Several hours after discharge, the man committed suicide with a gun. Which people should participate in a root cause analysis of this sentinel event? *(Select all that apply.)*
    1. The wife and all immediate family members
    2. Only the physician who discharged the patient
    3. Any nurse who cared for the patient during hospitalization
    4. The case manager who arranged home visits for the patient
    5. Only the nurse who discharged the patient
    6. Any physician who was involved in the care of the patient

An adolescent girl (Ms. C) is admitted to your medical-surgical unit for diagnostic evaluation and nutritional support related to anorexia nervosa. She is mildly dehydrated, her potassium level is 3.5 mEq/L, and she has experienced weight loss of more than 25% within the past 3 months.

25. At this time, what is the primary collaborative goal for the treatment of Ms. C?
    1. Assist her to increase feelings of control
    2. Decrease power struggles over eating
    3. Resolve dysfunctional family roles
    4. Restore normal nutrition and weight

26. For Ms. C, which route for delivery of nutrition and fluids will the health care team try first?
    1. Nasogastric
    2. Oral
    3. Intravenous
    4. Hypodermoclysis

27. In caring for this patient with anorexia nervosa, which task can be delegated to the UAP?
    1. Sitting with the patient during meals and for 1 to 1½ hours after meals
    2. Observing for and reporting ritualistic behaviors related to food
    3. Obtaining special food for the patient when she requests it
    4. Weighing the patient daily and reinforcing that she is underweight

28. You find Ms. C in her room jogging in place and doing jumping jacks "for about the last 20 minutes." What is the best response to give at this time?
    1. "You can jog for a few more minutes, but then you will tell me why you are exercising."
    2. "If you continue to exercise like this, you are just going to have to eat more at mealtime."
    3. "Stop jogging right now. This is unacceptable behavior and you will lose all privileges."
    4. "We have talked about exercise, and you agreed to reach your target weight goal first."

29. Ms. C's self-esteem and weight have gradually improved, but she continues to refer to herself as "fatty." She is able to appropriately verbalize an appropriate diet and exercise plan. What is the priority nursing diagnosis?
    1. Imbalanced Nutrition: Less than Body Requirements
    2. Disturbed Body Image
    3. Risk for Situational Low Self-Esteem
    4. Ineffective Health Maintenance

Answer Key for this chapter begins on p. 207.

CASE STUDY 1

Chest Pressure, Indigestion, Nausea, and Vomiting

Ms. S is a 58-year-old African-American woman who is admitted to the coronary care unit (CCU) from the emergency department (ED) with reports of chest pressure and indigestion associated with nausea and vomiting. She started feeling ill about 3 hours before admission. She told the nurse that she tried drinking water and took some bismuth subsalicylate (Pepto-Bismol) that she had in her bathroom medicine cabinet. She also tried lying down to rest, but none of these actions helped. She says, "It just gets worse and worse." Ms. S has been under a physician's care for the past 12 years for management of hypertension and swelling in her ankles. She was a smoker, but quit 1 year ago.

In the ED, admission laboratory tests, including levels of cardiac markers, were performed and a 12-lead electrocardiogram (ECG) was taken.

Ms. S's CCU vital sign values on admission are as follows:

Blood pressure	174/92 mm Hg
Heart rate	120 to 130 beats/min, irregular
O₂ saturation	94% on room air
Respiratory rate	30 to 34 breaths/min
Temperature	99.8° F (37.7° C) (oral)

1. Which action may you delegate to a UAP caring for Ms. S?
   1. Placing the client on a cardiac telemetry monitor
   2. Drawing blood to test cardiac marker levels and sending it to the laboratory
   3. Obtaining a 12-lead ECG
   4. Monitoring and recording the client's intake and output

2. Which physician order takes first priority at this time?
   1. Measure vital signs every 2 hours.
   2. Obtain a 12-lead ECG every 6 hours.
   3. Place the client on a cardiac monitor.
   4. Check levels of cardiac markers every 6 hours.

3. The client's cardiac telemetry monitor shows a rhythm of sinus tachycardia with frequent premature ventricular contractions (PVCs). Which drug should you prepare to administer first?
   1. Amiodarone (Cordarone) IV push
   2. Nitroglycerin (Nitrostat) sublingually
   3. Morphine sulfate IV push
   4. Atenolol (Tenormin) IV push

4. All of these laboratory values were obtained in the ED. Which value has immediate implications for the care of this client?
   1. Potassium level of 3.4 mEq/L
   2. Troponin T level of more than 0.20 ng/mL
   3. Glucose level of 123 mg/dL
   4. Slight elevation of white blood cell count

5. Ms. S reports worsening chest discomfort. The cardiac monitor shows ST-segment elevation, and you notify the health care provider. Which order takes priority at this time?
   1. Administer morphine sulfate 2 mg IV push.
   2. Schedule an echocardiogram.
   3. Draw blood for coagulation studies.
   4. Administer ranitidine (Zantac) 75 mg orally every 12 hours.

6. Because Ms. S continues to experience chest pain and has elevated levels of cardiac markers, the following interventions have been ordered. Which interventions may you assign to an experienced UAP? *(Select all that apply.)*
   1. Measuring vital signs every 2 hours
   2. Accurately recording intake and output
   3. Administering tenecteplase (TNKase) IV push
   4. Drawing blood for coagulation studies
   5. Assessing the cardiac monitor every 4 hours
   6. Assisting the client to the bedside commode

Complex Health Scenarios

PART 3

7. You assign the UAP the task of taking the client's vital signs every 2 hours and recording the vital sign values in the electronic chart. Later you check the client's chart and discover that vital sign measurements have not been recorded. What is your best action?
   1. Take the vital signs because the UAP is not competent to complete this task.
   2. Notify the nurse manager immediately.
   3. Reprimand the UAP at the nurses' station.
   4. Speak to the UAP privately to determine why the values were not recorded.

8. Ms. S's condition is stable, and she has been transferred to the cardiac step-down unit. What should you instruct the UAP to report immediately?
   1. Temperature of 99° F (37.2° C) with morning vital sign monitoring
   2. Chest pain episode occurring during morning care
   3. Systolic blood pressure increase of 8 mm Hg after morning care
   4. Heart rate increase of 10 beats/min after ambulation

9. The health care provider orders captopril (Capoten) 12.5 mg by mouth (PO) twice daily and hydrochlorothiazide (HCTZ [Microzide]) 25 mg PO daily. Which information would you be sure to include when teaching the client about these drugs?
   1. "Take your HCTZ in the morning."
   2. "If you miss a dose of captopril, take two tablets next time."
   3. "Avoid foods that are rich in potassium, such as bananas and oranges."
   4. "You should expect an increase in blood pressure with these drugs."

10. Ms. S is returning from a cardiac catheterization procedure. Which follow-up care orders could you delegate to an experienced LPN/LVN? *(Select all that apply.)*
    1. Reminding the client to remain on bed rest with the insertion site extremity straight
    2. Preparing a teaching plan that includes activity restrictions and risk factor modification
    3. Measuring the client's vital signs every 15 minutes for the first hour
    4. Assessing the catheter insertion site for bleeding or hematoma formation
    5. Monitoring peripheral pulses, skin temperature, and skin color with each measurement of vital signs
    6. Administer 2 tablets of acetaminophen (Tylenol) for back pain

11. Which instruction would you be sure to include in a discharge plan for Ms. S after her cardiac catheterization?
    1. "Avoid heavy lifting and exercise today."
    2. "Report any hematoma, even a small one, to the physician."
    3. "Leave the dressing in place for the first day that you are at home."
    4. "Keep your affected extremity straight while sleeping for several days."

12. Before discharging Ms. S, the health care provider orders an ECG. This test reveals normal sinus rhythm with a heart rate of 88 beats/min. What is your best action at this time?
    1. Delay the client's discharge until she is seen by the health care provider.
    2. Administer the client's next dose of atenolol 3 hours early before she goes home.
    3. Contact the health care provider and ask about drawing an additional set of cardiac markers.
    4. Document this finding as the only action.

Answer Key for this case study begins on p. 209.

CASE STUDY 2

Dyspnea and Shortness of Breath

Mr. W is an 83-year-old man who was brought to the hospital from a long-term care facility by the paramedics after reporting severe dyspnea and shortness of breath. He has been experiencing coldlike symptoms for the past 2 days. He has a productive cough with thick greenish sputum. When Mr. W awoke in the nursing home, it was found that he was having difficulty breathing even after using his albuterol (Proventil) metered-dose inhaler (MDI). He appears very anxious and is in respiratory distress. His history includes chronic obstructive pulmonary disease (COPD) related to smoking 2 packs of cigarettes per day since he was 15 years old. Mr. W has been incontinent of urine and stool for the past 2 years.

In the emergency department, the Mr. W undergoes chest radiography, and admission laboratory tests are performed, including electrolyte levels and a complete blood count. A sputum sample is sent to the laboratory for culture and sensitivity testing and Gram staining.

Mr. W's vital sign values are as follows:

Blood pressure	154/92 mm Hg
Heart rate	118 beats/min
O_2 saturation	88% on 1 L/min oxygen by nasal cannula
Respiratory rate	38 breaths/min
Temperature	100.9° F (38.3° C) (oral)

1. What is the priority nursing diagnosis for this patient?
   1. Decreased Cardiac Output
   2. Ineffective Airway Clearance
   3. Risk for Electrolyte Imbalance
   4. Anxiety

2. The health care provider's orders for this patient include all of the following. Which intervention should you complete first?
   1. Send an arterial blood gas sample to the laboratory.
   2. Schedule pulmonary function tests.
   3. Repeat chest radiography each morning.
   4. Administer albuterol via MDI 2 puffs every 4 hours.

Mr. W's arterial blood gas results include the following: pH, 7.37; arterial partial pressure of carbon dioxide ($PaCO_2$), 55.4 mm Hg; arterial partial pressure of oxygen (PaO_2), 51.2 mm Hg; bicarbonate (HCO_3^-) level, 38 mEq/L.

3. What is your interpretation of these results?
   1. Compensated metabolic acidosis with hypoxemia
   2. Compensated metabolic alkalosis with hypoxemia
   3. Compensated respiratory acidosis with hypoxemia
   4. Compensated respiratory alkalosis with hypoxemia

4. Based on the patient's arterial blood gas results, what are your priority actions at this time? *(Select all that apply.)*
   1. Administer oxygen at 2 L/min via nasal cannula.
   2. Initiate a rapid response.
   3. Teach the patient how to cough and deep breathe.
   4. Begin IV normal saline at 100 mL/hr.
   5. Arrange a transfer to the intensive care unit (ICU).
   6. Remind the patient to practice incentive spirometry every hour while awake.

5. Which intervention would you assign to an experienced LPN/LVN?
   1. Drawing a sample for arterial blood gas determination
   2. Administering albuterol by hand-held nebulizer
   3. Measuring vital signs every 2 hours
   4. Increasing oxygen delivery to 2 L/min via nasal cannula

6. Which interventions could you delegate to the new UAP? *(Select all that apply.)*
   1. Helping the patient get up to use the bedside commode
   2. Performing pulse oximetry every shift
   3. Teaching the patient to cough and deep breathe
   4. Reminding the patient to use incentive spirometry every hour while awake
   5. Assessing the patient's breath sounds every shift
   6. Encouraging the patient to drink adequate oral fluids

7. During morning rounds, you note all of these assessment findings. Which finding indicates a worsening of the patient's condition?
   1. Barrel-shaped chest
   2. Clubbed fingers on both hands
   3. Crackles bilaterally
   4. Frequent productive cough

8. You report your morning assessment findings (see question 7) to the health care provider. Which order is most directly related to your findings?
   1. Administer furosemide (Lasix) 20 mg IV push now.
   2. Keep accurate records of intake and output.
   3. Administer potassium 20 mEq orally every morning.
   4. Weigh the patient every morning.

9. Which assessment finding would you instruct the UAP to report immediately?
   1. Incontinence of urine and stool
   2. 1-lb weight loss since admission
   3. Increased temperature elevation
   4. Eating only half of breakfast and lunch

10. The UAP takes morning vital signs and immediately reports the following values to the nurse. Which takes priority when notifying the health care provider?
    1. Heart rate of 96 beats/min
    2. Blood pressure of 160/90 mm Hg
    3. Respiratory rate of 34 breaths/min
    4. Oral temperature of 103.5° F (39.7° C)

11. An LPN/LVN tells you that the patient is now receiving oxygen at 2 L/min via nasal cannula and his pulse oximetry reading is now 91%. What intervention should you assign to the LPN/LVN?
    1. Begin creating a plan for discharging the patient.
    2. Administer furosemide 20 mg orally each morning.
    3. Get a baseline weight for the patient now.
    4. Administer cefotaxime (Claforan) IV piggyback every 6 hours.

12. You observe the patient's use of the albuterol MDI. The patient takes 2 puffs from the inhaler in rapid succession. Which intervention takes priority at this time?
    1. Call the pharmacy to request a spacer for the patient.
    2. Notify the provider that the patient will need to continue receiving nebulizer treatments.
    3. Ask the UAP to help get the patient into a chair.
    4. Instruct the patient about proper techniques for using an MDI inhaler.

13. Mr. W has lost 15 pounds over the past year. On assessment, he tells you that his appetite is not what it used to be and he becomes short of breath while eating. Which interventions should be included in his nursing care plan? *(Select all that apply.)*
    1. Initiate a dietary consult.
    2. Stress that he must eat all of his meals or he'll become malnourished.
    3. Monitor serum prealbumin levels.
    4. Suggest 4 to 6 small meals per day.
    5. Instruct the patient to use his bronchodilator 30 minutes before meals.
    6. Encourage dry foods to avoid coughing.

14. The UAP tells you that Mr. W is unable to complete his AM care without assistance and wonders if he is being lazy. What is your best response?
    1. "Encourage the patient to do as much as he can, as quickly as he can."
    2. "If the patient is short of breath, increase his oxygen flow."
    3. "Tell the patient to take his time and not to rush his morning care."
    4. "He may not need as much help as he is asking for, so try to get him to do more."

Answer Key for this case study begins on p. 210.

Multiple Clients on a Medical-Surgical Unit

You are the leader of a team providing care for six clients. Your team includes yourself (an RN), an LPN/LVN, and a newly hired UAP who is undergoing orientation to the unit. The clients are as follows:

- *Mr. C, a 68-year-old with unstable angina who needs teaching for a cardiac catheterization scheduled this morning*
- *Ms. J, a 45-year-old experiencing chest pain scheduled for a graded exercise test later today*
- *Mr. R, a 75-year-old who had a left-hemisphere stroke 4 days ago*
- *Ms. S, an 83-year-old with heart disease, a history of myocardial infarction, and mild dementia*
- *Ms. B, a 93-year-old newly admitted from a long-term care facility, with decreased urine output, altered level of consciousness, and an elevated temperature of 99.5° F (37.5° C)*
- *Mr. L, a 59-year-old with mild shortness of breath and chronic emphysema*

1. For which clients should you assign the LPN/LVN to perform nursing care tasks, under your supervision? *(Select all that apply.)*
   1. Mr. C
   2. Ms. J
   3. Mr. R
   4. Ms. S
   5. Ms. B
   6. Mr. L

2. Which client should you assess first?
   1. Mr. C
   2. Ms. J
   3. Ms. B
   4. Mr. L

3. Which key point would you be sure to include when teaching the client about the postprocedure care after cardiac catheterization?
   1. "There are no restrictions after the procedure."
   2. "We will get you out of bed within 2 hours after the procedure."
   3. "You will have to stay almost flat in bed with limited position changes for 4 to 6 hours."
   4. "Family visitors will be restricted until the next day."

4. The health care provider's orders for Ms. J, who is currently experiencing chest pain, are as follows. List the orders in the sequence in which they should be completed. *(Answers may be used more than once.)*
   1. Obtain a 12-lead electrocardiogram (ECG) when the client experiences chest pain.
   2. Administer nitroglycerin (Nitrostat) 0.6 mg sublingually every 5 minutes as needed for chest pain.
   3. Administer morphine 2 mg IV push as needed for chest pain.
   4. Monitor blood pressure and heart rate.
   5. Place on a telemetry monitor. _____, _____, _____, _____, _____, _____, _____, _____, _____, _____

5. Which task should you delegate to the newly-hired UAP?
   1. Asking Ms. S memory-testing questions
   2. Teaching Ms. J about treadmill exercise testing
   3. Performing pulse oximetry for Mr. L
   4. Monitoring urine output for Ms. B

6. The UAP is delegated the task of measuring morning vital signs for all six clients. What would you instruct the UAP to report immediately?
   1. Oral temperature higher than 102° F (38.9° C)
   2. Blood pressure higher than 140/80 mm Hg
   3. Heart rate lower than 65 beats/min
   4. Respiratory rate lower than 18 breaths/min

7. The UAP asks you why it is important to notify someone whenever a client with heart disease reports chest pain. What is your best response?
   1. "It's important to keep track of the chest pain episodes so we can notify the health care provider."
   2. "The client may need morphine to treat the chest pain."
   3. "Chest pain may indicate coronary artery blockage and heart muscle damage that will need treatment."
   4. "Our unit policy includes specific steps to take in the treatment of clients with chest pain."

8. The health care provider's orders for Mr. R, who had a stroke 4 days ago, include assisting the client with meals. Which person should be assigned to this task?
   1. Physical therapist
   2. UAP
   3. LPN/LVN
   4. Occupational therapist

9. The UAP tells you that Mr. L, the client with chronic emphysema, says he is feeling short of breath after walking to the bathroom. What action should you take first?
   1. Notify the health care provider.
   2. Increase oxygen flow to 4 L/min via nasal cannula.
   3. Assess oxygen saturation by pulse oximetry.
   4. Remind the client to cough and deep breathe.

10. The oral temperature of Ms. B, the client newly admitted from a long-term care facility with decreased urine output and altered level of consciousness, is now 102.6° F (39.2° C). What is your best action?
   1. Notify the health care provider.
   2. Administer acetaminophen (Tylenol) 2 tablets orally.
   3. Ask the LPN/LVN to give an acetaminophen suppository.
   4. Remove extra blankets from the client's bed.

11. Which factor most likely precipitated Ms. B's elevated temperature?
   1. Bladder infection
   2. Increased metabolic rate
   3. Kidney failure
   4. Nosocomial pneumonia

12. You are working on a nursing care plan for Ms. B. Which nursing intervention is most appropriate to delegate to the UAP?
   1. Checking the client's level of consciousness every shift
   2. Assisting the client with ambulation to the bathroom to urinate
   3. Teaching the client the side effects of antibiotic therapy
   4. Administering sulfamethoxazole/trimethoprim (Bactrim) orally every 12 hours

13. The UAP reports that Mr. L's heart rate, which was 86 beats/min in the morning, is now 98 beats/min. What would be the most appropriate question for the nurse to ask Mr. L?
   1. "Have you just returned from the bathroom?"
   2. "Did you recently use your albuterol inhaler?"
   3. "Are you feeling short of breath?"
   4. "How much do you smoke?"

14. The LPN/LVN reports that Ms. S will not leave the chest leads for her cardiac monitor in place and asks if the client can be restrained. What is your best response?
   1. "Yes, this client had a heart attack and we must keep her on the cardiac monitor."
   2. "Yes, but be sure to use soft restraints so that the client's circulation is not compromised."
   3. "No, we must have a physician's order before we can apply restraints in any situation."
   4. "No, but try covering the lead wires with the sheet so that the client does not see them."

15. Close to the end of the shift, the LPN/LVN reports that the UAP has not totaled clients' intake and output for the past 8 hours. What is your best action?
   1. Confront the UAP and instruct her to complete this assignment at once.
   2. Delegate this task to the LPN/LVN.
   3. Ask the UAP if she needs assistance completing the intake and output records.
   4. Notify the nurse manager to include this on the UAP's evaluation.

16. The "Five Rights" guide delegation of nursing care tasks. As the team leader, list the Five Rights.

   _____
   _____
   _____
   _____
   _____

Answer Key for this case study begins on p. 211.

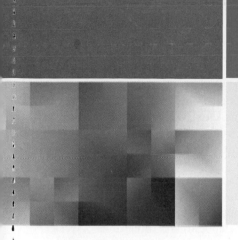

Shortness of Breath, Edema, and Decreased Urine Output

Ms. J is a 63-year-old woman who is admitted directly to the medical unit after visiting her health care provider because of shortness of breath and increased swelling in her ankles and calves. She is being admitted to rule out a diagnosis of chronic kidney disease (CKD). Ms. J states that her symptoms have become worse over the past 2 to 3 months and that she uses the bathroom less often and urinates in smaller amounts. Her medical history includes hypertension (30 years), coronary artery disease (18 years), and type 2 diabetes (14 years).

Ms. J's vital sign values on admission were as follows:

Blood pressure	*162/96 mm Hg*
Heart rate	*88 beats/min*
O₂ saturation	*91% on room air*
Respiratory rate	*28 breaths/min*
Temperature	*97.8° F (36.6° C)*

Admission laboratory tests for which patient samples are to be collected on the unit include serum electrolyte levels, kidney function tests, complete blood count, and urinalysis. A 24-hour urine collection for determination of creatinine clearance has also been ordered.

1. During admission assessment, Ms. J has all of these findings. For which finding should you notify the health care provider immediately?
   1. Bilateral pitting ankle and calf edema rated 2+
   2. Crackles in both lower and middle lobes
   3. Dry and peeling skin on both feet
   4. Faint but palpable pedal and post-tibial pulses

2. Which task associated with 24-hour urine collection is appropriate to delegate to the UAP?
   1. Instructing Ms. J to collect all urine with each voiding
   2. Teaching Ms. J the purpose of collecting urine for 24 hours
   3. Ensuring that all urine obtained for the test is kept on ice
   4. Assessing Ms. J's urine for color, odor, and sediment

3. You review Ms. J's laboratory results. Which laboratory finding is of most concern?
   1. Serum potassium level of 7.1 mmol/L
   2. Serum creatinine level of 15 mg/dL
   3. Blood urea nitrogen level of 180 mg/dL
   4. Serum calcium level of 7.8 mg/dL

4. Which medication should you be prepared to administer to lower the patient's potassium level?
   1. Furosemide (Lasix) 40 mg IV push
   2. Epoetin alfa (Epogen), 300 units/kg subcutaneously
   3. Calcium, 1 tablet by mouth (PO)
   4. Sodium polystyrene sulfonate (Kayexalate), 15 g PO

5. You are the team leader supervising an LPN/LVN. Which nursing care action for Ms. J should you delegate to the LPN/LVN?
   1. Inserting a catheter intermittently to assess for residual urine
   2. Planning restricted fluid amounts to be given with meals
   3. Assessing breath sounds and noting increased presence of crackles
   4. Discussing renal replacement therapies with the patient

6. As team leader, you observe the UAP perform all of these actions for Ms. J. For which action must you intervene?
   1. Assisting her to replace the oxygen nasal cannula
   2. Measuring vital signs after the patient drinks fluids
   3. Ambulating with the patient to the bathroom and back
   4. Washing her back, legs, and feet with warm water

7. Ms. J's nursing care plan includes the nursing diagnosis Excess Fluid Volume. What interventions are appropriate for this nursing diagnosis? *(Select all that apply.)*
   1. Measure weight daily.
   2. Review daily intake and output.
   3. Restrict sodium intake with meals.
   4. Restrict fluid to 1500 mL plus urine output.
   5. Assess for crackles and edema every shift.

8. After discussing renal replacement therapies with the health care provider and nurse, Ms. J is considering hemodialysis (HD). Which statement indicates that Ms. J needs additional teaching about HD?
   1. "I will need surgery to create an access route for HD."
   2. "I will be able to eat and drink what I want once I start dialysis."
   3. "I will have a temporary dialysis catheter for a few months."
   4. "I will be having dialysis three times every week."

9. You are supervising a new nurse on orientation to the unit who is providing care for Ms. J after her return from surgery to create a left forearm access for dialysis. Which action by the nurse requires that you intervene?
   1. Monitoring the patient's operative site dressing for evidence of bleeding
   2. Obtaining a blood pressure reading by placing the cuff on the right arm
   3. Drawing blood for laboratory studies from the temporary dialysis line
   4. Administering oxycodone (Roxicodone) PO for moderate postoperative pain

10. Assessment of Ms. J after dialysis reveals all of these findings. Which assessment finding necessitates immediate action?
    1. Weight decrease of 4.5 lb
    2. Systolic blood pressure decrease of 14 mm Hg
    3. Decreased level of consciousness
    4. Small blood spot near the center of the dressing

11. Six months later, Ms. J is readmitted to the unit. She has just returned from HD. Which nursing care action should you delegate to the UAP?
    1. Measuring vital signs and postdialysis weight
    2. Assessing the HD access site for bruit and thrill
    3. Checking the access site dressing for bleeding
    4. Instructing the patient to request assistance getting out of bed

12. Ms. J is preparing for discharge. You are supervising a student nurse, who is teaching the patient about her discharge medications. For which statement by the student nurse will you intervene?
    1. "Sevelamer prevents your body from absorbing phosphorus."
    2. "Take your folic acid after dialysis on dialysis days."
    3. "The docusate is to prevent constipation that may be caused by ferrous sulfate."
    4. "You must take the epoetin alfa three times a week by mouth to treat anemia."

Ms. J is admitted for a kidney transplantation 6 months later. Her son is the kidney donor.

13. You are caring for Ms. J 1 day postoperatively. On assessment, her temperature is 100.4° F (38° C), her blood pressure is 168/92 mm Hg, and the patient tells you she has pain around the transplant site. What is the best interpretation of these findings?
    1. Hyperacute rejection
    2. Acute rejection
    3. Chronic rejection
    4. Transplant site infection

14. What intervention is required at this time?
    1. Increased doses of immunosuppressive drugs
    2. IV antibiotics
    3. Conservative management including dialysis
    4. Immediate removal of the transplanted kidney

Answer Key for this case study begins on p. 212.

Complex Health Scenarios — PART 3

CASE STUDY 5

Diabetic Ketoacidosis

Mr. D, a 19-year-old college student, has been brought to the emergency department (ED) by his roommate. He reports abdominal pain, polyuria for the past 2 days, vomiting several times before arrival, and thirst. He appears flushed, and his lips and mucous membranes are dry and cracked. His skin turgor is poor. He has deep, rapid respirations, and there is a fruity odor to his breath. He has type 1 diabetes and "may have skipped a few doses of insulin because of cramming for finals." He is alert and conversant but is having trouble focusing on your questions.

Mr. D's vital sign and glucose values are as follows:

Blood glucose level (fingerstick)	685 mg/dL
Blood pressure	100/60 mm Hg
Heart rate	120 beats/min
Respiratory rate	32 breaths/min
Temperature	100.8° F (38.2° C)

1. To clarify pertinent data, what questions are appropriate to ask Mr. D? *(Select all that apply.)*
   1. "When did your symptoms start?"
   2. "How many times have you vomited?"
   3. "What was your last blood sugar reading?"
   4. "Why didn't you go to see your physician?"
   5. "Where does your abdomen hurt?"
   6. "Did you take any insulin today?"
   7. "Do you have any allergies?"

2. You have completed the triage assessment and history taking. Now, what is your priority action?
   1. Page the ED physician to come immediately to triage.
   2. Call the client's parents for permission to treat.
   3. Notify the client's primary care physician.
   4. Take the client immediately to a treatment room.

3. What is the priority nursing diagnosis for Mr. D?
   1. Ineffective Breathing Pattern related to acidosis
   2. Anxiety related to the uncertainty of the outcome
   3. Deficient Fluid Volume related to hyperglycemia
   4. Noncompliance related to medications and treatment plan

4. Which tasks are appropriate to assign to an experienced UAP? *(Select all that apply.)*
   1. Measuring and reporting Mr. D's vital signs every 15 minutes
   2. Checking and reporting Mr. D's blood glucose level
   3. Bagging and labeling Mr. D's belongings
   4. Updating the roommate regarding Mr. D's status
   5. Measuring and recording the volume of Mr. D's vomitus

5. In the initial emergency care for Mr. D, which orders would you question? *(Select all that apply.)*
   1. Start a peripheral IV line with a large-bore catheter.
   2. Insert a Foley catheter with a urinometer.
   3. Administer regular insulin subcutaneously.
   4. Maintain the client in a semi-Fowler position.
   5. Initiate continuous electrocardiographic (ECG) monitoring.
   6. Encourage intake of oral fluids as tolerated.

6. What do you anticipate the physician will order for initial fluid replacement?
   1. Normal saline (0.9% sodium chloride)
   2. Half-strength saline (0.45% sodium chloride)
   3. Dextrose 5% in water and half-strength saline
   4. Normal saline with potassium chloride

7. You are reviewing the potassium values that were obtained when Mr. D first arrived in the ED. Which serum potassium level would concern you the most?
   1. 3.5 mEq/L
   2. 2.0 mEq/L
   3. 5.8 mEq/L
   4. 6.0 mEq/L

8. An insulin infusion is ordered for Mr. D to begin at 0.1 units/kg/hr. Mr. D weighs 155 lb. The pharmacy delivers a premixed bag of 100 units of regular insulin in 100 mL of normal saline. Another nurse has calculated the infusion pump setting as 10 mL/hr. What will you do next?
   1. Tell the nurse to obtain a pump and start the infusion as calculated.
   2. Advise the nurse to recalculate the infusion rate.
   3. Call the physician and ask for the exact pump setting to be clarified.
   4. Allow the nurse to independently administer the infusion using her own best judgment.

9. Mr. D says to you, "Please don't call my mother. If she knows I'm in the hospital, she'll make me quit school and move back home. I know I messed up, but I really don't want to move back in with my parents." What is the best therapeutic communication response?
   1. "None of the staff will say anything, but you should tell her yourself."
   2. "Your mom loves you, and she is just concerned about your well-being."
   3. "It sounds like you want to be independent and responsible for yourself."
   4. "You are an adult and you have a right to make your own decisions."

10. You overhear one of the UAPs talking to someone on the phone. The UAP says, "Yes, Mr. D is doing much better than when he first got here. I will tell him that you called and I will give him your message." What will you do first?
    1. Ask the UAP about the phone conversation that you just overheard.
    2. Remind the UAP that release of information is outside her scope of practice.
    3. Report the UAP to the nurse manager for a HIPAA violation.
    4. Give positive feedback for trying to help the client and the caller.

11. You are reviewing the intensive care unit (ICU) admission orders. There is an order for an IV potassium infusion. Related specifically to the order for potassium, which information would the ICU nurse be most interested in knowing?
    1. Mental status has improved with therapy.
    2. Urinary output is 60 mL/hr and urine is a clear yellow color.
    3. Blood pressure was 100/60 mm Hg on admission and is now 125/76 mm Hg.
    4. One IV site showed infiltration, but the current IV line flushes easily.

12. You are trying to call a report to the ICU but are told, "We were not notified about the admission." You call the admitting clerk, but she says, "I was never notified." You ask the unit secretary and he tells you, "I forgot to do it." What should you do first?
    1. Report the unit secretary to the manager.
    2. Ask the secretary to call the admissions office now.
    3. Take the secretary aside and allow him to explain his actions.
    4. Ask the ICU to take the report regardless of the clerical omission.

13. You are preparing to transfer Mr. D to the ICU, and you observe the cardiac monitor pattern. Which finding is of greatest concern?
    1. P wave precedes every QRS complex.
    2. Ventricular dysrhythmias are occurring.
    3. QRS complexes are occurring more frequently.
    4. The isoelectric line shows an artifact.

14. In caring for Mr. D, you are vigilant for signs and symptoms of hypokalemia. What are you watching for? (Select all that apply.)
    1. Fatigue
    2. Seizure activity
    3. Hallucinations
    4. Muscle weakness
    5. Hypotension
    6. Weak pulse
    7. Shallow respirations
    8. Cold, clammy skin

15. Which tasks can you delegate to an experienced UAP to facilitate Mr. D's transfer to the ICU? (Select all that apply.)
    1. Giving Mr. D's roommate directions to the ICU waiting room
    2. Independently transporting Mr. D to the ICU
    3. Collecting and organizing the chart and laboratory reports
    4. Obtaining a portable oxygen tank and cardiac monitor
    5. Connecting Mr. D's ECG leads to the portable cardiac monitor
    6. Obtaining the last set of vital sign values

Answer Key for this case study begins on p. 213.

CASE STUDY 6
Home Health

You are working as a staff nurse for the home health division of a public health agency. You arrive for the day with plans to make home visits to six patients:

Ms. A
Diagnosis: Chronic obstructive pulmonary disease (COPD)
Data:
- *Called reporting increased dyspnea*
- *Has been increasing home oxygen flow rate*

Mr. D
Diagnoses: Diabetic, Chronic leg infection
Data:
- *Needs weekly assessment of leg infection*
- *Daily home health aide visits*

Ms. F
Diagnosis: Chronic kidney disease with peritoneal dialysis
Data:
- *Daughter assists patient with dialysis*

Mr. I
Diagnosis: Lung cancer
Data:
- *Last chemotherapy 1 week ago*
- *Needs to have blood drawn today at nadir for complete blood count (CBC) with differential*

Ms. R
Diagnosis: Acute myocardial infarction (MI) with percutaneous coronary intervention
Data:
- *Hospital discharge yesterday*
- *Needs home health admission assessment*

Mr. W
Diagnosis: Schizophrenia
Data:
- *Receives risperidone (Risperdal) injection every 4 weeks*
- *Risperidone dose scheduled today*

1. Soon after you arrive, your manager tells you about a required case management in-service training session today at 2:00 PM. You realize that you will only have time to make four visits before the in-service session. Which four patients will you schedule to see today?
   1. Ms. A
   2. Mr. D
   3. Ms. F
   4. Mr. I
   5. Ms. R
   6. Mr. W

2. You have adjusted your schedule to visit the following four patients today. Which patient will you see first?
   1. Ms. A, the patient who has COPD and increased shortness of breath
   2. Mr. I, the patient receiving chemotherapy who will need blood drawn
   3. Ms. R, the patient with a recent MI who will need an initial assessment
   4. Mr. W, the patient with schizophrenia who will need a risperidone injection

3. You call the four patients to confirm the visits and schedule times. All goes well until you call Ms. R to schedule a visit. She says that she doesn't have much time today but will be available for longer tomorrow. What is the best response?
   1. "The visit will not take very long, so I will plan on seeing you today."
   2. "I have rescheduled other patients because it is essential that I assess you today."
   3. "Perhaps you are feeling that you do not really need any help at home."
   4. "Because of your recent heart attack, I would like to visit as soon as possible."

After obtaining Ms. R's consent for a visit later today, you head off to see Ms. A. Her husband answers the door and tells you that Ms. A is resting so comfortably that he does not want you to disturb her. He explains, "She has been so short of breath lately that this is the best sleep she has had in a while."

You talk him into allowing you to assess Ms. A and find that she is very difficult to awaken. She tries to respond to your questions, but her speech is so slurred that you are unable to understand her. The flow meter on her home oxygen unit is set at 6 L/min.

4. Which nursing action is most appropriate next?
   1. Auscultate Ms. A's anterior and posterior lung sounds.
   2. Check Ms. A's oxygen saturation using pulse oximetry.
   3. Continue to stimulate Ms. A until she can respond to you.
   4. Notify the health care provider (HCP) about Ms. A's change in status.

5. You obtain an oxygen saturation of 99% with the pulse oximeter. Which action is appropriate now?
   1. Discontinue the patient's oxygen.
   2. Draw a sample for arterial blood gas analysis.
   3. Call the HCP and obtain an order to transport Ms. A to the hospital.
   4. Remind the patient's husband about the reasons for using oxygen at low flow rates.

When you call the HCP to discuss Ms. A's status and your actions, you receive an order to have her admitted to the hospital medical unit for further evaluation.

After calling a brief report to the charge nurse on the hospital medical unit, you leave to make the scheduled visit to Ms. R. On the way, you receive a phone call from Mr. D's home health aide. Mr. D is reporting generalized aches and pains. In addition, his morning blood glucose level was 306 mg/dL, and he has a temperature of 100.1° F (37.8° C).

6. You realize that Mr. D will require an assessment today and that you need to reschedule one of your planned patient visits. Which one of the three patients that you were planning to visit today is best to reschedule for tomorrow?
   1. Mr. I
   2. Ms. R
   3. Mr. W

7. After rescheduling your patient, you arrive at Ms. R's home as arranged, and she greets you at the door. Her respiratory effort seems a little labored, and she looks anxious. After you introduce yourself to Ms. R, you ask her how she has been feeling since her discharge from the hospital yesterday. Which response indicates a need for immediate intervention?
   1. "I have been a bit short of breath."
   2. "I feel a slight chest pressure."
   3. "I don't understand why I need to take all these pills."
   4. "I am confused about why you are here to see me."

8. Five minutes after taking a nitroglycerin (Nitrostat) sublingual tablet, Ms. R tells you that the chest pressure is "almost gone." Which action should you take next?
   1. Proceed with assessing her and completing the admission documentation.
   2. Have her rest for another 5 minutes and then reassess the chest pressure.
   3. Check her blood pressure and administer another nitroglycerin tablet.
   4. Call the HCP, anticipating an order to readmit her to the hospital.

After taking a second nitroglycerin tablet, Ms. R says that the chest pressure is completely gone, and you proceed to obtain a health history and perform an admission assessment. She lives alone, but her daughter visits her about twice a week. Her daughter arrives while you are assessing Ms. R and stays for the rest of the visit. The house is cluttered, and Ms. R's hair is uncombed. She says she is too tired to get in and out of the bathtub, so she tried to clean up at the bathroom sink today.

You find that Ms. R has crackles at the bases of both lungs and 2+ pedal edema. She has felt the chest pressure twice since her discharge yesterday, but says, "I just waited and it went away after an hour or so." She has not been taking her prescribed medications, because "I can't remember which ones I have taken and I don't want to take an overdose." She has many questions about her medications. Her medications include:

- *Nitroglycerin (Nitrostat) 0.4 mg sublingually as needed for chest pain*
- *Transdermal nitroglycerin (Nitro-Dur) 0.2 mg/hr every morning*
- *Metoprolol (Toprol-XL) 25 mg by mouth (PO) daily*
- *Clopidogrel (Plavix) 75 mg PO daily*
- *Aspirin (Ecotrin) 81 mg PO daily*
- *Enalapril (Vasotec) 2.5 mg PO daily*

9. Based on the information you have obtained, you develop a care plan. Which nursing activities will you delegate to a home health aide? *(Select all that apply.)*
   1. Setting up Ms. R's medications in a multidose pill box twice a week
   2. Instructing the daughter how to set up Ms. R's daily medications
   3. Teaching Ms. R and her daughter the purpose of each medication
   4. Assisting Ms. R with a bath and personal hygiene every day
   5. Measuring vital signs daily
   6. Weighing the patient daily
   7. Auscultating lung and heart sounds weekly
   8. Checking for any peripheral edema weekly

You assist Ms. R with taking her scheduled medications for today and remind the patient and her daughter to use the nitroglycerin tablets if Ms. R develops any more chest pressure or pain. The daughter says she will stay with Ms. R for the rest of the day. You instruct the patient and her daughter that Ms. R should go to the emergency department (ED) if she develops more dyspnea or has chest pressure or pain that is unrelieved by nitroglycerin.

10. When will you schedule the next home visit with Ms. R?
    1. Later today, because Ms. R's condition is very unstable and she may require hospital readmission
    2. Tomorrow, because Ms. R's assessment indicates that she needs frequent evaluation and/or interventions
    3. In 3 days, because the home health aide will see Ms. R every day and will call you if there are any further problems
    4. Early next week, so that there will be enough time to evaluate the effect of the medications on Ms. R's symptoms

11. You still have visits to make to Mr. D and Mr. I before the mandatory in-service session. Which patient will you visit first?
    1. Mr. D
    2. Mr. I

While driving to your next home visit, you receive a telephone call from your nurse manager. The manager tells you about a newly referred 70-year-old patient with emphysema who will need an initial visit today to evaluate the need for home oxygen therapy.

12. Since you will not have time today to visit a new patient, which of your colleagues will you suggest as the best staff member to assign to make the home visit?
    1. An experienced and knowledgeable LPN/LVN who has worked for 10 years in home health
    2. A respiratory therapist who regularly works with patients who are receiving home oxygen therapy
    3. An RN who usually works in the maternal-child division of the public health agency
    4. An on-call RN who works in the home health agency for a few days each month on an as-needed basis

13. When you arrive at Mr. I's condominium, his wife answers the door and tells you that Mr. I is very lethargic and a little confused today. Usually he is well oriented and cheerful, in spite of his diagnosis of right-sided lung cancer. Which information noted during your assessment is the best indicator that rapid nursing action is needed?
    1. Breath sounds are decreased on the right posterior chest.
    2. Mr. I says that his appetite has not been very good recently.
    3. Mr. I's oral temperature is 101° F (38.3° C).
    4. The oral mucosa is pale and dry.

14. You call the oncologist to discuss Mr. I's condition and obtain an order to call an ambulance to transport him to the hospital ED for evaluation. Which information is most important to communicate when you call a report to the ED?
    1. Mr. I has lung cancer and decreased breath sounds.
    2. Mr. I's appetite and oral intake are decreased.
    3. Mr. I has an order for a CBC blood sample to be drawn today.
    4. Mr. I is receiving chemotherapy and has a fever.

It is 12:30 PM, and you are on your way to make your final visit of the day to Mr. D. You check your laptop for the patient data that the home health aide has entered into the electronic record for this week:

Day	Temperature	Heart Rate (beats/min)	Respiratory Rate (breaths/min)	Blood Pressure (mm Hg)	Weight (kg)	Capillary Blood Glucose Level (mg/dL)
Monday	98° F (36.7° C)	78	22	152/72	77	142
Tuesday	97.9° F (36.6° C)	82	20	140/66		140
Wednesday	99.5° F (37.5° C)	74	18	138/72	77.2	256
Thursday	100.5° F (38° C)	76	22	144/80		300
Friday	101.2° F (38.4° C)	88	24	146/78	77.5	326

15. Which data in the table above are most important to report to the HCP? *(List all that apply.)*

_____

While you are assessing Mr. D, you change his left foot dressing and find that the wound on his left heel looks about the same as it did last week when you assessed it. It is dry appearing and pale pink, with no wound drainage.

You hear scattered coarse crackles and wheezes over the left posterior chest when you listen to his lung sounds. He says he feels short of breath with activity, but "my breathing is fine when I rest." He tells you that he has been coughing up some thick green mucus for the last few days. He has been voiding the usual amounts with no problems. He has been using his regular insulin with sliding-scale dosing as prescribed for his elevated blood glucose levels.

16. You call the HCP to report Mr. D's status and receive orders for these interventions. In which order will you implement the prescribed interventions?
   1. Give ciprofloxacin (Cipro) 500 mg orally now and instruct patient to take Cipro every 12 hours.
   2. Obtain blood specimens for culture from two separate sites.
   3. Check oxygen saturation level.
   4. Teach the patient about the use of antibiotics and to increase fluid intake to 2000 mL/day. _____,

   _____, _____, _____

You plan to visit Mr. D again early tomorrow and reassess his lung sounds, shortness of breath, temperature, blood pressure, oxygen saturation, and capillary blood glucose level. After discussing Mr. D's plan of care with him and with the home health aide, you head back to your agency, where the mandatory in-service topic is how to prioritize care in the home health setting.

Complex Health Scenarios   PART 3

Spinal Cord Injury

Mr. M is a 32-year-old man brought to the emergency department by paramedics after a fall from the second-story roof of his home. He was placed on a spinal board with a cervical collar to immobilize his spine. After spinal radiographs are obtained, the physicians determine that he has a vertebral compression injury at the C4–C5 level.

After Mr. M undergoes endotracheal intubation and is placed on mechanical ventilation, his oxygen saturation increases to 96% and respirations decrease to 18 breaths/min (10 ventilator breaths per minute). On auscultation, he has breath sounds present in all lung lobes bilaterally.

1. What is your priority concern at this time?
    1. Spinal immobilization to prevent additional injuries to the client
    2. Airway status due to interruption of spinal innervation to the respiratory muscles
    3. Potential for injuries related to the client's decreased sensation
    4. Dysrhythmias caused by disruption of the autonomic nervous system

2. Mr. M is stabilized and moved to the neurologic intensive care unit with a diagnosis of spinal cord injury (SCI) at level C4–C5. You are the admitting nurse, working with an experienced UAP. When frequent respiratory assessments are performed, which actions can you delegate to the UAP? *(Select all that apply.)*
    1. Auscultating breath sounds every hour to detect decreased or absent ventilation
    2. Ensuring that oxygen is flowing at 5 L/min via the nasal cannula
    3. Teaching the client to breathe slowly and deeply and use incentive spirometry
    4. Checking the client's oxygen saturation by pulse oximetry every 2 hours
    5. Assessing the client's chest wall movement during respirations

3. An hour later, Mr. M's oxygen saturation drops to 88%, and his respirations are rapid and shallow. On auscultation, he has decreased breath sounds bilaterally. What is your best action at this time?
    1. Increase the oxygen flow to 10 L/min.
    2. Suction the client's airway for oral secretions.
    3. Notify the health care provider immediately.
    4. Call the respiratory therapist for a nonrebreather mask.

4. The client's cervical injury has been immobilized with cervical tongs and traction to realign the vertebrae, facilitate bone healing, and prevent further injury. Which occurrence necessitates your immediate intervention?
    1. The traction weights are resting on the floor after the client is repositioned.
    2. The traction ropes are located within the pulley and are hanging freely.
    3. The insertion sites for the cervical tongs are cleaned with hydrogen peroxide.
    4. The client is repositioned every 2 hours by using the logrolling technique.

5. Mr. M has a nursing diagnosis of Impaired Physical Mobility. Which nursing actions should you delegate to the nursing student on the unit? *(Select all that apply.)*
    1. Administering intravenous ranitidine (Zantac) 50 mg in 50 mL normal saline to prevent gastric ulcers
    2. Monitoring traction ropes and weights while the client is repositioned
    3. Assessing the client's neurologic status for changes in movement and strength
    4. Providing pin site care using hydrogen peroxide and normal saline
    5. Initiating the nursing care plan for the client with SCI

6. Which action to prevent complications associated with Mr. M's nursing diagnosis of Impaired Physical Mobility should you delegate to the experienced UAP?
    1. Turning and repositioning the client in bed every 2 hours
    2. Inspecting the client's skin for reddened areas
    3. Performing range-of-motion exercises every 8 hours
    4. Administering enoxaparin (Lovenox) subcutaneously every 12 hours

7. The nursing student asks you how best to assess Mr. M's motor function. What is your best response?
   1. "Apply resistance while the client plantar flexes his feet."
   2. "Apply resistance while the client lifts his legs from the bed."
   3. "Apply downward pressure while the client shrugs his shoulders upward."
   4. "Make sure the client is able to grasp objects firmly and forms a fist."

8. Mr. M's condition has stabilized, and he has been removed from the ventilator. His cervical injury is now immobilized with a halo fixation device with jacket. He has regained the use of his arms and partial movement in his legs. Which instruction should you give the UAP providing help to Mr. M in activities of daily living?
   1. "Feed, bathe, and dress the client so that he does not become fatigued."
   2. "Encourage the client to perform all of his own self-care."
   3. "Allow the client to do what he can, and then assist with what he can't."
   4. "Let the client's wife do the bathing and dressing."

9. Mr. M continues to be incontinent. You plan to establish a bladder retraining program for him. Which actions are important points for this program? *(Select all that apply.)*
   1. Remove the indwelling Foley catheter.
   2. Use intermittent catheterization every 4 hours.
   3. Gradually increase intervals between catheterizations.
   4. Teach the patent to initiate voiding by tapping on his bladder every 4 hours.
   5. Teach the client to perform self-catheterization if necessary.
   6. Administer bethanechol chloride (Urecholine) 20 mg orally twice a day.
   7. Encourage the client to limit fluid intake to 1000 mL of fluid every day.

10. Mr. M is to be transferred to a rehabilitation facility. Which statement indicates that the client needs additional teaching?
    1. "After rehabilitation I may be able to achieve control of my bladder."
    2. "With rehabilitation I will regain all of my motor functions."
    3. "Rehabilitation will help me to become as independent as possible."
    4. "After rehabilitation I hope to return to gainful employment."

Answer Key for this case study begins on p. 216.

Multiple Patients with Adrenal Gland Disorders

Ms. B is admitted through the emergency department (ED) after being hit in the abdomen by an automobile. An 18-gauge IV catheter is inserted in the left forearm and normal saline is started at 100 mL/hr. The UAP reports that her blood pressure has dropped to 92/58 mm Hg and she is reporting weakness, fatigue, and abdominal pain. When you assess Ms. B, you also discover that she is nauseated and has just vomited 560 mL.

Laboratory values from the ED are as follows:

Aldosterone level	3 ng/dL (low)
Cortisol level	2 mcg/dL (low)
Potassium level	3.7 mEq/L
Sodium level	136 mEq/L

1. What is your first action?
   1. Administer an antiemetic.
   2. Measure abdominal girth.
   3. Notify the health care provider.
   4. Hang an IV bag of normal saline.

2. Ms. B's blood pressure is now 84/50 mm Hg. Which order from the health care provider would you implement first?
   1. Infuse normal saline at 250 mL/hr.
   2. Type and cross-match for 2 units of packed red blood cells.
   3. Insert a second large-bore IV catheter.
   4. Administer prednisone (Deltasone) 10 mg orally.

3. Which actions will you delegate to the UAP in providing care for Ms. B? *(Select all that apply.)*
   1. Encouraging the patient to take in adequate fluids
   2. Measuring vital signs every 15 minutes
   3. Recording intake and output accurately every hour
   4. Getting a baseline weight to guide therapy
   5. Administering oral antinausea medication

4. Ms. B develops diaphoresis, increased heart rate (124 beats/min), and tremors. She also reports an increasing headache. Which action should you take first?
   1. Check fingerstick glucose level.
   2. Check serum potassium level.
   3. Place the patient on a cardiac monitor.
   4. Decrease IV fluids to 100 mL/hr.

Ms. H is admitted to the medical-surgical unit for a workup for Cushing disease.

5. Which vital sign value reported by the UAP is of most concern for a patient with Cushing disease (hypercortisolism)?
   1. Heart rate of 102 beats/min
   2. Respiratory rate of 26 breaths/min
   3. Blood pressure of 156/88 mm Hg
   4. Oral temperature of 101.8° F (38.8° C)

6. Which factor reported by Ms. H supports the diagnosis of Cushing disease?
   1. Cessation of menses at age 33
   2. Increased craving for salty foods
   3. Weight loss of 25 lb
   4. Nausea, diarrhea, and loss of appetite

7. A nursing student will assess Ms. H. Which findings will you teach the student nurse to expect if a patient has Cushing disease? *(Select all that apply.)*
   1. Truncal obesity
   2. Weight loss
   3. Bruising
   4. Hypertension
   5. Thickened skin
   6. Dependent edema

Complex Health Scenarios

PART 3

8. Cushing disease is diagnosed in Ms. H because of increased secretion of adrenocorticotropic hormone (ACTH), and she is scheduled for an adrenalectomy. Which preoperative actions should the nurse delegate to the LPN/LVN? *(Select all that apply.)*
   1. Assessing the patient's cardiac rhythm
   2. Reviewing the patient's laboratory results
   3. Checking the patient's fingerstick glucose results
   4. Administering insulin on a sliding scale as needed
   5. Discussing goals and outcomes of care with the patient

9. A nursing diagnosis of Risk for Infection related to immunosuppression and inadequate primary defenses has been identified for Ms. H. Which nursing care actions should you delegate to the UAP? *(Select all that apply.)*
   1. Providing the patient with a soft toothbrush
   2. Instructing the patient to avoid activities that can result in skin trauma
   3. Reminding the patient to change positions in bed every 2 hours
   4. Assessing the patient's skin for reddened areas, excoriation, and edema
   5. Teaching the patient to avoid crowded areas and people with cold symptoms

10. Ms. H had a complete adrenalectomy, and you are preparing to educate her about cortisol replacement therapy. Which key points will you include in the teaching plan? *(Select all that apply.)*
    1. "Take your medication in divided doses, with the first dose in the morning and the second dose between 4 and 6 pm."
    2. "Take your medications on an empty stomach to facilitate absorption."
    3. "Weigh yourself daily using the same scale and wearing the same amount of clothes."
    4. "Never skip a dose of medication."
    5. "Call your doctor if you experience persistent nausea, severe diarrhea, or fever."
    6. "Report any rapid weight gain, round face, fluid retention, or swelling to your doctor."

Ms. L is a 59-year-old who is admitted after experiencing intermittent episodes of high blood pressure accompanied by headaches, diaphoresis, and chest pain. She tells the admitting nurse that she gets frightened and feels a "sense of doom" when these episodes occur. The endocrinologist has ordered hospitalization to rule out pheochromocytoma.

11. Which assessment actions should you avoid when admitting Ms. L?
    1. Palpating the patient's abdomen
    2. Checking the patient's extremity reflexes
    3. Testing the pupillary reaction to light
    4. Measuring baseline weight with the patient standing

12. The health care provider orders a 24-hour urine collection for vanillylmandelic acid (VMA), metanephrine, and catecholamine testing. Which instruction given to Ms. L by a nursing student would cause you to intervene?
    1. "You will be on a special diet for 2 to 3 days before the urine collection for this test."
    2. "You should not drink caffeinated beverages or eat citrus fruits, bananas, or chocolate."
    3. "You will take your usual medications, including the aspirin and the beta-blocker for your high blood pressure."
    4. "In 2 to 3 days you will begin the 24-hour urine collection after discarding the first void in the morning."

13. In providing nursing care for Ms. L, which action should you delegate to the UAP?
    1. Working with the patient to identify stressful situations that may lead to a hypertensive crisis
    2. Reminding the patient not to smoke, drink caffeinated beverages, or change positions suddenly
    3. Assessing the patient's hydration status and report manifestations of dehydration or fluid overload
    4. Telling the patient to limit activity and remain in a calm, restful environment during headaches

14. You are the charge nurse. Which patients would be appropriate to assign to a newly graduated nurse who has just completed orientation to the unit? *(Select all that apply.)*
    1. Ms. L with pheochromocytoma, who is scheduled for adrenalectomy and needs preoperative teaching
    2. Ms. B with adrenal gland hypofunction, whose blood pressure is dropping and who is experiencing addisonian crisis
    3. Ms. H with Cushing disease, who is very anxious and fearful about her scheduled adrenal surgery
    4. Mr. J with hyperaldosteronism, whose current serum potassium level is 3.2 mEq/L
    5. Mr. M with rule-out Addison disease, who is newly admitted with muscle weakness, weight loss, and hypotension

Answer Key for this case study begins on p. 217.

Multiple Clients with Gastrointestinal Problems

You are the leader of a team caring for clients with gastrointestinal (GI) disorders on a medical-surgical unit. In addition to yourself (an RN), the team includes a newly graduated RN who has recently completed hospital orientation, an experienced UAP, and a nursing student. At the beginning of the shift, there are six clients as follows:

- *Ms. H, a 36-year-old woman, has right upper quadrant pain that radiates to the right shoulder. She has a history of gallstones. She was admitted through the emergency department (ED) last night with acute cholecystitis. The night shift nurse reports, "She had a good night."*
- *Ms. D, a 60-year-old woman, was admitted with vomiting and pain in the midabdomen related to a bowel obstruction. She reports abdominal pain that has gradually improved since the insertion of a nasogastric (NG) tube. She is receiving IV fluids and is currently on "nothing by mouth" (NPO) status.*
- *Ms. T, a 29-year-old woman, appears wasted and malnourished. She has severe diarrhea and reports predefecation abdominal pain and generalized tenderness to palpation. She is receiving total parenteral nutrition (TPN) through a central line.*
- *Mr. A, a 26-year-old man, will be discharged in the afternoon. He had discharge teaching from the enterostomal therapist yesterday regarding his infected wound secondary to a ruptured appendix; he wants a review of the wound care instructions before he leaves.*
- *Mr. K, an 85-year-old man, is frail but alert and oriented × 2. He was transferred from an extended-care facility to receive a percutaneous endoscopic gastrostomy (PEG) tube that was placed 5 days ago. He has a large family. They ask a lot of questions and argue continuously among themselves and with the staff. His vital signs are stable.*
- *Mr. R, a 57-year-old man, has periumbilical pain. The pain is very severe, despite medication, and radiates to the back. Mr. R was admitted with acute pancreatitis. He is on NPO status and has an NG tube and IV line. He is belligerent and confused. White blood cell count (WBC) and blood glucose level are increased.*

1. The night shift nurse has just finished giving you a report on the six clients. Which client has the highest acuity level and is at greatest risk for shock during your shift?
   1. Ms. H
   2. Ms. D
   3. Ms. T
   4. Mr. A
   5. Mr. K
   6. Mr. R

2. Which clients would be best to assign to the new RN? *(Select all that apply.)*
   1. Ms. H
   2. Ms. D
   3. Ms. T
   4. Mr. A
   5. Mr. K
   6. Mr. R

3. Which tasks will you delegate to the UAP? *(Select all that apply.)*
   1. Assisting Ms. T with perineal care after diarrheal episodes
   2. Measuring vital signs every 2 hours for Mr. R
   3. Transporting Ms. H off the unit for a procedure
   4. Gently cleansing the nares around Ms. D's NG tube
   5. Removing Mr. A's dressing

4. Which reporting tasks are appropriate to delegate to the UAP? *(Select all that apply.)*
   1. Reporting on the condition of Ms. T's perineal area after application of ointment
   2. Reporting the quality and color of NG drainage for Ms. D
   3. Reporting whether Mr. R's blood pressure is below 100/60 mm Hg
   4. Reporting if any of the clients indicate pain
   5. Reporting if Mr. A is seen leaving the unit to smoke a cigarette

5. The night nurse gives a brief and incomplete report. Which question should you pose to the night shift nurse to help determine the priority actions for Ms. H?
   1. "What are her vital signs?"
   2. "Is she going to surgery or radiology this morning?"
   3. "Is she still having pain?"
   4. "Does she need any morning medications?"

6. Ms. H's physician told her that she would probably need a laparoscopic cholecystectomy; however, the hepatobiliary iminodiacetic acid scan and laboratory results are still pending. Ms. H asks, "What should I expect?" What is the best intervention at this point?
   1. Describe the surgical procedure.
   2. Call the physician to come and speak with her.
   3. Provide some written material about gallbladder disease and options.
   4. Explain general postoperative care, such as coughing and deep breathing exercises.

7. All of these clients must receive their routine morning medications. Which client should receive his or her medication last?
   1. Ms. H
   2. Ms. D
   3. Ms. T
   4. Mr. A
   5. Mr. K

8. You are observing the nursing student perform an abdominal assessment on Ms. D. For which actions will you intervene? *(Select all that apply.)*
   1. Palpating for abdominal distention with the index finger
   2. Auscultating for bowel sounds with the NG tube attached to low wall suction
   3. Performing the physical assessment before asking about pain
   4. Checking the NG collection canister for quantity and quality of drainage
   5. Inspecting for visible signs of peristaltic waves or abdominal distention
   6. Checking for skin turgor over the lower abdominal area

9. You are unable to locate Ms. D's morning vital signs. The new nurse who is assigned to the client says that she assumed that the UAP would take and record them. The UAP tells you that she thought that the nursing student was supposed to do that. The nursing student says that no one told her to take Ms. D's vital signs. What should you do first?
   1. Take Ms. D's vital signs yourself, reassess the client, and write an incident report.
   2. Talk to the nursing instructor and find out if the student was expected to take Ms. D's morning vital signs.
   3. Ask the UAP to take Ms. D's vitals now, record them, and report the values to the new nurse.
   4. Advise the new nurse to take Ms. D's vital signs herself and remind her that the nurse is ultimately responsible.

10. Ms. D reports feeling weak. She seems more confused compared with her baseline. You observe that the NG drainage container has a large amount of watery bile-colored fluid. Which laboratory values will you check first?
    1. Blood urea nitrogen and creatinine levels
    2. Platelet count and WBC count
    3. Sodium level, potassium level, and pH of blood
    4. Bilirubin level, hematocrit, and hemoglobin level

11. Ms. T is discouraged and dispirited about her ulcerative colitis. She is resistant to TPN because "I'm being kept alive with tubes." Which explanation will encourage Ms. T to continue with the TPN therapy?
    1. "It will help you regain your weight."
    2. "It will create a positive nitrogen balance."
    3. "Your physician has ordered this important therapy for you."
    4. "Your bowel can rest and the diarrhea will decrease."

12. Ms. T is receiving sulfasalazine (Azulfidine) 500 mg by mouth every 6 hours for treatment of ulcerative colitis. Which assessment finding concerns you the most?
    1. Urine discoloration
    2. Nausea and vomiting
    3. Decreased urine output
    4. Headache

13. The UAP asks, "Why can't Ms. T get out of bed and do things for herself? She's only 29." What is your best response?
    1. "The physician ordered bed rest for a few days."
    2. "Decreasing activity helps to decrease the diarrhea."
    3. "Acute exacerbations require decreased GI motility."
    4. "She is too depressed and malnourished."

14. Mr. A reluctantly discloses to you that his financial and social situations are problematic. Which aspect of his situation has the most impact on the discharge teaching on wound care and other follow-up issues?
    1. He is homeless and has no family in the city.
    2. He has no money for the prescribed medications.
    3. He has no transportation to the follow-up appointment.
    4. He cannot read or write very well.

15. While you are teaching Mr. A about dressing changes, he says, "When you live on the street, you can't do everything the way you nurses do in the hospital." What is the most important thing to emphasize in helping him to accomplish self-care?
    1. "Use new sterile gloves every time."
    2. "Maintain a sterile field for supplies."
    3. "Wash your hands before a dressing change."
    4. "Discard any opened packages of unused gauze."

16. You are teaching the nursing student about enteral feedings for clients such as Mr. K, who has a PEG tube. In the postoperative period, when can enteral feedings be started?
    1. Within 6 to 8 hours after the procedure
    2. When bowel sounds are present, usually within 24 hours
    3. When the client reports feeling hungry
    4. On a schedule determined by the pharmacy

17. Because of Mr. K's advanced age, which complications of enteral feedings may occur? *(Select all that apply.)*
    1. Hyperglycemia
    2. Hypotension
    3. Aspiration
    4. Diarrhea
    5. Fluid overload

18. During the shift, the following events happen at the same time. Indicate the order in which you will attend to these issues.
    1. Ms. H calls for an antiemetic after vomiting bile.
    2. Mr. A wants to know when he will be discharged.
    3. Mr. K's family wants to speak to the physician.
    4. Mr. R is walking down the hall, threatening to leave.

    _____, _____, _____, _____

19. You find the new RN in the bathroom crying. She tells you, "I'm a terrible nurse. I'm so disorganized and so far behind. I'm going to quit. I hate this job." What is the best thing to do?
    1. Send her on a break off the unit.
    2. Offer to take one of her clients.
    3. Ask the UAP to help her.
    4. Calm her down and help her prioritize.

20. What information regarding Mr. R, who has acute pancreatitis, is appropriate to report to the physician? *(Select all that apply.)*
    1. Hematocrit is decreased by more than 10%.
    2. Calcium level is less than 9 mg/dL.
    3. Partial oxygen pressure (P_{O_2}) is less than 60 mm Hg.
    4. Pain is unrelieved by medication.
    5. Blood type is O positive.

21. The physician has been paged and is en route to see Mr. R *with acute pancreatitis.* The client is increasingly agitated and confused. He pulls out his IV line and NG tube and removes the oxygen nasal cannula. His skin is pale and clammy. Pulse rate is 140 beats/min, and blood pressure is 140/60 mm Hg. List in order of priority the following steps in caring for Mr. R.
    1. Restart the IV line.
    2. Reinsert the NG tube.
    3. Stay with the client.
    4. Replace the nasal cannula for supplemental oxygen.
    5. Have a colleague gather equipment, including a pulse oximeter and nonrebreather mask.
    6. Check the blood glucose level.
    7. Continuously monitor vital signs.

    _____, _____, _____, _____, _____, _____, _____

22. The physician arrives while you are caring for Mr. R. Based on Mr. R's change of status (refer to questions 20 and 21), before the physician leaves, which order should you advocate for?
    1. Perform additional laboratory tests and continue monitoring.
    2. Prepare Mr. R for emergency surgery.
    3. Prepare Mr. R for transfer to the intensive care unit.
    4. Reestablish NG suction and apply restraints.

23. What tasks should be accomplished toward the end of the shift before leaving for the day? *(Select all that apply.)*
    1. Complete documentation on all assigned clients.
    2. Admit a new client from the ED.
    3. Check all IV sites and total IV fluids.
    4. Ask the UAP to obtain repeat vital sign values for all clients.
    5. Briefly check and assess every client.
    6. Thank ancillary staff for their help.
    7. Complete Mr. R's transfer to the intensive care unit.

PART 3 Complex Health Scenarios

Answer Key for this case study begins on p. 218.

Multiple Patients with Pain

You are the leader of a team caring for patients on a medical-surgical unit. Your team includes yourself (an RN), a newly-graduated RN who has recently completed hospital orientation, and a UAP. Your patients are as follows:

- Ms. R, a 55-year-old woman with rheumatoid arthritis, underwent shoulder arthroplasty 3 days ago. She reports morning stiffness in her joints. Swelling is noted in both wrists and proximal interphalangeal joints.

- Mr. L, a 35-year-old man with a history of kidney stones, reports severe back and right-sided flank pain intermittently (rating of 3 to 8 on a scale of 10). The night shift nurse reports episodic nausea and vomiting with hematuria and dysuria. Mr. L was admitted through the emergency department (ED) at 10:00 PM. He is using a patient-controlled analgesia (PCA) pump.

- Mr. O, an 18-year-old man, sustained a right tibia-fibula fracture in a motorcycle accident 7 hours ago. He has extensive skin abrasions underneath the cast and on the right anterolateral body. Although obvious chest and abdominal trauma were ruled out in the ED, he is being monitored for occult trauma. He is receiving an analgesic via PCA pump.

- Mr. H, a 28-year-old man, is currently in the operating room (OR) for an inguinal hernia repair. He should return from the OR later in the shift.

- Ms. J, a 65-year-old woman with end-stage multiple myeloma, is receiving palliative pain management. The family is considering hospice care. She has been on the unit for 2 weeks. Her physician signed the do-not-resuscitate order 3 days ago.

- Mr. A, a 55-year-old man, has been on the unit for 3 weeks. He is receiving IV antibiotics for bacterial pneumonia. He has a history of IV drug abuse and chronic back pain and has tested positive for human immunodeficiency virus (HIV) infection. Mr. A's oxygen saturation was decreasing during the night shift.

1. You decide to do a brief round of all the patients before shift report, to ensure safety and to help determine acuity and assignments. List the order in which you should briefly check in on these patients.
   1. Ms. R
   2. Mr. L
   3. Mr. O
   4. Mr. H
   5. Ms. J
   6. Mr. A

   _____, _____, _____, _____, _____, _____

2. Which of the six patients can be assigned to the new RN? (Select all that apply.)
   1. Ms. R
   2. Mr. L
   3. Mr. O
   4. Mr. H
   5. Ms. J
   6. Mr. A

3. You are talking to Ms. R (rheumatoid arthritis) about discharge plans and follow-up appointments. She begins to cry and says, "I was so active and athletic when I was younger." What is the most therapeutic response?
   1. "Your shoulder will get progressively better with time and patience. Don't cry."
   2. "I can see that you are really upset. Is your shoulder hurting a lot right now?"
   3. "I know what you mean. I used to be able to do a lot more when I was younger too."
   4. "It is difficult to deal with changes. What types of activities did you used to do?"

4. Which nonpharmacologic pain measure to help Ms. R relieve her early morning stiffness should be delegated to the UAP?
   1. Assisting Ms. R to get in a bathtub full of warm water
   2. Sharing some relaxation techniques with Ms. R
   3. Assisting Ms. R to take a warm shower
   4. Evaluating the effectiveness of paraffin therapy

5. The new nurse tells you that she cannot find any documentation that shows the time of Mr. L's (kidney stone) last dose of pain medication. What action should occur first?
   1. Help the new nurse look at the chart and medication administration record.
   2. Tell the new nurse to ask the night nurse before she leaves.
   3. Speak to the night shift nurse about the documentation.
   4. Have the new nurse ask Mr. L when he last had medication.

6. Which morning tasks can be delegated to the UAP? *(Select all that apply.)*
   1. Assisting Ms. R, who has rheumatoid arthritis, with morning care
   2. Reinforcing to Mr. L, who has a kidney stone, the need to save urine for straining
   3. Preparing Mr. H's room for his return from the OR for hernia repair
   4. Reporting on the condition of Mr. O's skin resulting from his motorcycle accident
   5. Getting coffee for Ms. J's (end-stage multiple myeloma) family
   6. Checking on the pulse oximeter reading for Mr. A, who has bacterial pneumonia

7. Which tasks related to pain management can you delegate to the UAP? *(Select all that apply.)*
   1. Reporting on grimacing seen in unresponsive patients
   2. Asking about the location, quality, and radiation of pain
   3. Reminding patients to report pain as necessary
   4. Observing for relief after medication is given
   5. Asking patients directly, "Are you having pain?"
   6. Determining if position change relieves pain

8. During the shift, the following events occur at the same time. Prioritize the order for addressing these problems.
   1. Mr. L is calling out loudly about right-sided flank pain caused by his kidney stone.
   2. Mr. O, who was in a motorcycle accident, is calling, "The pump tipped over and it's broken."
   3. Another nurse needs opioids wastage witnessed.
   4. Mr. A, with bacterial pneumonia, is urinating in the corner of his room.

   _____, _____, _____, _____.

9. Mr. L calls for pain medication. He describes the pain caused by his kidney stone as excruciating. He is crying, diaphoretic, and pacing around the room. What is your priority action?
   1. Instruct Mr. L to do deep breathing exercises.
   2. Remind Mr. L to use the PCA pump.
   3. Give Mr. L an "as needed" IV bolus dose as ordered.
   4. Call the physician immediately.

10. You are preparing to give Mr. L pain medication, but you note that the IV site is infiltrated, so you inform him that the IV catheter will have to be reinserted. He yells at you, "What's wrong with you people?! Can't you do anything right?!" What is the best response?
    1. "Let me call the physician, and I can get an order for an oral medication."
    2. "This is not my fault, but if you will just give me a couple of minutes I can fix it."
    3. "Let me call the nursing supervisor and you can talk to her about the situation."
    4. "I know you are having pain. Let me restart your IV line right now."

11. Mr. L reports that the pain has decreased compared with earlier, but now he is having other symptoms. Which symptom is of greatest concern?
    1. Painless hematuria with small clots
    2. Dull pain that radiates into the genitalia
    3. Absence of pain but scant urine output
    4. Sensation of urinary urgency

12. For Mr. O, in addition to pain medication, which action will help the most to relieve pain associated with the tibia-fibula fracture caused by his motorcycle accident?
    1. Instruct him to periodically move his toes.
    2. Use diversional therapy.
    3. Elevate the injured leg above the heart.
    4. Place the patient in high Fowler position.

13. Mr. O is at risk for compartment syndrome because of the cast. Which pain assessment finding would alert you to compartment syndrome?
    1. Pain on passive motion
    2. Sudden increase in pain
    3. Intense discomfort related to an itching sensation
    4. Absence of pain despite no recent medication

14. Mr. O reports an increasing pain in the right abdomen. On physical examination, you note hyperactive bowel sounds, a tense abdomen with guarding, and exquisite tenderness with gentle palpation. What is your priority action?
    1. Give a PRN pain medication.
    2. Notify the physician of your findings.
    3. Take the complete set of vital signs.
    4. Assist him to change positions.

15. Mr. H returns from the OR following a hernia repair. He says that he is "afraid to walk because it will make the pain really bad." What will you explain as being the best option?
    1. Pain medication every 4 hours if he needs it
    2. Medication 45 minutes before ambulation or dressing changes
    3. Around-the-clock pain medication even if he has no report of pain
    4. Talking to the physician for reassurance about the treatment plan

16. Mr. H is asking for pain medication, and the health care provider has ordered 10 mg of oxycodone controlled-release (OxyContin) as needed. The pharmacy has stocked 5-mg tablets of oxycodone immediate-release in the medication cabinet. What is your first action?
    1. Call the health care provider for clarification of the order.
    2. Call the pharmacy and obtain the controlled-release form of the drug.
    3. Ask the patient if the immediate- or controlled-release action is preferred.
    4. Give two of the 5-mg tablets to achieve the correct dose.

17. Mr. H is given a dose of pain medication. One hour later he is anxious and appears uncomfortable and asks, "What's the matter? Is something wrong? I'm still hurting." What action should you take first?
    1. Call the physician for a change in medication or dose.
    2. Initiate "nothing by mouth" status in case surgery is needed.
    3. Check for bladder distention and last voiding.
    4. Reassure the patient that the hernia is not recurring.

18. One of the staff members is talking about Mr. A, who has bacterial pneumonia, in the medication room. "He complains all the time about pain everywhere. Well, he is going to have pain. He's a drug addict, so what does he expect?" What is your best response to this comment?
    1. "All patients have a right to care regardless of race, creed, or other traits."
    2. "I'll take Mr. A; I don't mind taking care of him."
    3. "You should think about how he really feels."
    4. "What can we do to help Mr. A cope with his pain?"

19. Which team members (RN, UAP, physical therapist) should perform the following tasks related to Mr. A's pain management?
    1. Instruct in and supervise use of a transcutaneous electrical nerve stimulation (TENS) unit.
    _____
    2. Administer nonopioid pain medication.
    _____
    3. Answer questions about medication side effects.
    _____
    4. Identify contributing factors such as fatigue or anxiety. _____
    5. Suggest that relatives bring personal comfort items.
    _____
    6. Assist the patient to change position every 2 hours.
    _____
    7. Reinforce the use of a pillow to splint when coughing. _____

20. Mr. A has a single-lumen peripherally inserted central catheter, and he has the following scheduled medications and IV solutions that need to be given now: vancomycin (Vancocin) 1.5 g in 250 mL of dextrose 5% over 90 minutes; levofloxacin (Levaquin) 750 mg in 150 mL of normal saline over 90 minutes; dextrose 5% and 0.45% saline 1000 mL with 20 mEq of potassium at 125 mL/hr; and an IV bolus dose of morphine 3 mg. What is your priority action?
    1. Call the physician and ask if the medication times can be staggered.
    2. Call the pharmacy and enquire about the compatibility of medications and solutions.
    3. Give the bolus dose of morphine, because it will take the least amount of time.
    4. Establish an additional peripheral IV site.

21. Mr. A reports left-sided anterior chest pain. What is your priority action?
    1. Obtain an order for an electrocardiogram and continuous telemetry monitoring.
    2. Auscultate the lung fields and compare to baseline assessments.
    3. Give a PRN pain medication and reevaluate after 30 minutes.
    4. Ask him to describe the pain and measure all vital signs.

22. The UAP reports that the new nurse is undermedicating the patients. What is the best way to handle this situation?
    1. Ignore her; the UAP is not qualified to judge an RN.
    2. Ask the UAP to give specific examples.
    3. Go to the new nurse and question her.
    4. Do an assessment on all of the nurse's patients.

PART 3 Complex Health Scenarios

23. Ms. J is receiving opiates to control her pain caused by end-stage multiple myeloma. Which side effect is the major concern for this patient?
    1. Constipation
    2. Respiratory depression
    3. Nausea and vomiting
    4. Sedation

24. Ms. J is having severe pain and admits to it; however, she becomes very anxious when certain family members come and go and refuses to take the pain medication. Which adjunct medication would be most useful to Ms. J to help her manage these episodes?
    1. Naproxen (Naprosyn)
    2. Doxepin (Sinequan)
    3. Lorazepam (Ativan)
    4. Dicyclomine (Bentyl)

25. Ms. J's son repeatedly insists that Ms. J is not getting enough pain medication. He threatens to sue. You have used therapeutic communication skills with the son and advocated for the patient with the physician. The physician says to you, "I'll be in tomorrow. Just tell the son to chill out." What is your best action?
    1. Call another physician.
    2. Continue to use the current orders.
    3. Have the son call the physician.
    4. Notify the unit manager.

26. It is the end of the shift, and the new nurse is trying to give pain medication to one patient, provide comfort measures for another patient, and redo pain assessments on all her patients. Her documentation is incomplete. What should you do?
    1. Offer to help her by performing the comfort measures.
    2. Let her struggle through so she can find her own way.
    3. Help her to prioritize and delegate the tasks.
    4. Ask someone from the oncoming shift to help her.

27. Which end-of-shift tasks can be delegated to the UAP? *(Select all that apply.)*
    1. Emptying Ms. J's (end-stage multiple myeloma) trash can and placing personal items within reach
    2. Checking Mr. A's (bacterial pneumonia) linens for moisture and soiling and changing as needed
    3. Asking Mr. L (kidney stone) if he needs a dose of pain medication prior to shift change
    4. Assisting Ms. R (rheumatoid arthritis) to change position in bed to relieve pressure on joints
    5. Ensuring Mr. O's leg is elevated and evaluating comfort
    6. Emptying Mr. A's (bacterial pneumonia) urinal and recording the output

28. At the end of the shift, the opioid count shows that two tablets of oxycodone (OxyContin) are unaccounted for. You have spoken to all of the nurses and pharmacists who had access to the medication cabinet during the shift, but no one will admit to removing those two tablets. What should you do? *(Select all that apply.)*
    1. Inform the staff that no one can leave until the matter is resolved.
    2. Fill out an incident report and include facts about what you found and what you did.
    3. Interview all of the patients who have orders for oxycodone (OxyContin).
    4. Discuss the matter with the unit manager and review potential problems of the current system.
    5. Review available records of access and medication retrieval for the past 24 hours.
    6. Ask the staff if they saw any other people (e.g., students, physicians, instructors) who may have accessed the cabinet during the shift.

29. You are giving the end-of-shift report about Ms. R (rheumatoid arthritis) to the oncoming nurse. Place the following information in the correct order.
    1. "She had shoulder pain (4 of 10) and was reluctant to move around."
    2. "Do you have any questions for me?"
    3. "Ms. R is a 55-year-old woman."
    4. "She had shoulder arthroplasty 3 days ago."
    5. "She received a PRN dose of Tylenol with codeine, and pain is now 1 of 10."
    6. "The physical therapist must speak to Ms. R's daughter, so page him when she arrives."

    _____, _____, _____, _____, _____, _____

Complex Health Scenarios — **PART 3**

CASE STUDY 11

Multiple Clients with Cancer

You are the leader of a team caring for clients on a medical-surgical oncology unit. In addition to yourself (an RN), the team includes an experienced chemotherapy-certified RN, a new UAP, and a first-semester nursing student. Your clients are as follows:

- Mr. N, a 68-year-old man, went to see his physician with fever, weight loss, and painless axillary nodes. After lymph node biopsy, non-Hodgkin lymphoma was diagnosed. He is receiving chemotherapy and is on neutropenic precautions. He currently is afebrile, is in good spirits, and feels reasonably well.

- Mr. L, a 50-year-old man, was transferred 6 days ago from the surgical intensive care unit (SICU) following a tracheostomy and partial laryngectomy. He has a soft, small-bore nasogastric tube and a tracheostomy tube and is currently receiving chemotherapy. He received radiation therapy before surgery.

- Mr. B, a 59-year-old man, went to his physician with painless hematuria, and bladder cancer was subsequently diagnosed. He was admitted for intravesical chemotherapy. He received procedure-related teaching before admission. He is alert and conversant, and independently performs activities of daily living (ADLs).

- Ms. C, a 70-year-old woman, went to her physician because of rectal bleeding and a change in bowel habits. She underwent a bowel resection and colostomy 5 days ago. She is progressing well, but needs and likes companionship at the bedside.

- Ms. G, a 65-year-old woman, was admitted for a right breast lumpectomy, scheduled for later in the day, which will be followed by radiation therapy. She appears nervous and tearful and is frequently asking questions.

- Mr. U, a 62-year-old man, has a history of cough, hemoptysis, fatigue, and dyspnea, and after bronchoscopy and sputum cytologic analysis, non–small cell lung cancer was diagnosed. He underwent pulmonary resection 5 days ago and has a chest tube drainage system.

1. You make very brief rounds to see each client before receiving the shift report to ensure client safety and to help you determine acuity and assignments. Which actions will these brief assessments entail? *(Select all that apply.)*
   1. Asking, "How are you feeling?"
   2. Noting mental status (alert and oriented?)
   3. Measuring vital signs and looking at intake and output
   4. Palpating chest and abdominal areas for pain
   5. Noting the presence and complexity of equipment
   6. Observing ease of respiratory effort

2. The first-semester nursing student tells you that her clinical assignment for the day is to take vital signs and obtain a client history that will take about 1 or 2 hours to complete. Which clients would you recommend she approach to fulfill her assignment? *(Select all that apply.)*
   1. Mr. N
   2. Mr. L
   3. Mr. B
   4. Ms. C
   5. Ms. G
   6. Mr. U

3. You must assign a UAP to help care for Mr. N with non-Hodgkin lymphoma. For this neutropenic client, which factor is most important in making this assignment?
   1. The UAP is in the first trimester of pregnancy.
   2. The UAP has had cold symptoms for 3 days.
   3. The UAP has no experience with neutropenic precautions.
   4. The UAP has a generalized fear of isolation clients.

4. The nursing student tearfully reports to you, "I took some flowers into Mr. N's room to cheer him up and he told me that he didn't think he was supposed to have flowers. I took them out of the room right away, and then I realized I had made a mistake." What should you do first?
   1. Direct the student to read the isolation precautions before entering the room.
   2. Call the nursing instructor and report the student for making an error.
   3. Acknowledge and praise the student for taking responsibility for the mistake.
   4. Write an incident report and have the student and instructor sign it.

5. You are reviewing new orders for Mr. N. Which order would you question?
   1. Administer filgrastim (Neupogen) 5 mcg/kg subcutaneously every day.
   2. Catheterize to obtain a urinalysis specimen.
   3. Flush the IV saline lock every shift.
   4. Monitor vital signs every 4 hours.

6. In the early postoperative period, what is the priority nursing diagnosis for Mr. L, who has a *tracheostomy and partial laryngectomy*?
   1. Risk for Infection related to chemotherapy and the surgical procedure
   2. Imbalanced Nutrition: Less than Body Requirements related to presurgical dysphagia and malignancy
   3. Impaired Verbal Communication related to the tracheostomy tube
   4. Risk for Aspiration related to secretions and removal of the epiglottis

7. Which assessment finding for Mr. L is of greatest concern?
   1. Pulsation of the tracheostomy tube in synchrony with the heartbeat
   2. Increased secretions in and around the tracheostomy
   3. Increased coughing, with difficulty in expectorating secretions
   4. Presence of food particles in tracheal secretions

8. You are teaching the nursing student about emergency respiratory equipment that should be available for Mr. L. Which piece of equipment is the most important to show to the student?
   1. Adult-sized endotracheal tube
   2. Laryngeal scope with blades of several sizes
   3. Bag-valve mask with extension tubing
   4. Tracheostomy insertion tray

9. Mr. B will receive intravesical chemotherapy consisting of bacille Calmette-Guérin (BCG) instillation for his bladder cancer. Place the following steps related to this therapy in the correct order.
   1. Clamp the tube distal to the injection port of the catheter.
   2. Insert a Foley catheter.
   3. Instill BCG fluid via the catheter.
   4. Change the client's position from side to side every 15 minutes for 2 hours.
   5. Direct the client to drink two glasses of water to flush the bladder.
   6. Unclamp the catheter at the end of 2 hours.

   _____, _____, _____, _____, _____, _____

10. Following the BCG treatment, you delegate disposal of Mr. B's Foley bag and fluid contents to the UAP. What instructions should you give?
    1. No special handling of the bag or its contents is required.
    2. "Wear a lead apron when you are emptying the drainage container."
    3. "Discard the fluid in the toilet and disinfect the toilet with bleach for 6 hours."
    4. "Wear sterile gloves when you are handling the bag and its contents."

11. The physician should be notified if a normal voiding pattern (i.e., pain free, symptom free) fails to resume within which time period after removal of Mr. B's catheter (after the BCG treatment)?
    1. 6 hours
    2. 12 hours
    3. 3 days
    4. 1 week

12. During the midmorning, the following events occur at the same time. Prioritize the events in the order in which they should be addressed.
    1. Mr. B, who has bladder cancer, reports dysuria.
    2. Mr. U's (pulmonary resection) chest drainage system has tipped over.
    3. Mr. N, with non-Hodgkin lymphoma, has a fever of 101° F (38.3° C).
    4. Mr. L's (*partial laryngectomy*) tracheostomy tube needs to be suctioned.
    5. Ms. C, who had a bowel resection, has a swollen, tender, red calf.

    _____, _____, _____, _____, _____

13. In helping a client such as Ms. C, who had a colostomy with a bowel resection, which team member (RN, UAP, wound, ostomy, continence nurse [WOCN]), under the appropriate supervision, should be assigned to perform each of these actions related to her postoperative care?
    1. Assist Ms. C with perineal care.

       _____

    2. Administer stool softeners and assess their effectiveness. _____

    3. Monitor wounds for drainage and infection.

       _____

    4. Provide initial information about ostomy care and management. _____

    5. Advise about the prevention of skin breakdown around the stoma site. _____

14. Ms. C repeatedly refuses to perform a return demonstration of any aspect of colostomy care. Despite steady improvement and independent resumption of other ADLs, she protests, "I'm too weak. You'll have to do it for me." What is the priority diagnosis for Ms. C?
    1. Activity Intolerance related to the disease process
    2. Risk for Impaired Skin Integrity related to the ostomy
    3. Deficient Knowledge related to the procedure
    4. Defensive Coping related to change in health and ADLs

15. The nursing staff are making suggestions about how to help Ms. C overcome her reluctance to perform colostomy care. Which suggestion will you try first?
    1. Verbally reexplain the procedure and give her written material.
    2. Have a family member come in and do it for her.
    3. Continue to do it for her until she is ready.
    4. Ask her to hold the clamp while the bag is being emptied.

16. Ms. C repeatedly calls for help during the shift with various small requests. She is talkative and pleasant, and she does everything she can to get you to "stay and chat." What is the best response?
    1. "I really do like talking to you, but I do have other clients."
    2. "You'll be okay for right now, and I will come back and check on you later."
    3. "I have 10 minutes right now. Later this afternoon, I'll have time to talk."
    4. "Let me call one of the hospital volunteers to come and sit with you."

17. You are working through the preoperative checklist and Ms. G, who has a breast lump, begins to cry. "What do you think about this breast surgery? My friend's arm got really swollen after she had the surgery. Can't I just take medication?" What is the priority diagnosis for Ms. G?
    1. Anxiety related to uncertainty about future outcomes
    2. Disturbed Body Image related to imminent loss of a body part
    3. Deficient Knowledge related to the treatment plan
    4. Noncompliance related to the surgical procedure

18. Ms. G continues to be anxious and tearful, and she tells you that she has changed her mind about the surgery, "I'm going to go home. I just can't deal with everything that is going on right now. I need some time to think about things." What is your best response?
    1. "It's okay to change your mind. You have the right to make your own decisions."
    2. "Please reconsider. This surgery is very important and your health is the priority."
    3. "Would you like me to call your physician, so that you can discuss your concerns?"
    4. "I see you are very concerned. What things are you dealing with and thinking about?"

19. Which assessment finding is the most critical?
    1. Mr. U has tracheal deviation after a pulmonary resection.
    2. Mr. B, with bladder cancer, has decreased urinary output.
    3. Mr. N, with non-Hodgkin lymphoma, is having dysrhythmias.
    4. Ms. C has severe abdominal pain after a bowel resection.

20. List at least three assessment findings of tension pneumothorax that help you identify this potentially life-threatening emergency.

    _____

    _____

21. You determine that Mr. U has developed a tension pneumothorax following surgery for a pulmonary resection 5 days ago. He is currently receiving high-flow oxygen via nonrebreather mask but continues to experience respiratory distress. What is the priority action?
    1. Remove the occlusive dressing around the chest wound.
    2. Perform a needle thoracotomy with a 14- to 16-gauge catheter needle.
    3. Initiate cardiopulmonary resuscitation (CPR).
    4. Call for the crash cart and intubation equipment.

22. You are calling the physician to report events related to Mr. U's condition. Prioritize the following information according to the SBAR (situation, background, assessment, recommendation) format.

1. "Mr. U is 5 days postoperative for pulmonary resection for non–small cell lung cancer. He has a chest tube that has been draining progressively smaller amounts of dark red blood."

2. "Dr. S, this is Nurse C on the medical-surgical oncology unit. I am calling about Mr. U. About 15 minutes ago, he developed severe respiratory distress, and tracheal deviation was noted. We removed the occlusive dressing at the chest tube insertion site, and his breathing improved. The Rapid Response Team was called and is currently managing the airway. He is receiving 100% oxygen via a nonrebreather mask."

3. "The Rapid Response Team is recommending transfer to the intensive care unit, because the exact cause of the tension pneumothorax is undetermined. The radiology department is waiting to do a portable chest radiograph if we could get an order. Would you like us to get an arterial blood gas analysis or do anything else?"

4. "Mr. U is currently alert and anxious, and he is following commands. Blood pressure is 160/96 mm Hg, pulse rate is 110 beats/min, respiratory rate is 32 breaths/min, and pulse oximetry reading is 90% with the client on 100% oxygen via nonrebreather mask."

_____, _____, _____, _____

23. There are 2 hours left before the shift ends. The new UAP tells you that she has to leave now because she has a family emergency. What should you do? *(Select all that apply.)*

1. Ask her what tasks and duties are pending for the next 2 hours.
2. Call a UAP who is scheduled for the next shift to come early.
3. Remind the UAP that shift change is a busy time.
4. Allow her to leave, but remind her she is still on probation as a new staff member.
5. Call another unit and see if there is a UAP who could float to your unit.
6. Explain to her that her priority is to fulfill her work responsibilities.
7. Ask her to explain the nature of the family emergency, so that you can make a decision.
8. Check with the other staff members to see if they will be able to cover her duties.

24. The nursing student tells you that Ms. C has just asked her to stay after the shift ends, so that she can meet her granddaughter. What should you say to the student?

1. "What do you think your instructor would tell you to do?"
2. "What do you think about Ms. C's request?"
3. "It sounds like you really made a connection with Ms. C."
4. "Tell Ms. C that you have to go, but you will see her tomorrow."

CASE STUDY 12

Gastrointestinal Bleeding

Mr. S, a 50-year-old man, has driven himself to the emergency department (ED) after vomiting bright red blood twice within 6 hours. He arrives alert and oriented × 3 but appears anxious. He is able to provide only a vague history but admits to drinking "a few" last weekend. He knows that he is "supposed to stop drinking" and takes "something for his stomach," but he cannot recall the name of the medication. He reports intermittent dizziness and fatigue that has been worsening over the past 2 days. His skin is dry and pale. His abdomen is slightly distended. He reports pain (4 on a scale of 10) in the midepigastric area. Capillary refill is longer than 3 seconds, blood pressure is 140/90 mm Hg, pulse rate is 110 beats/min, respiratory rate is 24 breaths/min, and temperature is 99° F (37.2° C).

1. What is the priority nursing diagnosis for Mr. S?
   1. Risk for Aspiration related to active bleeding
   2. Anxiety related to the uncertainty of his health status
   3. Deficient Fluid Volume related to vomiting of blood and gastric secretions
   4. Noncompliance related to alcohol consumption and medication use

2. Which actions are appropriate in the care of this patient? *(Select all that apply.)*
   1. Start a peripheral IV line using a 22-gauge catheter.
   2. Initiate input and output monitoring with hourly urine measurements.
   3. Check emesis and stool for occult blood.
   4. Monitor hemoglobin level and hematocrit every 4 hours.
   5. Maintain the patient in a semi- or high Fowler position.
   6. Prepare the patient for surgery.

3. Which task is appropriate to assign to a UAP?
   1. Repeating measurement of vital signs every 2 hours
   2. Gathering equipment for nasogastric (NG) lavage
   3. Checking the blood glucose level every 2 hours
   4. Notifying the family (with the patient's permission)

4. The physician has ordered several immediate (STAT) interventions for Mr. S. To complete these interventions in a rapid and efficient manner, you ask several team members to assist. Which staff member (UAP, paramedic, RN, clergy, LPN/LVN), under the appropriate supervision, can be assigned to perform these tasks? *(More than one staff member may be qualified to perform each of these tasks.)*
   1. Place an automatic blood pressure cuff.

      _____

   2. Establish two peripheral IV lines with 16-gauge catheters. _____

   3. Place an NG tube and initiate saline lavage.

      _____

   4. Insert a Foley catheter attached to a urinometer.

      _____

   5. Set up blood transfusion equipment.

      _____

   6. Liaison with family members in the waiting room.

      _____

   7. Assess baseline breath and bowel sounds.

      _____

5. You are performing additional assessment and history taking for Mr. S. Which finding should you immediately report to the physician?
   1. Melena stools
   2. History of nonsteroidal anti-inflammatory drug use
   3. Tense, rigid abdomen
   4. Probable positive human immunodeficiency virus status

6. The physician orders an NG tube insertion with saline lavage. List the correct order of actions for this procedure.
   1. Measure tube from the tip of nose, to the earlobe, to the xiphoid process.
   2. Place the patient in a high Fowler position and provide an emesis basin.
   3. Ask the patient to sip water as you pass the tube.
   4. When tube is just above the oropharynx, instruct the patient to bend the chin forward.
   5. Obtain an order for a radiograph and check pH to verify tube placement.
   6. Inspect for the patient's most patent nostril.
   7. Insert the lubricated tube into the most patent nostril.

   _____, _____, _____, _____, _____, _____, _____

7. Despite your best efforts at therapeutic communication, Mr. S refuses to cooperate with the NG tube insertion. He threatens to leave "if you stick that tube down my nose again." What should you do first?
   1. Physically restrain him and insert the tube.
   2. Explain the "against medical advice" (AMA) form.
   3. Notify the nursing supervisor and patient advocate.
   4. Page the physician and document the attempt.

8. You discover that the phlebotomist drew the sample for STAT blood tests from another patient, not Mr. S. You are unsure how the sample was labeled. What should you do first?
   1. Call the phlebotomist to come back.
   2. Draw the blood sample yourself.
   3. Report the phlebotomist to his supervisor.
   4. Ask the phlebotomist to explain what happened.

9. The physician orders a STAT blood transfusion. In the event of an emergency, for a patient such as Mr. S, a type-specific non–cross-matched blood product could be used. What do you anticipate as the blood product in this case?
   1. O negative
   2. AB negative
   3. AB positive
   4. A negative

10. You are preparing to administer a blood transfusion to Mr. S. Place the steps of transfusion in the appropriate order.
    1. Prime the correct tubing and filter with normal saline.
    2. Take vital signs before starting the transfusion.
    3. Transfuse the first 10 to 24 mL slowly; monitor the patient closely.
    4. Inspect the bag for leaks, clots, or unusual color.
    5. Compare the bag label with the chart and blood bank forms.
    6. Have two nurses (or MDs) compare the blood band identification with the tag on the blood bag.
    7. Repeat vital sign measurement after 15 minutes and then every hour until the transfusion is complete.
    8. Document the outcomes, names of personnel, and starting and ending times. _____, _____, _____, _____, _____, _____, _____, _____

11. You are talking to Mr. S about his alcohol consumption. Which statement represents the most common defense mechanism that is used by people who have problems with alcoholism?
    1. "You would drink too if you were married to my wife."
    2. "My wife and I have a couple of beers after work. It's no big deal."
    3. "If you think I drink a lot, you should see my wife put it away."
    4. "I would rather talk to my wife about this situation when I get home."

12. Mr. S has been in the ED for about 8 hours. He is becoming increasingly anxious and irritated. He tells you that he has decided he wants to leave. What is your best response?
    1. "You are very sick today. Why do you want to leave?"
    2. "Let me call your wife, so that you can discuss this with her."
    3. "What will you do and where will you go if you decide to leave?"
    4. "You can leave if you want to, but I will have to notify the physician first."

13. You suspect that Mr. S may be at risk for alcohol withdrawal effects. What is an early manifestation?
    1. Startles easily
    2. Paranoid delusions
    3. Slurred speech
    4. Grand mal seizure

14. Which serious complications may result from alcohol withdrawal delirium? *(Select all that apply.)*
    1. Myocardial infarction
    2. Electrolyte imbalance
    3. Aspiration pneumonia
    4. Anaphylaxis
    5. Sepsis
    6. Suicide

15. Mr. S and his wife ask for privacy so that they can talk. Later, when you return to check on him, the NG tube is on the floor and there is a strong odor of alcohol on Mr. S's breath and he appears relaxed and groggy. What should you do first?
    1. Politely ask the wife to leave and call security to check the room for illicit substances.
    2. Assess the patient's mental status and ask what happened to the NG tube.
    3. Explain that his behavior is unacceptable and counterproductive to his therapy.
    4. Reinsert an NG tube and call the physician for an order for a STAT blood alcohol test.

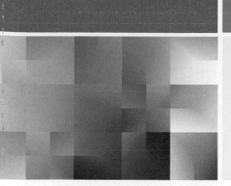

Ms. A, a 20-year-old college student who had been drinking at a fraternity party before she fell from a second-floor balcony, has just arrived in the emergency department (ED). A fellow college student who accompanies Ms. A tells you, "She was completely knocked out right after the fall. But then she woke up a little, so we thought she was okay—until she stopped moving again."

You are assigned as the ED triage nurse. When you assess Ms. A, there is no response to commands or to having her name called. She extends her arms and legs stiffly when nail bed pressure is applied, but there is no verbal response. Her eyes are shut, and she does not open them even with the nail bed pressure. When you open her eyelids, you see that her pupils are unequal, with the right pupil larger than the left. The pupil response when you shine a flashlight into her eyes is sluggish.

Ms. A's blood pressure is 70/30 mm Hg, she is in a sinus bradycardia with a rate of 40 beats/min, and her respiratory rate is 6 breaths/min. Her respirations are irregular, and she has 20-second periods of apnea. You note that she has a large occipital laceration and that her left leg is misaligned.

The paramedics have a cervical collar and backboard in place. A 16-gauge catheter has been inserted at the left antecubital area and lactated Ringer's solution is infusing at 150 mL/hr.

1. Which additional assessment information is most important to obtain at this time?
   1. Temperature
   2. Breath sounds
   3. Pedal pulses
   4. Oxygen saturation

2. Which is the best way to clearly document Ms. A's level of consciousness (LOC)?
   1. Client is comatose.
   2. Client is unresponsive.
   3. Client has a decreased LOC.
   4. Client Glasgow Coma Scale (GCS) score = 4.

3. When describing Ms. A's neurologic assessment, you will chart "Client demonstrates _____ posturing in response to nail bed pressure."

4. Based on Ms. A's vital signs, she appears to be in shock. Which types of shock are you most concerned about for this client? *(Select all that apply.)*
   1. Cardiogenic
   2. Hypovolemic
   3. Neurogenic
   4. Septic
   5. Anaphylactic

5. You are working with Dr. G, a new medical resident whose first day in the ED rotation is today. Which action by Dr. G indicates that you need to consult quickly with the supervising physician?
   1. Assessing for the Babinski sign
   2. Increasing the IV infusion rate to 200 mL/hr
   3. Ordering an electrocardiogram taken at once (STAT)
   4. Preparing to perform a lumbar puncture

6. After you perform triage for Ms. A, which ED staff member will you assign to take primary responsibility for Ms. A's ongoing care?
   1. RN from a temporary agency with extensive previous ED experience who has been in your ED for 3 days
   2. LPN/LVN with 10 years of experience in your ED who is in the last semester of an RN program
   3. RN who has worked in your ED for the last 5 years after transferring from the mother-baby unit
   4. RN who has 12 years of intensive care unit (ICU) experience and has floated to the ED today

7. Ms. A suddenly begins to vomit. Which action is best to take at this time?
   1. Utilize the backboard to log-roll Ms. A to her side.
   2. Suction Ms. A's airway with a Yankauer suction device.
   3. Hyperoxygenate Ms. A with a bag-valve mask system.
   4. Insert a nasogastric tube and connect to low suction.

8. The ED physician prescribes these actions. Which one will you implement first?
   1. Administer metoclopramide (Reglan) 10 mg IV.
   2. Obtain computed tomographic (CT) scan of head.
   3. Clean occipital laceration and apply antibiotic ointment.
   4. Infuse famotidine (Pepcid) 20 mg IV every 12 hours.

The results of laboratory tests that were performed when Ms. A arrived in the ED are faxed to the RN. Complete blood count results are as follows:

Hematocrit	42%
Hemoglobin level	12.6 g/dL
Platelet count	200,000/mm³
White blood cell count	7500/mm³

The metabolic profile shows the following:

Blood urea nitrogen level	13 mg/dL
Chloride level	102 mEq/L
Creatinine level	0.7 mg/dL
Glucose level	144 mg/dL
Magnesium level	1.5 mEq/L
Potassium level	4.1 mEq/L
Sodium level	133 mEq/L

The drug screen shows the following:

Blood alcohol level	0.14%
Tetrahydrocannabinol level	15 ng/mL

Arterial blood gas results are as follows:

Arterial partial pressure of carbon dioxide ($PaCO_2$)	56 mm Hg
Arterial partial pressure of oxygen (PaO_2)	65 mm Hg
Bicarbonate (HCO_3^-)	22 mEq/L
O_2 saturation	88%
pH	7.30

9. Based on the laboratory values, which collaborative intervention will you anticipate next?
   1. Type and cross-match for 3 units of packed red blood cells.
   2. Administer magnesium sulfate 1 g IV over the next 3 hours.
   3. Give insulin aspart (NovoLog) using the standard sliding scale.
   4. Obtain an endotracheal intubation tray and assist with intubation.

After being intubated and placed on mechanical ventilation, Ms. A is transported to the radiology department. The CT scans indicate that she has a large left frontoparietal lobe epidural hematoma. In addition, chest and left leg x-rays show that she has a left femur fracture and evidence of aspiration pneumonia.

When you reassess Ms. A after the CT scan, she is flaccid, with no response to verbal or painful stimulation. Her pupils are dilated and nonreactive to light. Vital sign values are as follows:

Blood pressure	190/40 mm Hg
Heart rate	40 beats/min (sinus bradycardia)
O_2 saturation	92%
Respiratory rate	14 breaths/min (ventilator controlled)
Temperature	96° F (35.6°C) (axillary)

10. Which complication are you most concerned about at present?
    1. Brainstem herniation
    2. Respiratory acidosis
    3. Hemorrhage
    4. Hypothermia

Ms. A is transported to the operating room, where the epidural hematoma is evacuated and an open reduction and internal fixation of her left leg fracture is completed.

After surgery, Ms. A is transferred to the ICU. She is attached to a cardiac monitor and has an arterial line in place in her left radial artery. She is making no spontaneous respiratory effort but is being mechanically ventilated with a ventilator in the assist/control mode at a rate of 14 breaths/min. Ms. A has an indwelling urinary catheter, which is draining large amounts of clear, pale yellow urine. An intracranial monitor is in place. Her vital sign values and intracranial pressure (ICP) are as follows:

Blood pressure	112/64 mm Hg (mean arterial pressure [MAP], 80 mm Hg)
Heart rate	50 to 56 beats/min (sinus bradycardia)
ICP	22 mm Hg
O_2 saturation	93%
Respiratory rate	14 breaths/min (ventilator controlled)
Temperature	97.4° F (36.3° C) (axillary)

11. Which of the assessment data listed above requires the most immediate nursing action?
    1. Cardiac rhythm
    2. Blood pressure
    3. O_2 saturation
    4. ICP

12. These collaborative and nursing interventions are included in the postcraniotomy plan of care. Which ones are used to meet the goal of maintaining Ms. A's cerebral perfusion pressure (CPP) at 60 mm Hg or more? *(Select all that apply.)*
    1. Keep the head of the bed elevated 30 degrees.
    2. Check pupil reaction to light every hour.
    3. Reposition the client at least every 2 hours.
    4. Perform endotracheal suctioning as necessary.
    5. Check GCS score hourly.
    6. Administer mannitol (Osmitrol) 100 mg IV as needed (PRN) if ICP is above 20 mm Hg.
    7. Titrate norepinephrine (Levophed) drip to maintain MAP above 80 mm Hg.

When you assess Ms. A on the first postoperative day, she is still receiving mechanical ventilation and has an oxygen saturation of 94% to 99%, with stable vital signs and an ICP of 12. Her GCS score is 5.

13. The postcraniotomy care plan for the first postoperative day includes all these nursing actions. Which actions can you delegate to an experienced LPN/LVN working with you in the ICU? *(Select all that apply.)*
    1. Checking the gastric pH every 4 hours
    2. Performing a neurologic status examination every 2 hours
    3. Assessing breath sounds every 4 hours
    4. Checking endotracheal tube cuff pressure each shift
    5. Turning the client side to side every 2 hours
    6. Monitoring intake and output hourly
    7. Sending a urine specimen to check specific gravity daily
    8. Giving acetaminophen (Tylenol) elixir 625 mg via orogastric tube for temperature above 101° F (38.3° C).

Arterial blood gas values at 7:00 AM on the first postoperative day are as follows:

$PaCO_2$	25 mm Hg
PaO_2	110 mm Hg
HCO_3^-	20 mEq/L
O_2 saturation	100%
pH	7.54

14. Which parameter indicates a need for an immediate change in the ventilator settings?
    1. $PaCO_2$
    2. O_2 saturation
    3. HCO_3^-
    4. PaO_2

15. At 10:00 AM, the LPN/LVN tells you that Ms. A's output for the last hour was 1200 mL and that her urine is very pale yellow. Which action is best to take next?
    1. Instruct the LPN/LVN to continue to monitor the urine output hourly.
    2. Send a urine specimen to the laboratory to check specific gravity.
    3. Notify the neurosurgeon and anticipate an increase in the IV rate.
    4. Assess the client's neurologic status for signs of increased irritability.

16. The neurosurgeon assesses Ms. A and then writes new orders. Which order is most important to clarify?
    1. Give hydroxypropyl methylcellulose (artificial tears) OU q 4 hours.
    2. Continue SS insulin aspart (NovoLog) for blood glucose >150 mg/dL.
    3. Increase normal saline infusion to 500 cc/hr for the next 2 hours.
    4. Administer heparin sodium (Heparin) 5000 U SC every 12 hours.

17. Ms. A's mother, who has been staying at the bedside, asks you why her daughter is receiving famotidine, stating that her daughter has no history of peptic ulcers. Which answer is best?
    1. "Famotidine will lower the chance that she will aspirate."
    2. "Famotidine decreases the incidence of gastric stress ulcers."
    3. "Famotidine will reduce the risk for gastroesophageal reflux."
    4. "Famotidine prevents gastric irritation caused by the orogastric tube."

18. About 20 minutes after Ms. A is positioned on her right side, you notice that her ICP has increased to 30 mm Hg. Which action should you take next?
    1. Administer the PRN mannitol 100 mg IV.
    2. Assess the alignment of Ms. A's head and neck.
    3. Elevate the head of the bed to 45 degrees.
    4. Check Ms. A's pupil size and response to light.

PART 3

Complex Health Scenarios

19. When you assess Ms. A at 2:00 PM, there is little change in her neurologic status. Her left leg, however, is pale, swollen, and very firm when you palpate it. The left leg pulses are only faintly audible using a Doppler flow meter. Which action is most appropriate at this time?
    1. Call the orthopedic surgeon to communicate your assessment.
    2. Elevate the left leg on two pillows to decrease the swelling.
    3. Continue to monitor the left leg appearance and pedal pulses.
    4. Assess the client for indications of pain, such as restlessness.

20. As your shift ends, you are preparing Ms. A for transfer to surgery for an emergency fasciotomy. What is your best choice for obtaining informed consent for the fasciotomy?
    1. Informed consent is not needed for emergency surgery.
    2. Permission for surgery can be given by Ms. A's mother.
    3. Consent for surgery is not required for unconscious clients.
    4. Authorization can be given by the nursing supervisor.

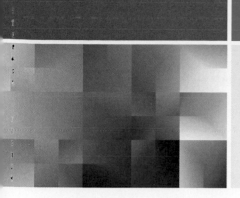

CASE STUDY 14

Septic Shock

Ms. D, a 54-year-old patient, is brought to the emergency department (ED) by her daughter because of weakness and a decreasing level of consciousness. The patient responds to brief commands to open her eyes and move her arms and legs, but she is unable to answer any of your questions. The daughter tells you that, when she stopped by her mother's house today for a visit, Ms. D was complaining about abdominal and back pain. She also was a little bit nauseated and vomited a small amount twice. Although usually she is very alert and oriented, today she seemed lethargic and became increasingly sleepy. Because of her lethargy and nausea, she has not had anything to eat or drink today.

Her medical history includes hypertension, peripheral arterial disease, and diabetes mellitus type 2. The daughter brings in a list of her usual home medications, which include enalapril (Vasotec) 40 mg daily, insulin lispro (Humalog) on a sliding scale for elevated glucose levels, metformin (Glucophage) 500 mg twice daily, and atorvastatin (Lipitor) 10 mg daily.

You obtain and document the initial vital sign values as follows:

Blood pressure	102/38 mm Hg
Heart rate	102 beats/min
O₂ saturation	76%
Respiratory rate	40 breaths/min
Temperature	102.4° F (39.1° C) (orally)

1. Based on the initial history and assessment, which action prescribed by the health care provider (HCP) will you implement first?
   1. Insert a Foley catheter and send a urine specimen for culture and sensitivity testing.
   2. Start oxygen and titrate to maintain oxygen saturation at 90% or higher.
   3. Place the patient on a cardiac monitor.
   4. Check the blood glucose level.

2. Which method of oxygen administration will be best to increase Ms. D's oxygen saturation?
   1. Nasal cannula
   2. Nonrebreather mask
   3. Venturi mask
   4. Simple face mask

3. Available staffing in the ED includes you and an experienced UAP. Which actions will be best for you to delegate to the UAP? (Select all that apply.)
   1. Measuring vital signs every 15 minutes
   2. Attaching the patient to a cardiac monitor
   3. Documenting a head-to-toe assessment
   4. Checking orientation and alertness
   5. Inserting an IV line
   6. Monitoring urine output hourly

4. The cardiac monitor shows atrial fibrillation with a rate of 90 to 114 beats/min. Routine treatment orders for dysrhythmias are included in the ED protocols. Which action will you prepare to take next?
   1. Continue to monitor cardiac rhythm.
   2. Administer metoprolol (Lopressor) 5 mg IV push.
   3. Prepare to perform cardioversion at 50 J.
   4. Administer adenosine (Adenocard) 6 mg IV push.

Arterial blood gas (ABG) analysis is performed and the following results are obtained:

Arterial partial pressure of carbon dioxide (PaCO₂)	62 mm Hg
Arterial partial pressure of oxygen (PaO₂)	50 mm Hg
Bicarbonate (HCO₃⁻)	22 mEq/L
O₂ saturation	87%
pH	7.23

5. Based on your analysis of these ABG values, which collaborative intervention do you anticipate?
   1. Sodium bicarbonate ($NaHCO_3$) bolus IV
   2. Endotracheal intubation and mechanical ventilation
   3. Continuous monitoring of Ms. D's respiratory status
   4. Nebulized albuterol (Proventil) therapy

6. You are preparing to assist with endotracheal intubation of Ms. D. In which order will these actions be accomplished?
   1. Use capnography to check for exhaled carbon dioxide.
   2. Tape the endotracheal tube in place.
   3. Preoxygenate with bag-valve mask device at 100% oxygen.
   4. Place the patient in a supine position.
   5. Briefly explain the intubation procedure to the patient and her daughter.
   6. Inflate the endotracheal tube cuff.
   7. Auscultate breath sounds bilaterally.
   8. Obtain a chest radiograph.
   9. Insert the endotracheal tube orally through the vocal cords.

   _____, _____, _____, _____, _____, _____, _____, _____, _____

After the successful intubation, you perform a rapid assessment of Ms. D and chart your findings: "Heart tones irregular and distant. Face flushed and warm. Extremities cool and mottled. Radial pulses faintly palpable. Pedal pulses nonpalpable. Breath sounds audible bilaterally with crackles present in left lung base. Grimaces with light abdominal palpation above pelvic bone. Urine is amber and cloudy, with red streaks. 100 mL urine output when Foley catheter inserted. Opens eyes and moves to command. Pupils equal, round, and reactive to light."

The patient's current vital sign values are as follows:

Blood pressure	*86/40 mm Hg*
Heart rate	*112 beats/min*
O_2 saturation	*93%*
Respiratory rate	*32 breaths/min*
Temperature	*103° F (39.4° C) (axillary)*

7. Which information in your assessment requires the most immediate action?
   1. Elevated temperature
   2. Left lung crackles
   3. Nonpalpable pulses
   4. Low blood pressure

8. Ms. D is admitted to the intensive care unit (ICU) with a diagnosis of probable sepsis and septic shock. Which data that you have collected in the health history and physical assessment are significant in developing and confirming the diagnoses of sepsis and septic shock? *(Select all that apply.)*
   1. Increased temperature
   2. Atrial fibrillation rhythm
   3. Cloudy, blood-streaked urine
   4. Decreased blood pressure
   5. Elevated heart rate
   6. Abdominal and back pain
   7. History of diabetes mellitus

9. Because the ICU is short staffed, the nursing supervisor assigns you to follow Ms. D to the ICU and care for her there. In which order will you implement the prescribed collaborative interventions?
   1. Draw blood for culture from three separate sites.
   2. Give acetaminophen (Tylenol) 650 mg rectally.
   3. Infuse 1 L of normal saline over 30 minutes.
   4. Start a dopamine (Intropin) drip at 15 mcg/kg/min.
   5. Administer gentamicin (Gentacidin) 60 mg IV.

   _____, _____, _____, _____, _____

10. When you are infusing the normal saline, which action is most important in evaluating for an adverse reaction to the rapid fluid infusion?
    1. Palpating for any peripheral edema
    2. Monitoring urine output
    3. Listening to lung sounds
    4. Checking for jugular venous distention

11. When you recheck the dopamine drip, you notice that you have miscalculated the dopamine dose and have mistakenly set the rate at 20 mcg/kg/min. Which action should you take first?
    1. Assess for toxic effects of the medication.
    2. Notify the HCP about the medication error.
    3. Complete a medication incident report per policy.
    4. Ask the pharmacist to recalculate the dopamine dose.

12. Which patient finding is most important to report to the HCP regarding the error in the dopamine infusion?
    1. The noninvasive blood pressure monitor shows a blood pressure of 102/48 mm Hg.
    2. The data screen on the ventilator indicates a respiratory rate of 44 breaths/min.
    3. The patient's pulse oximetry monitor shows an oxygen saturation of 90%.
    4. The cardiac monitor indicates a sinus tachycardia at a rate of 156 beats/min.

13. You are working with an experienced LPN/LVN in caring for Ms. D. Which nursing activities included in the care plan should be delegated to the LPN/LVN? *(Select all that apply.)*
    1. Documenting the nasogastric tube drainage and urinary output on the ICU flow sheet
    2. Notifying the laboratory after giving gentamicin so that gentamicin peak level can be measured
    3. Monitoring the dopamine infusion site for signs of extravasation
    4. Administering sliding-scale insulin lispro subcutaneously every 6 hours
    5. Completing and documenting a head-to-toe assessment every 4 hours
    6. Monitoring blood pressure and titrating dopamine to keep systolic pressure at 100 mm Hg

The ICU intensivist arrives to examine Ms. D and inserts an arterial line and a pulmonary artery (PA) pressure line (Swan-Ganz catheter). After a few hours, the dopamine drip has been decreased to 11 mcg/kg/min, and there are orders to titrate the dopamine to keep the systolic blood pressure 100 mm Hg or higher. Ms. D is receiving an infusion of normal saline running at 200 mL/hr. The current values for vital signs and other parameters are as follows:

Blood pressure	104/56 mm Hg
Heart rate	104 beats/min (atrial fibrillation)
O₂ saturation	95%
PA systolic pressure	15 mm Hg (normal = 15 to 30 mm Hg)
PA diastolic pressure	2 mm Hg (normal = 4 to 12 mm Hg)
PA wedge pressure	2 mm Hg (normal = 6 to 12 mm Hg)
Respiratory rate	26 breaths/min
Temperature	101.6° F (38.7° C) (rectal)

14. Which information about Ms. D is most important for you to communicate rapidly to the intensivist?
    1. Decreased blood pressure
    2. Ongoing atrial fibrillation
    3. Low PA wedge pressure
    4. Continued temperature elevation

Before calling the intensivist, you quickly look at Ms. D's latest laboratory test results, which have just arrived on the unit:

Hematocrit	32%
Hemoglobin level	10.9 g/dL
Platelet count	96,000/mm³
White blood cell count	26,000/mm³
Blood urea nitrogen level	56 mg/dL
Creatinine level	2.9 mg dL
Glucose level	330 mg/dL
Potassium level	5.2 mEq/L
Sodium level	140 mEq/L

15. Which laboratory value requires the most immediate action?
    1. Creatinine level
    2. Glucose level
    3. Potassium level
    4. Hemoglobin level

16. At the end of your shift, the ICU supervisor consults with you about which of these oncoming staff members is best to assign to care for Ms. D. Which RN is the best one to care for this patient?
    1. Travel RN with 20 years of ICU experience who has been working in this ICU for 4 months
    2. Newly graduated RN who worked in the ICU as a nursing assistant and has finished the precepted orientation
    3. Experienced ICU RN who has been called in on a day off to work for the first 4 hours of the shift
    4. RN who has been floated from the postanesthesia care unit (PACU) to the ICU for the shift

PART 3   Complex Health Scenarios

Answer Key for this case study begins on p. 227.

CASE STUDY 15

Heart Failure

You are admitting Ms. C, an 81-year-old client, to the coronary care unit (CCU). Ms. C, who has a history of mitral valve regurgitation and left ventricular enlargement, came to the emergency department (ED) with symptoms of increasing shortness of breath over the last week. The ED RN tells you that the client received furosemide (Lasix) 100 mg IV and that she is receiving oxygen via a nasal cannula at 3 L/min. According to the ED nurse, Ms. C has crackles in both lung bases, and her cardiac monitor shows a sinus rhythm, at a rate of 94 to 96 beats/min, with occasional premature ventricular contractions (PVCs).

1. You review the treatments prescribed by the ED physician. Which is most important to clarify at this time?
   1. Infuse D_5W at 10 cc/hr.
   2. Administer O_2 per CCU policy.
   3. Give MS 2-4 mg IV PRN dyspnea or pain.
   4. Start nitro drip per protocol PRN chest pain.

When Ms. C arrives in the CCU, you find that she is sitting up in bed at a 60-degree angle. She is pale, with circumoral cyanosis, and her respirations appear labored and rapid. You ask if she feels more short of breath. Because she is unable to catch her breath enough to speak, she nods her head yes.

2. What action should you take first?
   1. Listen to her breath sounds.
   2. Ask when the dyspnea started.
   3. Increase her oxygen flow rate to 6 L/min.
   4. Raise the head of the bed to 75 to 85 degrees.

When you assess her, you find that she has crackles audible throughout both lung fields and is coughing up pink, frothy sputum. Her oxygen saturation is 85% with the oxygen turned up to 6 L/min. Her respiratory rate is 38 breaths/min. She also has 3+ to 4+ pitting edema in her feet and up to midcalf. Even though you have the bed elevated to a 75-degree angle, you can see her jugular veins distended up to her jawline.

3. Which complication are you most concerned about, based on your assessment?
   1. Pulmonary edema
   2. Cor pulmonale
   3. Myocardial infarction
   4. Pulmonary embolus

4. Which action will you take next?
   1. Activate the hospital's Rapid Response Team.
   2. Switch to a nonrebreather mask at a flow rate of 15 L/min.
   3. Assist the client to cough and deep breathe.
   4. Administer the ordered morphine sulfate 2 mg IV to the client.

5. What additional assessment data are most important to obtain at this time?
   1. Skin color and capillary refill
   2. Orientation and pupil reaction to light
   3. Heart sounds and point of maximum impulse
   4. Blood pressure and apical pulse

6. Ms. C's blood pressure is 98/52 mm Hg and her apical pulse is 116 beats/min and irregular. The cardiac monitor shows sinus tachycardia at a rate of 110 to 120 beats/min, with frequent multifocal PVCs. After receiving orders from the health care provider, which intervention will you implement first?
   1. Give enalapril (Vasotec) 2.5 mg by mouth (PO).
   2. Administer furosemide (Lasix) 100 mg IV.
   3. Obtain a blood potassium level.
   4. Insert a no. 16 French Foley catheter.

7. Which prescribed action is best to delegate to the experienced LPN/LVN who is assisting you?
   1. Give enalapril 2.5 mg PO.
   2. Administer furosemide 100 mg IV.
   3. Obtain a blood potassium level.
   4. Insert a no. 16 French Foley catheter.

8. While you are waiting for the results of the potassium testing, you administer morphine sulfate 2 mg to Ms. C. A new RN graduate who has just started in CCU asks why you are giving the morphine. What is the best response?
   1. "To help prevent chest discomfort."
   2. "To slow Ms. C's respiratory rate."
   3. "To lower Ms. C's anxiety level."
   4. "To decrease venous return to the heart."

9. Ms. C's potassium level is 3.1 mEq/L. The health care provider prescribes potassium chloride (KCl) 20 mEq IV before the furosemide is administered. How will you administer the KCl?
   1. Use an infusion pump to give the KCl over 10 minutes.
   2. Dilute the KCl in 100 mL of 5% dextrose in water (D_5W) and infuse over 1 hour.
   3. Administer the KCl by IV push over at least 1 minute using a 10-mL syringe.
   4. Add the KCl to 1 L of D_5W and administer over 8 hours.

10. After you have infused the KCl, you administer the furosemide to Ms. C. Which nursing action will be most useful in evaluating whether the furosemide is having the desired effect?
    1. Weighing the client daily
    2. Measuring the hourly urine output
    3. Monitoring blood pressure
    4. Assessing lung sounds

11. Ms. C's health care provider arrives and, after assessing her status, prescribes nesiritide (Natrecor) 100 mcg (2 mcg/kg) IV bolus, followed by a continuous IV infusion of 0.5 mcg/min (0.01 mcg/kg/min). Which parameter is most important to monitor during the nesiritide infusion?
    1. Heart rate
    2. Blood pressure
    3. Peripheral edema
    4. Neurologic status

12. You are preparing to leave at the end of your shift. Which nurse is the best to assign to care for Ms. C?
    1. Float RN who has worked on the coronary step-down unit for 9 years and has floated to the CCU before
    2. RN from a staffing agency who has 5 years of CCU experience and is orienting to your CCU today
    3. Experienced CCU RN who is already assigned to care for a newly admitted client with chest trauma
    4. Newly-graduated RN who needs more experience in caring for clients with left ventricular failure

When you return a few days later, Ms. C has improved enough to transfer to the coronary step-down unit. Her weight has decreased 4 kg from the admission weight. She experiences no shortness of breath at rest, and she has crackles only at the lung bases. She is receiving oxygen at 1 L/min via nasal cannula. When taking her apical pulse, you notice that she does have a grade III/VI murmur at the apex of the heart and that her pulse is very irregular. The cardiac monitor shows atrial fibrillation at a rate of 80 to 100 beats/min. Ms. C reports no dizziness but says that her vision seems "fuzzy." She has 2+ pitting ankle edema. Her vital sign measurements are as follows:

Blood pressure	118/62 mm Hg
Heart rate	86 beats/min
O_2 saturation	95%
Respiratory rate	24 breaths/min
Temperature	97.8° F (36.6° C)

Her medications are the following:
- *Furosemide (Lasix) 40 mg PO twice daily*
- *Aspirin (Ecotrin) 81 mg PO daily*
- *KCl (K-Dur) 10 mEq PO daily*
- *Enalapril (Vasotec) 2.5 mg PO twice daily*
- *Digoxin (Lanoxin) 0.25 mg PO daily*

13. Which of the assessment findings described earlier are most important to report to the physician?
    1. Crackles and oxygen saturation
    2. Atrial fibrillation and fuzzy vision
    3. Apical murmur and pulse rate
    4. Peripheral edema and weight

14. All of Ms. C's medications are scheduled to be given at 9:00 AM. Which ones will you hold until you have discussed them with her physician? *(Select all that apply.)*
    1. Furosemide
    2. Aspirin
    3. KCl
    4. Enalapril
    5. Digoxin

15. Using the SBAR (situation, background, assessment, recommendation) format, indicate the order in which you will communicate this information to the physician.
    1. "Ms. C has been receiving digoxin and furosemide for several days. I think her symptoms may indicate digoxin toxicity."
    2. "I'd like to hold the scheduled digoxin and furosemide until digoxin and potassium levels are checked."
    3. "This is the nurse caring for Ms. C; I am calling because she has some new-onset atrial fibrillation and reports of fuzzy vision."
    4. "Ms. C was admitted several days ago with pulmonary edema and dyspnea. She has a history of mitral regurgitation." _____, _____, _____, _____

Ms. C is discharged 2 days later. Her discharge medications are:
- *Furosemide (Lasix) 40 mg PO twice daily*
- *Aspirin (Ecotrin) 81 mg PO daily*
- *KCl (K-Dur) 10 mEq PO three times daily*
- *Enalapril (Vasotec) 2.5 mg PO twice daily*
- *Digoxin (Lanoxin) 0.125 mg PO every other day*

In addition, the physician orders a new medication, carvedilol (Coreg) 3.125 mg PO twice daily. A home health referral is also ordered.

16. Which information will you include when developing the discharge teaching plan? *(Select all that apply.)*
    1. Plan to weigh yourself every day at the same time.
    2. Call if you feel more short of breath or have weight gain.
    3. Take the furosemide first thing in the morning and again at bedtime.
    4. Drink at least 2500 mL of fluids daily.
    5. Move slowly when changing from a lying to a standing position.
    6. You will need a follow-up appointment soon after being discharged.

When Ms. C is visited by the home health nurse the next week, she tells the nurse that she feels "tired enough to take a nap every afternoon." In addition, she is concerned because "even though I'm on a much lower dose of digoxin than I used to be, my pulse rate has been 58 to 62." She has called the physician's office and was told to continue all her medications as ordered.

17. Based on this information, what nursing action is indicated for Ms. C?
    1. Teach her about the expected effects of carvedilol.
    2. Tell her to restrict her fluid intake to 1000 mL/day.
    3. Arrange for transport to the ED for treatment.
    4. Encourage her to go to bed earlier in the evening.

PART 3

Complex Health Scenarios

Answer Key for this case study begins on p. 228.

Multiple Patients with Peripheral Vascular Disease

You are the RN team leader working with an LPN/LVN, an experienced UAP, and a nursing student to provide nursing care for six patients in a vascular surgery unit. The patients are as follows:

- *Ms. C, a 38-year-old woman with Raynaud disease, who reports numbness, tingling, and cold in wrists and hands bilaterally*
- *Mr. R, a 57-year-old man with chronic peripheral arterial disease, who reports severe pain due to an arterial ulcer on his left great toe*
- *Mr. Z, a 44-year-old man with Buerger disease, who wants to discuss enrolling in a smoking cessation program*
- *Ms. Q, a 69-year-old woman with chronic hypertension, whose blood pressure at the end of the night shift was 208/96 mm Hg*
- *Mr. S, a 72-year-old man in whom an abdominal aortic aneurysm (AAA) must be ruled out, who is reporting severe, worsening back pain*
- *Ms. A, a 65-year-old woman with peripheral venous disease and calf swelling, who is scheduled for Doppler flow studies this morning*

1. After the change-of-shift report, you make rounds. List the priority order for assessing your patients.
   1. Ms. C
   2. Mr. R
   3. Mr. Z
   4. Ms. Q
   5. Mr. S
   6. Ms. A

   ____, ____, ____, ____, ____, ____

2. When Mr. S is assessed, which assessment technique would you instruct the student nurse to avoid?
   1. Auscultating the abdomen for a bruit
   2. Palpating the abdomen to detect a mass
   3. Observing the abdomen for a pulsation
   4. Performing a pain assessment

3. Mr. S continues to report severe back pain. On assessment, you detect a bruit and notice pulsation in the left lower quadrant. What is your best first action?
   1. Measure abdominal girth.
   2. Place the patient in a high sitting position.
   3. Notify the patient's health care provider.
   4. Administer pain medication.

4. All of these orders for Mr. S are placed by the health care provider. Which action should you delegate to the LPN/LVN?
   1. Insert a Foley catheter.
   2. Administer morphine sulfate 2 mg IV push.
   3. Place a second IV saline lock line.
   4. Measure vital signs every 15 minutes.

5. A computed tomographic (CT) scan reveals that Mr. S has an aneurysm that is 7.5 cm in diameter. Which preoperative care tasks should you delegate to the nursing student under your supervision? *(Select all that apply.)*
   1. Teaching Mr. S about coughing and deep breathing
   2. Assessing all peripheral pulses for postoperative comparison
   3. Administering bowel preparation magnesium sulfate orally
   4. Drawing blood for the laboratory for typing and screening
   5. Discussing the reasons for the surgery

6. Mr. S underwent surgery yesterday. The student nurse reports that the patient has no bowel sounds present. What is your best action?
   1. Check the nasogastric tube for kinks.
   2. Notify the surgeon immediately.
   3. Obtain an abdominal radiograph at once (STAT).
   4. Document the finding in the chart.

7. At 8:30 AM, the UAP reports that Ms. Q, with chronic hypertension, has a blood pressure of 198/94 mm Hg. Which is the best task delegation?
   1. Have the LPN/LVN give Ms. Q's 9:00 AM furosemide (Lasix) and enalapril (Vasotec) now.
   2. Instruct the UAP to get Ms. Q back into bed immediately.
   3. Tell the UAP to remeasure Ms. Q's blood pressure every 15 minutes.
   4. Send the LPN/LVN to recheck Ms. Q's blood pressure to ensure that the reading is correct.

8. A nursing diagnosis of Chronic Pain has been identified for Mr. R, who has chronic peripheral arterial disease. Which action by the nursing student causes you to intervene?
   1. Administering a narcotic analgesic 45 minutes before an ulcer dressing change
   2. Asking the patient if he has ever tried progressive muscle relaxation
   3. Assessing the patient's response to pain medication administration
   4. Agreeing to hold the patient's docusate (Colace) at the patient's request

9. At noon, the LPN/LVN goes to cardiopulmonary resuscitation training and is replaced by an RN floated from the postanesthesia care unit (PACU). Which patients should you assign to the PACU RN? *(Select all that apply.)*
   1. Ms. C, who needs teaching about how to avoid exacerbation of symptoms for her condition
   2. Mr. Z, who still needs information about available smoking cessation programs
   3. Ms. Q, whose blood pressure is still elevated and needs frequent blood pressure monitoring
   4. Ms. A, who is worried because the health care provider just told her she has a deep vein thrombosis
   5. Mr. S, who reports that his back pain is getting much worse

10. You are preparing a teaching plan for Ms. C, who has Raynaud disease. Which key points should you include? *(Select all that apply.)*
    1. Avoid exposure to cold by wearing warm clothes.
    2. The nifedipine (Procardia) will help decrease and relieve your symptoms.
    3. Keep your home at a comfortably warm temperature.
    4. The problems you experience are due to vasoconstriction.
    5. Stress reduction techniques can help prevent symptoms.

11. A nursing diagnosis of Ineffective Peripheral Tissue Perfusion has been identified for Ms. C. Which actions should you delegate to the experienced UAP? *(Select all that apply.)*
    1. Assessing for peripheral pulses, edema, capillary refill, and skin temperature
    2. Inspecting the skin for the presence of tissue breakdown and arterial ulcers
    3. Reminding the patient to perform active range-of-motion exercises as tolerated
    4. Reinforcing with the patient the need to take in adequate fluids during the day
    5. Assisting the patient to sit at the bedside and then transfer to a chair

12. Ms. A, whose calf is swollen from peripheral venous disease, asks why she must have an injection of heparin. What is your best response?
    1. "Heparin will dissolve the clots in your legs."
    2. "Heparin will prevent new clots from forming."
    3. "Heparin will thin your blood and slow down clotting."
    4. "Heparin will prevent the clots from migrating to your lungs."

13. Ms. A has received a nursing diagnosis of Risk for Injury. Which action will you delegate to the UAP?
    1. Assisting the patient with morning care and ambulation to the bathroom
    2. Monitoring the patient's daily international normalized ratio (INR)
    3. Checking the patient every 4 hours for signs of bleeding
    4. Telling the patient to call for assistance when getting out of bed

14. The UAP reports to the RN that Mr. Z, with Buerger disease, awoke from a nap reporting pain in the arch of his left foot. Which actions should you take? *(Select all that apply).*
    1. Assess the patient's pain.
    2. Initiate a consult for smoking cessation.
    3. Place the patient in a supine position and elevate the foot.
    4. Administer oral analgesics.
    5. Instruct the patient to avoid cold temperatures.

15. You are reviewing the lipid profile for Ms. Q, who has been diagnosed with atherosclerosis. Which finding is of most concern?
    1. Total serum cholesterol level of 220 mg/dL
    2. Triglyceride level of 165 mg/dL
    3. Low-density lipoprotein (LDL) cholesterol level of 104 mg/dL
    4. High-density lipoprotein (HDL) cholesterol level of 25 mg/dL

Answer Key for this case study begins on p. 230.

Respiratory Difficulty After Surgery

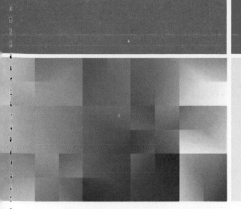

You have just received the change-of-shift report about Mr. E., a 26-year-old who had a ruptured appendix with emergency appendectomy 2 days ago. The report included this information about Mr. E's vital signs, assessments, and prescribed therapies:

Vital Signs
- *Temp: 101.4° F (38.6° C)*
- *Pulse: 108 (sinus tachycardia)*
- *Resp: 28*
- *BP: 148/76*
- *O_2 saturation 90% (decreased from 98% over the last 4 hours)*

Assessment
- *Respiratory: Breath sounds decreased throughout lungs; nonproductive cough*
- *GI: Bowel sounds present, brown purulent drainage from wound drain*
- *Neuro: Alert and oriented × 3*

Therapies
- *O_2 at 3 L/min*
- *Antibiotics: Gentamicin (Gentacidin) and ceftriaxone (Rocephin) IV*
- *ABGs, CBC, BUN, electrolytes, and glucose pending*
- *Gentamicin trough level ordered*

1. Based on the information you have been given during the change-of-shift report, what is your greatest concern for Mr. E?
   1. Purulent abdominal drainage
   2. Sinus tachycardia
   3. Decreased oxygen saturation
   4. Elevated temperature

2. You review Mr. E's medications and note that he has a dose of gentamicin scheduled at 10:00 AM. When will you ask the laboratory to draw blood for determining gentamicin trough level?
   1. 9:00 AM
   2. 9:45 AM
   3. 11:30 AM
   4. 2:00 PM

When you go into Mr. E's room to assess him, you find him sitting in a chair at the bedside. His respirations look labored, with a rate of 30 breaths/min. His continuous pulse oximetry readings indicate that his oxygen saturation is 88% to 89%. He looks anxious and says, "I'm having a little trouble catching my breath." His lung sounds are still decreased at the bases, with persistent fine crackles.

3. What action will you take next?
   1. Assist him back to bed.
   2. Increase the oxygen flow rate to 6 L/min.
   3. Administer the "as needed" (PRN) morphine IV.
   4. Finish the rest of his head-to-toe assessment.

The arterial blood gas (ABG) analysis is completed and the following results are faxed to the unit:

Arterial partial pressure of carbon dioxide ($PaCO_2$)	30 mm Hg
Arterial partial pressure of oxygen (PaO_2)	54 mm Hg
Bicarbonate (HCO_3^-)	20 mEq/L
O_2 saturation	88%
pH	7.34

4. Which action will you take next based on the ABG results?
   1. Place Mr. E on oxygen at 15 L/min via a nonrebreather mask.
   2. Obtain an order for sodium bicarbonate 50 mEq IV.
   3. Administer the PRN morphine to slow the respiratory rate.
   4. Continue to monitor Mr. E's respiratory status and vital signs.

5. The complete blood count (CBC) results are now also available. Which result causes you the most concern?
   1. Hematocrit of 37%
   2. Hemoglobin level of 10.5 g/dL
   3. White blood cell (WBC) count of 24,000/mm³
   4. Platelet count of 120,000/mm³

You realize that Mr. E's condition is unstable and that you will not have time to assess or provide care for your other assigned client, Ms. O. A client with diabetes, Ms. O was admitted yesterday with pyelonephritis and hyperglycemia. She is receiving a regular insulin infusion (Novolin R) using the hospital's standard insulin sliding-scale protocols and needs to have blood glucose monitoring every hour. Her temperature has decreased from 102° F to 100.6° F (38.9° C to 38.1° C) since IV ceftizoxime (Cefizox) was started yesterday.

6. Which staff member is best to assign to care for Ms. O?
   1. RN who has 10 years of experience on the pediatric unit and has floated to the step-down unit for the day
   2. Newly-graduated RN who has finished a 3-month orientation and is scheduled for the first day without a preceptor
   3. On-call RN with 5 years of experience on the step-down unit who will be able to arrive in about 1 hour
   4. Experienced RN from a staffing agency who is on orientation to the unit today in preparation for a 6-month assignment

7. After 15 minutes of oxygen administration using the nonrebreather mask, Mr. E's pulse oximeter still indicates that the oxygen saturation is 88% to 89%. What complication is Mr. E most likely experiencing, based on your ongoing assessments of this client?
   1. Aspiration pneumonia
   2. Pulmonary embolism
   3. Spontaneous tension pneumothorax
   4. Acute respiratory distress syndrome (ARDS)

8. Using the SBAR (situation, background, assessment, recommendation) format, indicate the order in which you will communicate your concerns about Mr. E to the physician.
   1. "Today, Mr. E's pulse oximetry reading is only 88% to 90%, although he is receiving oxygen by a nonrebreather mask. I am concerned he may be developing ARDS."
   2. "This is the nurse caring for Mr. E. I'm calling because the client is reporting dyspnea and has increasing hypoxemia."
   3. "I think that you need to come and evaluate this client as soon as possible; he may need mechanical ventilation."
   4. "Mr. E had an emergency appendectomy 2 days ago and has had purulent abdominal drainage, but has not had any respiratory difficulty until today." _____,
   _____, _____, _____

9. Mr. E's surgeon arrives and asks the hospital intensivist to consult. The intensivist gives these orders after assessing Mr. E. Which one will you implement first?
   1. Place the client on bilevel positive airway pressure (BiPAP) ventilation.
   2. Obtain an intubation tray and assist with client intubation.
   3. Administer nebulized albuterol (Proventil) every 4 hours.
   4. Obtain blood, urine, and abdominal drainage samples for culture.

The intensivist orders that Mr. E be transferred to the intensive care unit (ICU) and tells you to obtain the necessary equipment for intubation and mechanical ventilation. After the transfer, the intensivist proceeds to intubate Mr. E.

10. Which is the most accurate way to confirm correct placement of the endotracheal (ET) tube?
    1. Obtain a chest radiograph.
    2. Auscultate bilateral breath sounds.
    3. Use continuous wave-form capnography.
    4. Check pulse oximetry level.

Mr. E's ET tube placement is confirmed and the ET tube is secured. You note that the 23-cm mark on the ET tube is at the level of Mr. E's teeth. Mr. E is connected to a positive-pressure ventilator with the following settings:

Fraction of inspired oxygen (FIO$_2$)	70%
Mode	*Synchronized intermittent mandatory ventilation*
Positive end-expiratory pressure	*10 cm*
Respiratory rate	*30 breaths/min*
Tidal volume (V$_T$)	*400 mL*

The following ABG values are obtained 30 minutes after Mr. E is placed on the ventilator:

HCO$_3^-$	*20 mEq/L*
O$_2$ saturation	*94%*
PaCO$_2$	*47 mm Hg*
PaO$_2$	*60 mm Hg*
pH	*7.31*

11. Which ventilator change do you anticipate based on your analysis of these ABG values?
    1. Increasing the V$_T$ to 600 mL
    2. Changing the rate on the ventilator to 35 breaths/min
    3. Decreasing the FIO$_2$ to 60%
    4. Changing to continuous mandatory ventilation (CMV) mode

You assist with the insertion of Mr. E's pulmonary artery catheter (Swan-Ganz catheter) so that pulmonary artery wedge pressure (PAWP) can be monitored. An arterial line is also inserted into the left radial artery. In addition, you insert a nasogastric (NG) tube and connect it to low intermittent suction.

When you reassess Mr. E, he has scattered crackles audible throughout both lung fields. He is restless and needs frequent reminding not to pull on the ET tube or NG tube. His urine output over the last 2 hours has been 50 mL of clear amber urine. His bowel sounds are slightly hypotonic but are audible in all four abdominal quadrants. His abdominal dressing is still dry and intact, and the drainage in the Jackson-Pratt drain is unchanged. You obtain the following vital signs and PAWP values for Mr. E:

Blood pressure (BP)	100/46 mm Hg
Heart rate	124 beats/min (sinus tachycardia)
O₂ saturation	90%
PAWP	3 mm Hg
Respirations	24 breaths/min
Temperature	102.1° F (38.9° C)

12. Based on these data, which collaborative interventions will you anticipate for Mr. E? *(Select all that apply.)*
    1. Increase the IV rate to 150 mL/hr.
    2. Administer furosemide (Lasix) 40 mg IV.
    3. Start norepinephrine (Levophed) infusion.
    4. Give diltiazem (Cardizem) 15 mg IV.
    5. Infuse total parenteral nutrition at 70 mL/hr.
    6. Administer high-calorie enteral feeding at 25 mL/hr.
    7. Obtain blood, sputum, and urine specimens for culture.

13. Although his oxygen saturation remains at 90%, Mr. E continues to be restless and needs frequent reminders to not pull at the ET tube. Which method to reduce his anxiety and decrease the risk for accidental extubation will you try first?
    1. Obtain an order to restrain his hands, and apply soft wrist restraints.
    2. Administer neuromuscular blockade medications and sedatives.
    3. Have a family member stay at Mr. E's bedside and reassure him.
    4. Remind Mr. E frequently that he needs the ET tube to breathe.

14. You are working with a student who is preparing to suction Mr. E's ET tube. Which action by the student requires that you intervene immediately?
    1. Increasing the Fio₂ to 100% for 5 minutes before suctioning
    2. Using an open-suction technique to perform the suctioning
    3. Administering morphine 2 mg IV per standing order before suctioning
    4. Applying suction to the catheter while inserting it into the ET tube

15. Which action is most important to implement to prevent Mr. E from developing ventilator-associated pneumonia (VAP)?
    1. Change the ventilator tubing and humidifier daily.
    2. Avoid giving intermittent bolus enteral feedings.
    3. Keep the head of the bed elevated to at least 30 degrees.
    4. Use continuous pulse oximetry monitoring.

16. All of these activities are included in the standard plan of care for a client with ARDS. Which activities can you delegate to an experienced LPN/LVN? *(Select all that apply.)*
    1. Provide oral care every 2 hours.
    2. Place the client in the prone position for 4 hours every shift.
    3. Check residuals for enteral feedings every 4 hours.
    4. Assess breath sounds every 4 hours.
    5. Check temperature every 4 hours.
    6. Suction the ET tube as needed.
    7. Educate the client and family about routine nursing care.
    8. Check the PAWP every 2 hours.
    9. Obtain arterial pressures from the arterial line every hour.

You are documenting the events of the morning at the ICU nurse's station when you hear the ventilator alarm. You enter the room and find that the high pressure alarm is sounding and that Mr. E appears very agitated, with a respiratory rate of 40 breaths/min. The continuous pulse oximeter indicates an oxygen saturation of 81%. The blood pressure displayed on the arterial line monitor is 98/44 mm Hg. Mr. E's cardiac monitor shows a sinus tachycardia with a rate of 142 beats/min.

17. What action will you accomplish first?
    1. Listen to Mr. E's breath sounds.
    2. Increase the Fio₂ setting to 100%.
    3. Check the ventilator settings and readouts.
    4. Suction Mr. E's ET tube after hyperoxygenating him.

PART 3   Complex Health Scenarios

18. You do not hear any breath sounds over Mr. E's right side, and the right side does not expand much with inspiration. When you check the location of the ET tube at the client's teeth, you find that it is still at the 23-cm mark. What complication of intubation and mechanical ventilation do you suspect?
    1. Inadvertent extubation
    2. Tension pneumothorax
    3. ET tube displacement
    4. Aspiration pneumonia

19. The intensivist arrives quickly and inserts a chest tube into the right anterior chest at the second intercostal space. You assess Mr. E after the chest tube insertion. Which finding is most important to report to the physician?
    1. A large number of air bubbles appear in the water-seal chamber during expiration.
    2. Continuous bubbling occurs throughout the respiratory cycle in the suction control chamber.
    3. 100 mL of blood drains into the collection chamber immediately after the chest tube insertion.
    4. The client indicates that he has pain with every ventilator-assisted inspiration.

20. Just before you prepare to give a change-of-shift report to the oncoming RN, you review Mr. E's other laboratory test results for today. Which information is most important to communicate to the physician?
    1. Blood glucose level of 140 mg/dL
    2. Potassium level of 5.1 mEq/L
    3. Sodium level of 134 mEq/L
    4. Blood urea nitrogen (BUN) level of 52 mg/dL

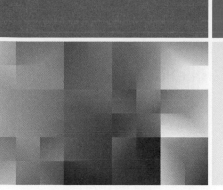

CASE STUDY 18

Long-Term Care

You are the nursing supervisor for the evening shift at a 30-bed long-term care facility (nursing home). Your staff for the evening includes an LPN/LVN and three UAPs. During change-of-shift report, you receive reports on the following six patients:

- *Mr. B is a 79-year-old man who underwent hip replacement surgery 3 days ago. He needs help getting out of bed, getting dressed, and ambulating. He was admitted yesterday from the hospital for rehabilitation.*
- *Ms. R is an 86-year-old woman who has heart failure and type 2 diabetes and is recovering from a recent myocardial infarction (MI). She has an indwelling Foley catheter. She is usually alert, but she has become confused over the past 12 hours.*
- *Mr. K is a 53-year-old man with a diagnosis of amyotrophic lateral sclerosis (ALS). He is totally dependent with regard to activities of daily living (ADLs) and has an indwelling percutaneous endoscopic gastrostomy (PEG) tube through which he receives intermittent feedings. He has a living will requesting that no heroic measures be used to prolong his life.*
- *Ms. L is an 81-year-old woman with diagnoses of hypertension and Alzheimer disease. She is pleasantly confused, wanders off the unit when not watched, and needs reminders for ADLs.*
- *Mr. W is a 68-year-old man who has chronic kidney disease, coronary artery disease, and chronic obstructive pulmonary disease (COPD). He is currently reporting shortness of breath and is receiving oxygen at 2 L/min via nasal cannula while lying in bed with his head elevated. He needs help with ADLs.*
- *Ms. Q is a 95-year-old woman with a diagnosis of osteoarthritis. She needs help getting out of bed, bathing, and dressing.*

1. The care of which patients can be assigned to the UAPs? *(Select all that apply.)*
   1. Mr. B
   2. Ms. R
   3. Mr. K
   4. Ms. L
   5. Mr. W
   6. Ms. Q

2. Which patient should you see first?
   1. Ms. R
   2. Mr. K
   3. Mr. W
   4. Ms. Q

3. Which aspect of patient care is most appropriately delegated to the LPN/LVN?
   1. Assisting Mr. B to ambulate to the end of the hall and back
   2. Administering Mr. K's 6:00 PM tube feeding
   3. Reminding Ms. L to use the bathroom every 4 hours
   4. Assessing Mr. W's oxygenation status

4. Mr. W continues to report shortness of breath when you assess him. You hear bilateral crackles with auscultation. He has a productive cough with thick greenish sputum. What should you check next?
   1. Oxygen saturation
   2. Blood pressure
   3. Heart rate
   4. Urine output

5. What is the priority nursing diagnosis for Mr. W?
   1. Ineffective Peripheral Tissue Perfusion
   2. Risk for Excess Fluid Volume
   3. Impaired Comfort related to chest pain
   4. Impaired Gas Exchange

6. Mr. W's arterial oxygen saturation (Sao₂) by pulse oximetry is now 85%. What is your best first action?
   1. Increase his oxygen flow rate to 8 L/min via nasal cannula.
   2. Attempt to suction the patient's airway by the nasotracheal route.
   3. Assist the patient to lie down in bed.
   4. Notify the health care provider.

The RN has received the following orders from Mr. W's health care provider:

- *Obtain a sputum sample for culture and sensitivity testing.*
- *Have the patient use incentive spirometry every 2 hours while awake.*
- *Check pulse oximeter oxygen saturation (SpO$_2$) every 4 hours.*
- *Administer levofloxacin (Levaquin) 250 mg by mouth (PO) twice daily.*

7. To which staff member would it be appropriate to delegate carrying out these orders from the provider?
   1. Experienced UAP
   2. Experienced LPN/LVN
   3. Newly graduated LPN/LVN
   4. RN supervisor

8. Your next patient to assess is Ms. R, who has become confused during the past 12 hours. You find that she does not recognize you or know where she is. The UAP tells you that Ms. R has been incontinent with liquid stool for the past 2 days. The urine in her Foley catheter collection bag is dark with a strong odor. What is the priority nursing diagnosis for Ms. R?
   1. Risk for Impaired Skin Integrity
   2. Impaired Verbal Communication
   3. Acute Confusion
   4. Risk for Infection

9. You notify Ms. R's health care provider about your assessment findings. Which provider and nursing orders will you assign to the UAP? *(Select all that apply.)*
   1. Obtain a urine sample for culture and sensitivity testing.
   2. Administer diphenoxylate (Lomotil) 5 mg PO every 6 hours until liquid stools resolve.
   3. Give ciprofloxacin (Cipro) 250 mg PO every 12 hours for 3 days.
   4. Reorient the patient to time, date, and place as needed.
   5. Check the patient for liquid stools at least every 2 hours.
   6. Perform catheter care every shift.
   7. Obtain a stool sample for ova and parasite testing.

10. Which provider and nursing orders are most appropriately delegated to the LPN/LVN? *(Select all that apply.)*
    1. Obtain a urine sample for culture and sensitivity testing.
    2. Administer diphenoxylate 5 mg PO every 6 hours until liquid stools resolve.
    3. Give ciprofloxacin 250 mg PO every 12 hours for 3 days.
    4. Reorient the patient to time, date, and place as needed.
    5. Check the patient for liquid stools at least every 2 hours.
    6. Perform catheter care every shift.
    7. Obtain a stool sample for ova and parasite testing.

11. Near the end of your shift, you reassess Mr. W. He reports that his breathing is better. The UAP tells you that his latest pulse oximetry reading is 90%. What is your best action?
    1. Notify the health care provider.
    2. Decrease the oxygen flow.
    3. Document the findings as the only action.
    4. Instruct the night shift UAP to wake Mr. W every hour for incentive spirometry.

12. The UAP reports that Mr. B, who had hip replacement surgery 3 days ago, refuses to get out of bed to walk in the hall as ordered. What is your best first action?
    1. Ask the LPN/LVN to administer "as needed" (PRN) pain medication.
    2. Tell the UAP that Mr. B must get up to prevent pneumonia.
    3. Remind the UAP the Mr. B has the right to refuse.
    4. Assess Mr. B for the reason he does not want to get up.

13. Mr. B tells you that he was taking a nap when the UAP woke him to get up and walk. He reports that he did not sleep well last night because of being in a strange setting and was angry at being awakened. What are your best actions at this time? *(Select all that apply.)*
    1. Ask Mr. B if he is willing to get up and walk now.
    2. Remind Mr. B that there are 30 patients who need care.
    3. Offer Mr. B PRN pain medication before he gets up to walk.
    4. Instruct the UAP never to wake a patient from a nap.
    5. Discuss strategies to help Mr. B achieve good rest at night.
    6. Teach Mr. B the importance of preventing respiratory problems.

14. Ms. Q, with osteoarthritis, refuses to take her evening dose of calcium because it makes her stomach upset. What is the priority teaching for the LPN/LVN at this time?

    1. Tell the LPN/LVN that Ms. Q must take her calcium because she is at risk for fractures.
    2. Suggest rescheduling the dose time so that Ms. Q receives the calcium with food.
    3. Remind the LPN/LVN that calcium is best absorbed on an empty stomach.
    4. Instruct the LPN/LVN to hold the dose and notify the provider.

15. Ms. L, with Alzheimer disease, wanders into Mr. K's room. The LPN/LVN finds her disconnecting Mr. K's tube feeding. "Hello, dearie, I was just cleaning this up for you," Ms. L tells the LPN/LVN. What is the best action for the LPN/LVN to take at this time?

    1. In a loud and stern voice, tell Ms. L that this is not her room.
    2. Ask the UAP to escort Ms. L back to her room and keep her there.
    3. Gently reorient Ms. L and reconnect Mr. K's tube feeding.
    4. Remind Ms. L that she is not a nurse but a patient and should never bother other patients.

16. Mr. K's mother comes running out of his room yelling, "He's dying! Call 911! Hurry, hurry!" What is your best action at this time?

    1. Call the life squad, because the mother's wishes supersede Mr. K's.
    2. Call the health care provider to ask what you should do.
    3. Begin cardiopulmonary resuscitation and continue until the life squad arrives.
    4. Assess Mr. K's status and respect his wishes.

Answer Key for this case study begins on p. 233.

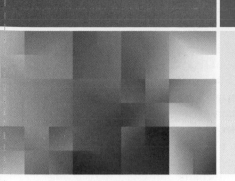

You are working in a large urban pediatric walk-in clinic that offers well-baby care, provides immunizations, and is an educational resource for child health topics. In addition, the clinic also accommodates walk-in clients and offers basic diagnostic testing and emergency care. The staff includes a pediatrician, a graduate student who is working toward an advanced practice nursing (APN) degree, an experienced RN, an experienced LPN/LVN, a pediatric social worker, a new graduate nurse (GN), and a UAP. Today, you are the charge nurse. This morning, in addition to scheduled appointments, there is an immunization clinic. You receive two phone calls, and there is one walk-in client.

1. Which member(s) of the staff (pediatrician, APN student, RN, LPN/LVN, pediatric social worker, GN, and/or UAP) should perform each of these tasks and duties to ensure that the general work flow of the clinic is efficient and that each team member is being used in the most effective manner? *(More than one staff member may be appropriate to list for some tasks.)*
   1. Perform well-baby physical examinations, including assessment of growth and developmental milestones.
      _____
   2. Perform triage for walk-in clients. _____
   3. Give routine immunizations. _____
   4. Obtain weight and height measurements. _____
   5. Ensure that the play therapy area is stocked and organized. _____
   6. Stock the treatment rooms with linens and supplies.
      _____
   7. Perform a physical assessment of walk-in clients.
      _____
   8. Supervise the APN student. _____

2. A mother brings her 12-month-old child to the clinic for an influenza vaccination. The nurse tells the mother that the child is also due for doses of measles-mumps-rubella, varicella, and hepatitis A vaccines. The mother declines the nurse's advice because "he has already had enough of those." What is the priority action?
   1. Encourage a follow-up appointment and notify Child Protective Services.
   2. Assess the mother's concerns and current level of knowledge about immunization.

3. Emphasize the benefits of immunization; explain the purpose and schedule.
4. Respect the mother's decision and alert the pediatrician to the situation.

3. Before giving a child an immunization, you note that the child is flushed and warm, is acting fussy, and has rhinorrhea. What is the priority action?
   1. Notify the pediatrician and obtain an order for an antipyretic.
   2. Assess the child for additional symptoms of febrile illness.
   3. Advise the mother that fever is a contraindication and reschedule the appointment.
   4. Give cool fluids to reduce fever and apply an anesthetic cream to the injection site.

4. A parent calls in for advice because her 18-month-old toddler has stumbled and bumped his head on the coffee table. Which symptom is cause for the greatest concern?
   1. A swelling the size of a golf ball that is tender to the touch
   2. Two episodes of vomiting a small amount of undigested food
   3. Continuous crying for 2 hours, unrelieved by familiar comfort measures
   4. Gaping 4-cm laceration on the forehead, with bleeding controlled by pressure

5. A parent calls in for advice because "Missy is 5 years old and she just won't sleep in her own bed. For the past 4 months, she wakes and comes to sleep with me and my husband. She cries and cries if we take her back to her own room." What is the priority action?
   1. Send the mother a brochure of things she can try to assist the child to sleep independently.
   2. Advise the mother that this is a normal behavior that will eventually pass with time.
   3. Suggest that the child be put back into her own bed and allowed to cry herself to sleep.
   4. Schedule an appointment with the APN student for assessment and management.

6. Six-year-old Billy woke last night with dyspnea, restlessness, wheezing, and cough. Mother and child spent the night in a reclining chair. His mother declares, "He is having an asthma attack." What is the priority nursing diagnosis?
   1. Disturbed Sleep Pattern related to difficulty breathing
   2. Impaired Gas Exchange related to thickening of bronchial wall and mucus
   3. Caregiver Role Strain related to duration of a chronic health condition
   4. Fatigue related to inadequate tissue oxygenation

7. As you approach Billy, which presentation would concern you the most and require immediate intervention?
   1. Alert and irritable, lying recumbent on the examination table
   2. Awake and nervous, sitting upright and crying, skin pale and dry
   3. Agitated, sweating, and sitting upright with shoulders hunched forward
   4. Asleep in a side-lying position breathing through open mouth

8. Which assessment finding for Billy is the most urgent and requires immediate intervention and notification of the pediatrician?
   1. Sudden increase in respiratory rate and decreased breath sounds
   2. Rattling cough productive of frothy, clear, gelatinous sputum
   3. Prodromal itching localized over the upper back
   4. Restlessness and wheezing auscultated at the end of expiration

9. As you care for Billy and address his asthmatic condition, in what sequence should the following orders be implemented?
   1. Administer IV methylprednisolone (Solu-Medrol).
   2. Contact the hospital about admission for 23-hour observation.
   3. Give nebulized albuterol (Proventil) every 30 minutes.
   4. Teach about measuring peak expiratory flow rate to determine personal best.
   5. Obtain a chest radiograph and a complete blood count (CBC).
   6. Administer humidified oxygen to maintain saturation above 90%.
   7. Schedule a radioallergosorbent test.

   _____, _____, _____, _____, _____, _____, _____

10. Billy is going to be transferred from the clinic to the hospital for 23-hour observation of his asthmatic condition. Which member(s) of the health care team (pediatrician, RN, LPN/LVN, UAP, and unit secretary) should perform each of these tasks needed to safely transfer this client? *(More than one staff member may be appropriate to list for some tasks.)*
    1. Give a report to the attending physician at the hospital. _____
    2. Give a report to the charge nurse at the receiving hospital. _____
    3. Notify radiology that a copy of the chest radiograph is needed. _____
    4. Help the parent and child to collect personal items. _____
    5. Determine that the client's condition is stable enough for transport to the hospital. _____
    6. Assess the response to treatment and summarize the client's condition. _____
    7. Check the patency of the IV line and convert to a saline lock as needed. _____
    8. Assist the client to transfer to the ambulance stretcher. _____

11. In the afternoon, several clients come to the clinic for walk-in care. Prioritize the following clients in the order in which they should be seen to ensure safe care and efficiently manage client load.
    1. Daisy is 4 years old; she is alert and irritable with pale, sweaty skin. An elderly neighbor who was temporarily watching Daisy reports that she was running around and playing and then she got "grumpy." Daisy has diabetes, but the neighbor "was not sure how to give her the insulin."
    2. Sarah is 11 months old; she is dirty and crying, and her right arm is swollen and red. Sam is Sarah's 2-year-old brother; he is dirty and hungry and signals you to pick him up. Ms. A, their mother, is 19 years old and single. She is thin and disheveled and seems somewhat confused. She is having trouble answering your questions. Ms. A says, "Those kids play too rough! The older one is always pushing the baby off the bed."
    3. Terry is 7 months old; he rubs at his ears, acts fussy, refuses to suck, and has a temperature of 101.2° F (38.4° C). He has had three episodes of otitis in the past. Social history includes being bottle-fed and having parents who are both smokers.
    4. James is 3 years old. He awakened last night with a sore throat, difficulty swallowing, and a fever. He is flushed, anxious, and drooling. You observe a thick, muffled quality to his voice and slow, quiet breathing. You note that James looks sick.

    _____, _____, _____, _____

12. What is the priority diagnosis for James (refer to question 11)?
    1. Hyperthermia related to an infectious process and decreased fluid intake
    2. Ineffective Airway Clearance related to swelling of tissues
    3. Anxiety related to respiratory difficulties and the clinic environment
    4. Impaired Swallowing related to discomfort in the throat

13. What is the priority action for James (refer to question 11)?
    1. Visually inspect the throat with a tongue blade and auscultate the lungs.
    2. Administer humidified oxygen and have the child sit upright on a parent's lap.
    3. Notify the pediatrician and prepare intubation equipment.
    4. Reassure the parents that the symptoms will readily resolve with breathing of cool moist air.

14. The APN student and the physician are at the bedside. Which two additional team members would be the best combination to provide the initial care for James (refer to question 11)?
    1. The experienced RN and the experienced LPN/LVN
    2. The experienced RN and the UAP
    3. The experienced RN and the GN
    4. The experienced LPN/LVN and the GN

15. The pediatrician examines James and determines that he should be taken immediately to the Children's Hospital emergency department (ED). The child is breathing slowly and quietly; humidified oxygen is being administered. What is the priority action?
    1. Instruct the parents to drive the child to the hospital immediately and call the ED.
    2. Contact a private ambulance service and prepare the client for transport.
    3. Call 911, ask for advanced emergency medical services (EMS), and monitor the child.
    4. Assist the pediatrician to intubate the child and then arrange for transport.

16. Daisy (from question 11) has type 1 diabetes. She is currently alert but irritable. She looks pale and her skin is clammy. What is the priority action for Daisy?
    1. Locate the mother to obtain a history and permission to treat.
    2. Administer supplemental oxygen, alert the physician, and establish IV access.
    3. Ask the child to describe how she feels and use simple questions to obtain a history.
    4. Perform blood glucose testing and then give the child a carton of milk.

17. Daisy's mother arrives at the clinic, and she is relieved to find Daisy happy and smiling, but the mother bursts into tears and begins to yell at the elderly neighbor and the nursing staff for "not taking care of her!" What is the best way to handle her anger and tears?
    1. Remind the mother that the child is okay and that the neighbor was doing what she thought was best based on the information that she had.
    2. Allow the mother to express her feelings and then take the neighbor aside and explain that the mother is just temporarily upset.
    3. Teach the mother about ways to communicate the child's needs to all caregivers and help her make a list of specific instructions.
    4. Direct the mother to a private area and encourage her to ventilate feelings, then gently assess how she typically manages Daisy's diabetes.

18. What is the priority nursing diagnosis for Terry, who is rubbing at his ears, acting fussy, refusing to suck, and has a temperature of 101.2° F (38.4° C)?
    1. Acute Pain related to accumulation of fluid behind the tympanic membrane
    2. Imbalanced Nutrition: Less than Body Requirements related to refusal to feed
    3. Deficient Knowledge about risk factors for recurrent ear infections in infants
    4. Hyperthermia related to infection, inflammation, and dehydration

19. For 7-month old Terry, which task would be appropriate to assign to the LPN/LVN?
    1. Teach parents that passive smoking and bottle feeding contribute to ear infections.
    2. Explain the concept of "watchful waiting" for 72 hours for uncomplicated otitis.
    3. Gently irrigate ears to remove cerumen, for assessment of the tympanic membrane.
    4. Administer an antihistamine, a decongestant, a steroid, and an antibiotic as prescribed.

20. The pediatrician writes an order for PRN ibuprofen (Advil) 100 mg by mouth every 6 hours for Terry (weight, 7 kg). According to your drug information book, the appropriate dosage range is 20 to 40 mg/kg/24 hr in four divided doses. What is the priority action?
    1. Give the medication as ordered, because it is within the appropriate dosage range.
    2. Contact the pediatrician, because the dosage is lower than the recommend dosage range.
    3. Call the pharmacist about special circumstances related to dosage alterations.
    4. Calculate the dosage, then ask another RN to recheck the order and the math.

PART 3   Complex Health Scenarios

Complex Health Scenarios

PART 3

21. The GN is preparing to give an antibiotic tablet to 7-month-old Terry. She checks a drug reference book, crushes the tablet, and then mixes it into 3 oz of applesauce. As the supervising nurse, what is your priority action?
    1. Accompany the nurse into the room and observe while she administers the drug.
    2. Allow her to proceed independently and ask her to report on the outcome.
    3. Suggest that she reconsider the client's circumstances and developmental needs.
    4. Suggest that she recheck the drug reference book before administering the drug.

22. What is the priority nursing diagnosis in caring for the A family? (Refer to question 11 for a description of the A family's circumstances.)
    1. Imbalanced Nutrition: Less than Body Requirements related to socioeconomic status
    2. Deficient Knowledge about the developmental needs of children
    3. Risk for Injury to the children related to lack of appropriate parenting
    4. Risk for Impaired Parenting related to the mother's youth and judgment

23. Which member(s) of the health care team (RN, LPN/LVN, UAP, pediatric social worker) should perform each of these tasks in caring for Sarah, Sam, and Ms. A? (More than one staff member may be appropriate to list for some tasks.)
    1. Perform an initial physical assessment of the infant and toddler. _____
    2. Obtain a history of the infant's injury, including the sequence of events. _____
    3. Observe the children for behavioral signs of abuse. _____
    4. Report any findings to Child Protective Services if appropriate. _____
    5. Assist by holding one child while the other is being examined. _____
    6. Accompany the infant to the radiology department. _____
    7. Administer an oral pain medication to the infant. _____
    8. Assist the toddler to eat an age-appropriate meal. _____

24. The pediatric social worker has just informed Ms. A that Child Protective Services has been notified and that a representative will arrive shortly to speak with her about the family's situation. Ms. A starts to cry and threatens to leave. What is the priority action?
    1. Obtain an "against medical advice" (AMA) form and have her sign it.
    2. Notify the pediatrician of the mother's intent to leave.
    3. Inform the mother that the police will be notified if she leaves.
    4. Encourage Ms. A to remain and to express feelings and fears.

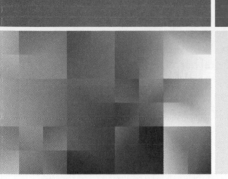

Note: In this case study, the term "mental health assistant" is used, rather than the more familiar "UAP." Different facilities and localities will use different titles for assistive personnel. The key point to remember in assigning tasks or making patient assignments is that UAPs who routinely work on a medical-surgical unit will have different skill sets than mental health assistants, who usually work on a psychiatric unit.

You are the charge nurse caring for psychiatric patients on an acute admission unit. The team includes an experienced male RN, a female RN who has floated from a medical-surgical unit, an experienced female LPN/LVN, and two experienced mental health assistants. There is also a male nursing student on the unit today. The patients are as follows:

- *Ms. G, an 82-year-old woman, has a history of dementia and depression. She has been admitted because her daughter feels that "Mom is getting more depressed and confused." She is oriented to self and believes it is 1985. She is continuously trying to "find my coat so I can go to work." She is ambulatory with an unsteady gait and can perform self-care with step-by-step coaching. Her daughter would like her transferred to a long-term geropsychiatric unit.*
- *Ms. B, a 32-year-old woman, has borderline personality disorder and a history of frequent admissions to the psychiatric unit. Five days ago she was admitted for suicidal gesture after self-infliction of cuts to the posterior forearm. She is extremely flirtatious with all males. She can independently perform activities of daily living (ADLs), but will dress in an excessively provocative manner.*
- *Mr. D, a 58-year-old man, has a long history of major depression. He appears lethargic and disinterested in the environment or in others. He responds appropriately when asked a direct question, but does not initiate any social interaction. He requires verbal prompting for all ADLs, which he can perform himself; however, he says, "I would rather not."*
- *Mr. S, a 38-year-old homeless man, was found wandering naked on a busy street. He has been on the unit for 7 weeks with minimal improvement, but he has not been aggressive toward anyone. He frequently giggles to himself, and if allowed he weaves bits of garbage into his hair. He demonstrates word salad (schizophasia) and looseness of associations. He requires repetitive coaching to perform all ADLs.*
- *Mr. V, a 62-year-old man, voluntarily committed himself 2 days previously for recurrent thoughts of suicide since the death of his wife several months ago. He reports frequently sitting at her graveside with a gun and a bottle of whiskey. He is alert and oriented × 3 (i.e., knows who he is, where he is, and what day and year it is) and answers questions appropriately, but he is preoccupied with thoughts of death. He is on one-to-one suicide precautions.*
- *Ms. M, a 40-year-old woman, was admitted after a verbal altercation in an expensive department store when her credit cards were declined because she was over the $10,000 limit. She is talkative, grandiose, and emotionally labile. She can accomplish ADLs, but will change her clothes repeatedly throughout the day.*
- *Mr. P, a 20-year-old man, was admitted yesterday through the emergency department (ED) after causing a disturbance on a public bus. He appears disheveled and acts suspicious. He has been refusing to eat or sleep because he believes that "those guys have been trying to kill me because I know who they are!"*

1. Which two of the seven patients would be best to assign to the nurse who has floated from the medical-surgical unit? _____, _____

2. Which three of the seven patients would be best to assign to the experienced female LPN/LVN? _____, _____, _____

3. Which two of the seven patients would be best to assign to the experienced male RN? _____, _____

4. A new mental health assistant is being temporarily floated to your unit for 2 hours to assist with morning hygiene. Select one patient of the seven who would be best to assign to this assistant for hygienic care. _____

5. The nursing student tells you that his clinical assignment for the day is to obtain a patient history and perform a mental status examination that will take about 1 or 2 hours to complete. Which two patients would you suggest to the student? _____, _____

6. You are receiving a report from a relatively new night shift nurse. She tells you that Ms. G (elderly patient with dementia) was confused during the evening and kept getting out of bed. Because of this, an "as needed" (PRN) sedative was administered and a temporary chest restraint was placed to prevent falls. What is your priority action?
   1. Report the nurse to the supervisor for violating the patient's rights.
   2. Assess the patient and obtain additional information about the incident.
   3. Advise the nurse to seek out the unit manager and discuss the incident.
   4. Check to see if physician orders were obtained for medication and restraints.

7. The nursing student is assisting Ms. G. You would intervene to assist the student if he did which action?
   1. Made a seasonally appropriate decoration to hang on the patient's wall
   2. Cleaned and rearranged the patient's room and put personal items in the closet
   3. Identified the patient by looking at her armband and asking the patient to state her name
   4. Displayed current pictures of the patient's family on the bedside table

8. Ms. G's daughter says, "I'm tired of waiting for my mother to be transferred to a geropsychiatric unit. I'm taking her home today!" What is the priority action?
   1. Obtain an "against medical advice" (AMA) form, explain the consequences to the daughter, and have her sign the form.
   2. Call the health care provider about the situation and encourage the daughter to call the provider directly.
   3. Encourage the daughter to allow the patient to remain and reassure her that the transfer to the geropsychiatric unit will occur soon.
   4. Verify the psychiatric unit's AMA policies and check on the status of the patient's transfer and explain your findings to the daughter.

9. A psychiatric social worker is conducting a community meeting. You are the co-leader. All patients are attending because there has been theft of personal items. Ms. M (manic phase bipolar disorder) continuously interrupts and loudly announces, "Ms. B (borderline personality) stole my lipstick. Look at her lips!" What is your best response to this situation?
   1. Walk over to Ms. M and quietly escort her out of the meeting.
   2. Allow the psychiatric social worker to control the meeting and the patients' behaviors.
   3. Instruct Ms. B to give an honest response to Ms. M's accusations.
   4. Tell Ms. M that there will be an investigation of the lipstick and to stop interrupting.

10. A health care provider verbally directs you to seclude Ms. M for several hours because "she was belligerent and argumentative" during an interview. You request a written order, but he declines because "it is just temporary and I already explained the consequences of the behavior to the patient." What is the best approach in dealing with this situation?
    1. Assess the patient for signs of aggressive or dangerous behavior and discuss your findings and concerns with the provider.
    2. Refuse to follow the verbal order because you are violating the patient's rights if you do not have a written order.
    3. Recognize that setting limits and enforcing consequences are part of the treatment plan, so seclude and monitor accordingly.
    4. Document the situation, seclude the patient, and continue to care for her to the best of your ability.

11. Which laboratory result causes you the most concern for Ms. M, who is receiving lithium?
    1. Serum chloride level of 100 mmol/L
    2. Serum sodium level of 125 mEq/L
    3. Serum potassium level of 5 mEq/L
    4. Serum glucose level of 140 mg/dL

12. Ms. B (borderline personality disorder) says that the male nursing student was flirting and trying to kiss her and touch her breasts. The student denies the accusation but says, "She asked me if I thought she was attractive, and I said yes." What is the best way to handle this situation?
    1. Advise the student that this type of behavior is typical for Ms. B, but suggest that he contact the instructor and fill out an incident report.
    2. Tell the student that this is a learning experience, but he should remember to carefully consider the impact of casual comments when working with psychiatric patients.
    3. Go with the student to confront Ms. B so that the details of the incident can be clarified and then write an incident report.
    4. Tell the student that the incident will have to be reported to the board of nursing, but that nothing is likely to come of it.

13. Ms. B requests that you "talk to her in private about a serious personal issue." You agree to spend 10 minutes with her, and during that time she tells you that her stepfather has raped her several times in the past and that she plans to "buy a gun and shoot him the next time I see him coming at me!" What is the best approach in responding to this information?
    1. Recognize that this is the patient's attempt to manipulate you to gain sympathy and gently but firmly set limits.
    2. Spend additional time with the patient and gather more information about the incident and her feelings.
    3. Acknowledge her underlying feelings of anger and powerlessness and say that you must report the conversation to the psychiatric team.
    4. Assess the patient for any physical evidence and offer to contact a rape crisis counselor.

14. Mr. D has major depression, and in addition to receiving pharmacologic and milieu therapy, he is to undergo electroconvulsive therapy (ECT). Which members of the team (RN, mental health assistant, nurse anesthetist, and psychiatrist) are the most appropriate to perform the following tasks related to the ECT? *(Select only one staff member for each task.)*
    1. Before the procedure: Explain the risks associated with the procedure (i.e., increased intracranial pressure, increased blood pressure) and obtain informed consent._____
    2. Before the procedure: Perform patient education about short-term memory loss, occasional headaches, and confusion, which will resolve in minutes to hours after the procedure. _____
    3. Before the procedure: Ensure that the patient has nothing by mouth for 6 to 8 hours. _____
    4. Before the procedure: Remove jewelry and assistive devices such as dentures, contact lenses, and hearing aids._____
    5. Before the procedure: Give a preoperative medication such as atropine. _____
    6. During the procedure: Administer a short-acting general anesthetic. _____
    7. After the procedure: Measure and report vital sign values. _____
    8. After the procedure: Reorient the patient and remind the family about temporary short-term memory loss. _____
    9. After the procedure: Assist the patient to eat a meal. _____

15. You are talking to Mr. S, who has disorganized schizophrenia with obvious thought disorder. The patient says, "I am god Jesus god. I will pray pray, say pray, say pray say day a pray for you." What is the most therapeutic response?
    1. "Thank you, Jesus, I need all the prayers I can get."
    2. "Praying is a good thing to do, but you are not Jesus."
    3. "Let's talk about something else right now."
    4. "Your offer to pray for me is kind and generous."

16. The nursing student asks, "How do I start therapeutic communication with a schizophrenic patient like Mr. S? With his thought disorder, word salad (schizophasia), inappropriate giggling, and the loose associations, I can't understand him." Which option would you recommend as best for the student to use with this patient?
    1. "Come and join us in a card game. We would enjoy your company."
    2. "My name is _____. I am a nursing student. What is your name?"
    3. "I have 15 minutes. Would you like to sit down and talk for awhile?"
    4. "I heard you were walking down the street. What do you remember about that?"

17. Mr. V is a quiet, polite, and cooperative patient; however, he has been placed on suicide precautions with one-to-one observation because "my [dead] wife explained to me in a dream how I could be with her." Which member(s) of the team (RN, mental health assistant, nursing student, LPN/LVN), under the appropriate supervision, should perform each of these actions? *(More than one staff member may be appropriate to list for some tasks.)*
    1. Assist Mr. V with hygiene while he shaves his face and takes a shower. _____
    2. Administer an antidepressant by mouth and observe for swallowing of each dose. _____
    3. Explain the need for one-to-one observation. _____
    4. Use active listening and encourage verbalization of feelings. _____
    5. Go through the patient's belongings and remove potentially harmful objects. _____
    6. Maintain an arm's length distance from Mr. V at all times. _____
    7. Ask Mr. V to sign a "no-suicide" contract for safety. _____
    8. Evaluate mood, statements, and behavior every 15 to 30 minutes. _____

18. Mr. P (paranoid schizophrenia) is screaming at the medication nurse, "You are trying to poison me!" You note that the nurse is gently trying to calm him down, but the patient is yelling, "It's the wrong pill! It's wrong!" What is your priority action?
    1. Support the medication nurse's efforts to administer the medication.
    2. Advise the medication nurse to double-check the physician's order.
    3. Advise that the medication be held and then notify the physician.
    4. Try to get Mr. P to take the medication by giving it to him yourself.

19. Mr. P is pacing in the day room. His fists are clenched, he appears tense and suspicious, and he periodically yells at an empty chair. What is the priority action?
    1. Quickly step between Mr. P and any other patients who are nearby.
    2. Gather several staff members for a show of force and unity.
    3. Administer a PRN anxiolytic to Mr. P.
    4. Use a calm, clear tone of voice to verbalize options.

20. Mr. P has a nursing diagnosis of Risk for Self-Directed and Other-Directed Violence related to fear and paranoid behavior. Which task can be delegated to the mental health assistant?
    1. Observing his interactions and behavior toward the other patients
    2. Following him around the day room to prevent occurrences of aggression toward other patients
    3. Serving his food tray and pointing out that all items are wrapped and sealed in original packaging
    4. Checking all his personal belongings for items that are potentially dangerous

21. You are in the day room and the following events are evolving at the same time. Which member(s) of the team (experienced mental health assistant, experienced LPN/LVN, experienced RN) should you delegate or assign to deal with each situation? *(More than one staff member may be appropriate to assign for some tasks.)*
    1. Ms. B (borderline personality disorder) locks herself in the bathroom and yells, "I'll drown myself in the toilet!" _____
    2. Mr. D (depression) has fecal incontinence in the day room and makes no effort to clean up. _____
    3. Ms. M (mania) is outside in the courtyard removing her clothes. _____
    4. Mr. S (disorganized schizophrenia) needs his routine medication and must be observed for "pouching." _____
    5. Mr. V (suicidal thoughts) is sitting at a table and writing letters to his family and friends. _____
    6. Ms. G (dementia) is looking for her coat and trying to get out the front door. _____

22. You are giving an SBAR (situation, background, assessment, recommendation) report to the health care provider about Ms. B (borderline personality disorder), who locked herself in the bathroom and threatened to drown herself in the toilet. Place the following information about the incident in the correct order using the SBAR format.
    1. "She did not verbalize suicidal intent before the incident, but this morning she had a verbal fight with another patient over a lipstick and claimed that a nursing student made sexually inappropriate advances toward her."
    2. "Ms. B was admitted 4 days ago for suicidal gesture of self-inflicted cuts to the arms and has a diagnosis of borderline personality disorder."
    3. "She is in her room, and we placed her on one-to-one observation. I need an order to continue the observation. And is there anything else you would like us to address at this time?"
    4. "She is currently alert, conversant, and uninjured. Her blood pressure is 120/80 mm Hg, pulse rate is 82 beats/min, and respiratory rate is 12 breaths/min."
    5. "She voluntarily opened the door when instructed to do so; her clothes, face, and hair were completely dry."
    6. "I talked to her, and she is apologetic about causing a commotion, but she refuses to sign a no-suicide contract for safety and she says that she'll probably try something else."
    7. "Dr. S, this is Nurse J from the acute psychiatric unit. I am calling about Ms. B. At 3:15 PM, she locked herself in the bathroom and threatened to drown herself in the toilet." _____, _____, _____, _____, _____, _____, _____

23. It is 6:30 PM and you receive a call from a newly hired nurse who is scheduled to work at 7:00 PM. She tells you (the charge nurse) that she is sick and will not be able to come in. What should you do?
    1. Inform her that 30 minutes is insufficient time to find a replacement, so that she will have to come in.
    2. Instruct her that she must speak to you the next time she comes in and attempt to find someone to replace her for this shift.
    3. Document in her file that she failed to give adequate notice for calling in sick.
    4. Tell the oncoming charge nurse that the new nurse called in, so the staffing will be short for the evening.

24. Which end-of-shift tasks should be delegated to one of the mental health assistants? *(Select all that apply.)*
    1. Assisting Ms. G (dementia) to change her soiled blouse before evening visitors arrive
    2. Accompanying Ms. B (borderline) to the bathroom to prevent a repeat of locking the door
    3. Encouraging Mr. D (depression) to finish a glass of water for the allotment of the shift
    4. Accompanying Mr. S (disorganized schizophrenia) to the gift shop before it closes
    5. Maintaining one-to-one observation with Mr. V (suicidal) until the oncoming shift takes over
    6. Explaining to Ms. M (manic phase) why she cannot independently go to the smoke break area
    7. Assisting Mr. P (paranoid schizophrenia) to straighten his room and pick up his belongings

25. As the charge nurse, which tasks should you complete at the end of the shift before leaving for the day? *(Select all that apply.)*
    1. Initiate a patient assignment sheet for the oncoming shift.
    2. Take brief summary information (from the admitting office) on a new patient who is being transferred from the ED.
    3. Call social services to search for the family of Mr. S (homeless, found wandering).
    4. Check with the mental health assistant who is performing one-to-one observation with Mr. V (suicidal thoughts).
    5. Briefly check and assess every patient.
    6. Thank the ancillary staff for their help.
    7. Call the family of Ms. G (elderly with dementia) to discuss alternative long-term care options.
    8. Talk to each RN and LPN/LVN about their concerns related to assigned patients.

Answer Key for this case study begins on p. 236.

Ms. N is a 20-year-old gravida 1, para 0 (G1P0) woman who begins her prenatal care today at 24 weeks' gestation. She says that she didn't know she was pregnant until now. Her prepregnancy body mass index was 23. She has gained 30 lb so far. She admits that she eats poorly and smokes a half-pack of cigarettes daily, but claims to use no other substances. She lives with her boyfriend and has no immediate family in the area. She reports no significant medical, surgical, or family history. You are the RN taking her history and drawing samples for laboratory work today on this first prenatal visit.

1. What would be your priority topics in client teaching today? *(Select all that apply.)*
   1. Smoking cessation methods
   2. Recommendation of a flu shot (if flu season)
   3. Danger signs during pregnancy
   4. Basics of nutrition
   5. Pain relief options in labor and birth

Ms. N returns for her second prenatal appointment 1 week later. You review her laboratory results with her and note the following abnormal findings: 1-hour glucose tolerance test, 190 mg/dL; Pap smear results, low-grade squamous intraepithelial lesion (LSIL) with high-risk human papillomavirus (HPV) present; chlamydia test, positive for the organism. The physician has written orders for a 3-hour glucose tolerance test and a colposcopy, and has provided a prescription for azithromycin (Zithromax) 1 g by mouth. Ms. N has increased her smoking to 1 pack/day because of stress.

2. What would be accurate and priority information to give Ms. N about the positive chlamydia test result?
   1. By taking the medication now and having her partner treated, she can help avoid complications in the pregnancy.
   2. The medication for chlamydia infection is not safe in pregnancy, and she should use condoms until she can be treated postpartum.
   3. Chlamydia infection cannot really be cured and may recur despite treatment.
   4. Chlamydia infection does no harm to the baby during the pregnancy or at delivery, but treatment is recommended to avoid pelvic inflammatory disease in the woman.

3. What else would be a priority given the scenario described earlier?
   1. Instruct Ms. N not to fast for the 3-hour glucose tolerance test because it is not safe to do so in pregnancy.
   2. Refer Ms. N to a social worker because her increased stress can be a risk factor for preterm birth.
   3. Instruct Ms. N that HPV infection can be effectively treated with colposcopy.
   4. Instruct Ms. N that, if HPV is present at the time of labor, a cesarean section will be needed.

Later that evening Ms. N calls the clinic and reports vaginal bleeding and cramping. You advise her to go to the emergency department (ED) and tell her that you will notify her provider and the RN in the ED.

4. Using the SBAR (situation, background, assessment, recommendation) format, how will you communicate priority information in your report to the ED RN?
   1. The client needs evaluation for preterm labor and bleeding. She smokes, has a chlamydia infection, and has had minimal prenatal care.
   2. The client is a 20-year-old G1P0 with a prepregnancy weight of 130 lb. Current weight is 160 lb. Has a family history of diabetes and twins. Takes a prenatal vitamin daily. Plans to breast-feed. Will arrive in the ED within 1 hour because of bleeding and cramping.
   3. The client is a 20-year-old G1P0 at 24 weeks' gestation who reports vaginal bleeding and cramping. She had an elevated 1-hour glucose level, tested positive for chlamydia and was given a medication prescription today, and had an abnormal Pap test result. She's had only two prenatal visits and no ultrasound yet. She is a smoker, reports a lot of stress, and is single, unemployed, and with little support. She is coming for evaluation for possible preterm labor and vaginal bleeding. Please be sure she also gets a social work consult and ensure that she has taken the medication for chlamydia infection.
   4. The client is a 20-year-old G1P0 coming to the ED with premature labor and placenta previa with bleeding. She was treated today for chlamydia infection and has been referred for colposcopy for an abnormal Pap test result. Her 1-hour glucose level was elevated. She has had minimal prenatal care, and a urine drug screen should be considered.

> *Ms. N arrives in the obstetrics triage area crying and accompanied by an agitated man who is speaking angrily to the client.*

5. Indicate the order in which the RN should take the following actions at this time.
   1. Apply a fetal monitor and measure vital signs.
   2. Obtain a thorough history from the client.
   3. Notify the physician.
   4. Instruct the man to wait in the waiting area and notify security.
   5. Call a social worker for a consult.

   _____, _____, _____, _____, _____

> *Ms. N relates that, when she told her partner about the positive chlamydia test result, he became violent and began hitting her in the face and abdomen. Upon examination, Ms. N's cervix is found to be 2 cm dilated and 50% effaced, she is contracting every 6 minutes, and she has a small amount of vaginal bleeding. Her ultrasound findings are normal and show no placenta previa. She is admitted to the hospital for treatment of preterm labor. The physician has ordered the following medications:*
> - *Nifedipine (Procardia) 30 mg by mouth (PO), followed by 10 mg PO every 4 hours*
> - *Betamethasone (Celestone Soluspan) 12 mg intramuscularly (IM) every 24 hours × 2 doses*

6. What priority information would be important to give Ms. N about this treatment?
   1. The nifedipine and betamethasone work together to help stop preterm labor.
   2. The nifedipine is to prevent neonatal heart problems after birth, and the betamethasone is to stop contractions.
   3. The betamethasone is to help the infant's lungs mature and to try to prevent other neonatal complications in case the infant is born early. The nifedipine is to attempt to stop the contractions.
   4. The nifedipine is to treat chlamydia infection and the betamethasone is to help the infant's lungs mature.

> *After treatment, Ms. N's contractions stop and there is no further cervical dilation. After a day of observation, Ms. N is being discharged today. Her discharge medications are as follows:*
> - *Prenatal vitamin 1 daily PO*
> - *Ferrous sulfate 325 mg PO 1 daily*

7. Which tasks to prepare for Ms. N's discharge could be delegated to a UAP?
   1. Teaching Ms. N the signs of preterm labor
   2. Discussing nutrition, smoking cessation, and stress reduction
   3. Calling the prenatal clinic to schedule the next prenatal appointment within 1 week
   4. Calling a social worker to discuss a plan of care given the history of domestic violence

8. A student nurse is helping you prepare for Ms. N's discharge. Which statement made to Ms. N by the student would require you to intervene and correct the information given?
   1. "The iron may cause constipation."
   2. "The iron should be taken daily with milk."
   3. "The iron may cause darkening of the stools."
   4. "The iron does not take the place of a high-iron diet, which should also be followed."

Ms. N's pregnancy continues uneventfully. She separates from her boyfriend and begins counseling, which she says makes her feel stronger and calmer. She has decreased her smoking to 1 to 2 cigarettes/day. Her mother comes from out of state to live with her and cooks healthy foods. She is now at 38 weeks' gestation and calls the RN to report that she has had uterine contractions for 6 hours.

9. What would be priority data for the RN to obtain before giving Ms. N advice by phone? *(Select all that apply.)*
   1. Did she take her vitamin and iron today?
   2. What are the frequency and intensity of the contractions?
   3. Is there vaginal bleeding?
   4. Did her water break?
   5. How far does Ms. N live from the hospital?

10. Which response by Ms. N would prompt the RN to notify the physician and advise Ms. N to go straight to the hospital?
    1. "The contractions are extremely painful."
    2. "I have vaginal bleeding that soaks about a pad an hour."
    3. "I have vaginal bleeding that is mixed with a lot of mucus."
    4. "My baby is moving a lot today."

Ms. N arrives at the hospital at 38 weeks' gestation in active labor. Her membranes are intact. Her contractions are every 3 minutes. Her mother is at the bedside assisting her with breathing and relaxation. A vaginal examination reveals that the cervix is 5 cm dilated and 100% effaced, with the fetal head at −1 station. Her vital sign values are as follows:

Blood pressure	*140/90 mm Hg*
Heart rate	*88 beats/min*
Respiratory rate	*24 breaths/min*
Temperature	*98.6° F (37° C)*

The fetal heart rate is 140 beats/min. There is average variability. Accelerations are present and no decelerations are noted.

11. Based on Ms. N's vital sign measurements, what are the priority questions that the RN should ask? *(Select all that apply.)*
    1. Is she having headaches?
    2. Is she having pain with urination?
    3. Is she having epigastric pain?
    4. Is she experiencing visual changes?
    5. Has her water broken?

The RN takes Ms. N's blood pressure a few more times and is careful to measure it in between contractions. All of the subsequent blood pressure values are normal, and Ms. N is admitted to the labor and delivery unit. She chooses not to receive pain medication at this time, and her mother continues to assist her with relaxation and breathing. She goes into the shower to help with the back pain she is feeling. When she comes out, there is a gush of fluid from the client, and the RN notes that the fluid is green.

12. Indicate the order in which the following nursing actions should be accomplished at this time.
    1. Prepare the infant bed for possible tracheal suctioning or intubation of the newborn.
    2. Assess the fetal heart rate.
    3. Notify the provider.
    4. Assess the contraction pattern and Ms. N's coping abilities. _____, _____, _____, _____

Ms. N is now moaning with her contractions, perspiring profusely, feeling nauseous, and experiencing an urge to push. A vaginal examination reveals that the cervix is 9.5 cm dilated and 100% effaced, and the fetal head is at +1 station.

13. A student nurse is working with Ms. N. Which is an inappropriate action by the student at this time that would require your intervention?
    1. Discussing with Ms. N the option of butorphanol (Stadol) for pain relief
    2. Reassuring Ms. N and her mother that these are normal reactions near the end of labor
    3. Applying firm pressure on Ms. N's lower back
    4. Encouraging Ms. N to continue breathing with her contractions and to refrain from pushing if possible

Ms. N's cervix is now completely dilated, and she pushes effectively and has a normal spontaneous delivery of a 7-lb male infant. The neonatologist is present to evaluate the infant because of the presence of meconium. The infant is initially limp and pale at birth. His heart rate is 90 and he is not breathing.

14. Indicate the order *in which the following actions should be taken with this newborn.*
    1. Provide positive-pressure ventilation to the infant.
    2. Provide the infant warmth.
    3. Open the infant's airway.
    4. Provide tactile stimulation to the infant.
    5. Perform endotracheal suctioning on the infant.

    _____, _____, _____, _____, _____

> *The newborn responds quickly to resuscitation, and by 3 minutes of age is breathing, is crying spontaneously, and has good color and tone. The neonatologist leaves and the RN continues to assess the newborn.*

15. Which finding would prompt the RN to call the neonatologist back to evaluate the infant further?
    1. Cyanosis of the hands and feet
    2. Heart rate of 160 beats/min
    3. Respiratory rate of 55 breaths/min
    4. Central cyanosis

16. Indicate the order in which the following nursing actions should be performed in the immediate care of a healthy normal newborn in the delivery room.
    1. Place identification bracelets on the mother and infant.
    2. Administer vitamin K to the infant.
    3. Assess the infant's airway and breathing.
    4. Perform bulb suctioning if excessive mucus is present.
    5. Assess the infant's heart rate.

    _____, _____, _____, _____, _____

17. Ms. N plans to breast-feed her infant. What evidence-based actions should the RN take in the delivery room to enhance the success of breast feeding? *(Select all that apply.)*
    1. Place the infant on the warming bed until his temperature is stable, then bring the infant to the mother and assist in breast feeding.
    2. Place the infant skin to skin with the mother as soon as possible after birth.
    3. Assist the mother to breast-feed in the first hour of life.
    4. Allow the mother to rest and give a first feeding of sterile water to assess infant sucking and swallowing, then assist with breastfeeding at the next feed.
    5. Instruct Ms. N to breast-feed for 5 minutes on each side.

18. After the placenta is delivered, Ms. N is noted to be bleeding profusely. Oxytocin (Pitocin) 20 units in 1000 mL of lactated Ringer's solution is infusing. The provider also orders carboprost (Hemabate) 250 mcg IM. Which finding would be a relative contraindication to administering carboprost?
    1. Temperature of 101° F (38.3° C)
    2. Blood pressure of 148/96 mm Hg
    3. Asthma
    4. Allergy to penicillin

19. Which nursing actions are most important at this time to prevent further hemorrhage? *(Select all that apply.)*
    1. Monitor vital signs.
    2. Assess and massage the uterine fundus every 15 minutes.
    3. Ensure that the maternal bladder is emptied.
    4. Assist Ms. N into a left lateral position.
    5. Provide a lunch tray with high-iron foods.

20. You are preparing to transfer Ms. N to the postpartum unit. Which statement by her would cause you to stop and reassess her before transfer?
    1. "My nipples are very sore."
    2. "I feel something gushing."
    3. "I feel dizzy if I walk."
    4. "I have bad cramping in my abdomen."

21. The RN receiving Ms. N on the postpartum unit is aware of her postpartum hemorrhage. What would be the first clinical sign of hypovolemia related to postpartum hemorrhage?
    1. Hypotension
    2. Tachycardia
    3. Mental status changes
    4. Decreased urine output

Answer Key for this case study begins on p. 239.

Answer Key

CHAPTER 1: Pain, pages 11-14

1. **Ans: 4** As charge nurse, you must assess the performance and attitude of the staff in relation to this client. After data are gathered from the nurses, additional information can be obtained from the records and the client as necessary. The educator may be of assistance if a knowledge deficit or need for performance improvement is the problem. **Focus:** Supervision, prioritization

2. **Ans: 3** Beliefs, attitudes, and familial influence are part of the sociocultural dimension of pain. Location and radiation of pain address the sensory dimension. Describing pain and its effects addresses the affective dimension. Activity level and function address the behavioral dimension. Asking about knowledge addresses the cognitive dimension. **Focus:** Prioritization

3. **Ans: 1** Gabapentin is an antiepileptic drug, but it is also used to treat diabetic neuropathy. Corticosteroids are for pain associated with inflammation. Hydromorphone is a stronger opioid, and it is not the first choice for chronic pain that can be managed with other drugs. Lorazepam is an anxiolytic that may be ordered as an adjuvant medication. **Focus:** Prioritization

4. **Ans: 3** Cancer pain generally worsens with disease progression, and the use of opioids is more generous. Fibromyalgia is more likely to be treated with nonopioid and adjuvant medications. Trigeminal neuralgia is treated with antiseizure medications such as carbamazepine (Tegretol). Phantom limb pain usually subsides after ambulation begins. **Focus:** Prioritization

5. **Ans: 4** In supervision of the new RN, good performance should be reinforced first and then areas of improvement can be addressed. Asking the nurse about knowledge of pain management is also an option; however, it would be a more indirect and time-consuming approach. Making a note and watching do not help the nurse to correct the immediate problem. In-service training might be considered if the problem persists. **Focus:** Supervision, delegation

6. **Ans:: 1, 3, 5, 6** These clients should be assigned to an experienced RN because all have acute conditions that require close monitoring for any developing complications. Abdominal cramps secondary to food poisoning is an acute condition; however, the cramping, along with vomiting and diarrhea, are usually self-limiting. The client with chronic back pain would be considered physically stable. While all clients will benefit from care provided by an experienced RN, the client with abdominal cramps and the client with back pain could be assigned to a new RN, an LPN/LVN, or a float nurse. **Focus:** Assignment

7. **Ans: 3** The client must be believed, and his or her experience of pain must be acknowledged as valid. The data gathered via client reports can then be applied to the other options in developing the treatment plan. **Focus:** Prioritization

8. **Ans: 3** The client with an acute myocardial infarction has the greatest need for IV access and is likely to receive morphine, which will relieve pain by increasing venous capacitance. Other clients may also need IV access for delivery of pain medication, other drugs, or IV fluids, but the need is less urgent. **Focus:** Prioritization

9. **Ans: 1** The goal is to control pain while minimizing side effects. For severe pain, the medication can be titrated upward until the pain is controlled. Downward titration occurs when the pain begins to subside. Adequate dosing is important; however, the concept of controlled dosing applies more to potent vasoactive drugs. **Focus:** Prioritization

10. **Ans: 2** Application of heat and cold is a standard therapy with guidelines for safe use and predictable outcomes; therefore, the LPN/LVN could implement and educate the client about this therapy under the supervision of an RN. Therapeutic touch requires additional training and practice. Meditation is not acceptable to all clients, and an assessment of spiritual beliefs should be conducted. TENS is usually applied by a physical therapist. **Focus:** Delegation

11. **Ans: 2** First assess the client. The UAP has correctly reported her findings, but the nurse is ultimately responsible to assess first and then determine the correct action. Based on your assessment findings, the other options may also be appropriate. **Focus:** Prioritization

12. **Ans: 4** At greatest risk are elderly clients, opiate-naive clients, and those with underlying pulmonary disease. The child has two of the three risk factors. **Focus:** Prioritization

13. **Ans: 1** This client has strong beliefs and emotions related to the issue of the sibling's addiction. First, encourage expression. This indicates to the client that

the feelings are real and valid. It is also an opportunity to assess beliefs and fears. Giving facts and information is appropriate at the right time. Family involvement is important, but it should be kept in mind that their beliefs about drug addiction may be similar to those of the client. **Focus:** Prioritization

14. **Ans: 3** Diaphoresis is one of the early signs that occur between 6 and 12 hours after withdrawal. Fever, nausea, and abdominal cramps are late signs that occur between 48 and 72 hours after withdrawal. **Focus:** Prioritization

15. **Ans: 1** The UAP is able to assist the client with hygiene issues and knows the principles of safety and comfort for this procedure. Monitoring the client, teaching techniques, and evaluating outcomes are nursing responsibilities. **Focus:** Delegation

16. **Ans: 4** Administering placebos is generally considered unethical. Consult the charge nurse as a resource person who can help you clarify the situation and locate and review the hospital policy. If the physician is insistent, suggest that he or she could give the placebo. (Note: Use "could," not "should" when talking to the physician. This provides a small opportunity to rethink the decision. "Should" is more commanding and elicits a more defensive response.) While following your own ethical code is correct, you must ensure that the client is not abandoned and that care continues. **Focus:** Prioritization

17. **Ans: 2** Complete information should be obtained from the family during the initial comprehensive history taking and assessment. If this information is not obtained, the nursing staff will have to rely on observation of nonverbal behavior and careful documentation to determine pain and relief patterns. **Focus:** Prioritization

18. **Ans: 5, 3, 1, 2, 4** All of the clients are in relatively stable condition. The client with the pneumothorax has priority, because chest tubes can leak or become dislodged or blocked. Lung sounds and respiratory effort should be evaluated. The woman who will be undergoing diagnostic testing should be assessed and medicated before she leaves for the procedure. In a client with meningitis, a headache is not an unexpected complaint, but neurologic status and pain should be assessed. The report of postoperative pain is expected, but this client is getting reasonable relief most of the time. Caring for and assessing the client with Alzheimer disease is likely to be very time consuming; checking on her last prevents delaying care for all the others. **Focus:** Prioritization

19. **Ans: 4** Assess the pain for changes in location, quality, and intensity, as well as changes in response to medication. This assessment will guide the next steps. **Focus:** Prioritization

20. **Ans: 4** The LPN/LVN is well trained to administer oxygen per nasal cannula. This client is considered unstable; therefore, the RN should take responsibility

for administering drugs and monitoring the response to therapy, which includes the effects on the respiratory system. The RN should also take responsibility to communicate with the physician for ongoing treatment and therapy. **Focus:** Delegation

21. **Ans: 4** If the pain is constant, the best schedule is around the clock, to provide steady analgesia and pain control. The other options may actually require higher dosages to achieve control. **Focus:** Prioritization

22. **Ans: 2, 3, 6** The clients with the cast, toe amputation, and arthritis are in stable condition and need ongoing assessment and pain management that are within the scope of practice of an LPN/LVN under the supervision of an RN. The RN should take responsibility for preoperative teaching, and the client with terminal cancer needs a comprehensive assessment to determine the reason for refusal of medication. The client with trauma needs serial assessments to detect occult trauma. **Focus:** Assignment

23. **Ans: 5, 2, 1, 3, 4** Using the SBAR format, the nurse first identifies himself or herself, gives the client's name, and describes the current situation. Next, relevant background information, such as the client's diagnosis, medications, and laboratory data, is stated. The assessment includes both client assessment data that are of concern and the nurse's analysis of the situation. Finally, the nurse makes a recommendation indicating what action he or she thinks is needed. **Focus:** Prioritization

24. **Ans: 2, 5, 6** The client who is second day postoperative, the client who has pain at the IV site, and the client with the kidney stone have predictable needs and require routine care that a new nurse can manage. The anxious client with chronic pain needs an in-depth assessment of the psychological and emotional components of pain and expert intervention. The client with HIV infection has complex complaints that require expert assessment skills. The client pending discharge will need special and detailed instructions. **Focus:** Assignment

25. **Ans: 3** Directly ask the client about the pain and perform a complete pain assessment. This information will determine which action to take next. **Focus:** Prioritization

26. **Ans: 2** This statement is a veiled suicide threat, and clients with pain disorder and depression have a high risk for suicide. New injuries must be evaluated, but this type of complaint is not uncommon for clients with pain disorder. Risk for substance abuse is very high and should eventually be addressed. He can threaten to sue, but current circumstances do not support his case. **Focus:** Prioritization

27. **Ans: 4** Measuring output and obtaining a specimen are within the scope of practice of the UAP. Insertion of the Foley catheter in this client should be done by the RN, because clients with obstruction and retention are usually very difficult to catheterize,

and the nurse must evaluate the pain response during the procedure. The UAP's knowledge of sterile technique is not the issue for this particular client. **Focus:** Delegation

28. **Ans: 3** Assessing the pain is the priority in this acute care setting, because there is a risk of infection or hemorrhage. The other options might be appropriate based on your assessment findings. **Focus:** Prioritization

29. **Ans: 2** Explain that insulin is a priority because life-threatening ketoacidosis is already in progress. If she is already aware of the dangers of an elevated blood glucose level, then her refusal suggests ongoing suicidal intent and the provider should be notified so that steps can be taken to override her refusal (potentially a court order). A blood glucose level of over 600 mg/dL is typically a criterion for transfer to intensive care, but making arrangements for transfer does not address the priority issue, which is refusal of therapy. Withholding pain medication is unethical, and merely documenting refusal of insulin is inappropriate because of possible ongoing suicidal intent. **Focus:** Prioritization

CHAPTER 2: Cancer, pages 15-18

1. **Ans: 1** Oral hygiene is within the scope of duties of the UAP. It is the responsibility of the nurse to observe response to treatments and to help the patient deal with loss or anxiety. The UAP can be directed to weigh the patient but should not be expected to know when to initiate that measurement. **Focus:** Delegation

2. **Ans: 4** The patient's physical condition is currently stable, but emotional needs are affecting his or her ability to receive the information required to make an informed decision. The other diagnoses are relevant, but if the patient leaves the clinic the interventions may be delayed or ignored. **Focus:** Prioritization

3. **Ans: 1** Pancreatic cancer is more common in African-Americans, males, and smokers. Other associated factors include alcohol use, diabetes, obesity, history of pancreatitis, exposure to organic chemicals, consumption of a high-fat diet, and previous abdominal irradiation. **Focus:** Prioritization

4. **Ans: 2, 3, 5, 6, 7** Mouthwash should not include alcohol, because it has a drying action that leaves mucous membranes more vulnerable. Insertion of suppositories, probes, or tampons into the rectal or vaginal cavity is not recommended. All other options are appropriate. **Focus:** Prioritization, knowledge

5. **Ans: 2** Administering enemas and antibiotics is within the scope of practice of LPNs/LVNs. Although some states an facilities may allow the LPN/LVN to administer blood, in general, administering blood, providing preoperative teaching, and assisting with central line insertion are the responsibilities of the RN. **Focus:** Assignment

6. **Ans: 1. Nurse practitioner, 2. Nutritionist, 3. LPN/LVN, 4. Nurse practitioner, 5. RN** The nurse practitioner is often the provider who performs the physical examinations and recommends diagnostic testing. The nutritionist can give information about diet. The LPN/LVN will know the standard seven warning signs and can educate through standard teaching programs. The RN has primary responsibility for educating people about risk factors. **Focus:** Assignment

7. **Ans: 3** Further assess what the patient means by having "control over my own life and death." This could be an indirect statement of suicidal intent. A patient who believes he will be cured should also be assessed for misunderstanding what the physician said; however, the patient may need to use denial as a temporary defense mechanism. The patient's acknowledgment that the treatments are for control of symptoms or plans for the immediate future suggest an understanding of what the physician said. **Focus:** Prioritization

8. **Ans: 3** The UAP can observe the amount that the patient eats (or what is gone from the tray) and report to the nurse. Assessing patterns of fatigue and skin reaction is the responsibility of the RN. The initial recommendation for exercise should come from the physician. **Focus:** Delegation

9. **Ans: 3** Paresthesia is a side effect associated with some chemotherapy drugs such as vincristine. The physician can modify the dosage or discontinue the drug. Fatigue, nausea, vomiting, and anorexia are common side effects of many chemotherapy medications. The nurse can assist the patient by planning for rest periods, giving antiemetics as ordered, and encouraging small meals containing high-protein and high-calorie foods. **Focus:** Prioritization

10. **Ans: 1** WBC count is especially important, because chemotherapy can cause decreases in WBCs, particularly neutrophils (known as neutropenia), which leave the patient vulnerable to infection. The other tests are important in the total management but are less directly specific to chemotherapy in general. **Focus:** Prioritization

11. **Ans: 3** Giving medications is within the scope of practice of the LPN/LVN. Assisting the patient in brushing and flossing should be delegated to the UAP. Explaining contraindications is the responsibility of the RN. Recommendations for saliva substitutes should come from the physician or pharmacist. **Focus:** Delegation

12. **Ans: 1** Chemotherapy drugs should be given by nurses who have received additional training in how to safely prepare and deliver the drugs and protect themselves and others from exposure. The other options express concerns, but the general principles of drug administration apply. **Focus:** Assignment

13. **Ans: 1, 3, 2, 4** Tumor lysis syndrome is an emergency involving electrolyte imbalances and potential

renal failure. A patient scheduled for surgery should be assessed and prepared for surgery. A patient with breakthrough pain needs assessment, and the physician may need to be contacted for a change of dosage or medication. Anticipatory nausea and vomiting has a psychogenic component that requires assessment, teaching, reassurance, and administration of antiemetics. **Focus:** Prioritization

14. **Ans: 1** Back pain is an early sign of spinal cord compression occurring in 95% of patients. The other symptoms are later signs. **Focus:** Prioritization

15. **Ans: 2, 7, 1, 3, 6, 4, 5** Determine level of consciousness and responsiveness, and changes from baseline. Oxygen should be administered immediately in the presence of respiratory distress or risk for decreased oxygenation and perfusion. Pulse oximetry can be used for continuous monitoring. Adequate pulse, blood pressure, and respirations are required for cerebral perfusion. Increased temperature may signal infection or sepsis. Blood glucose levels should be checked even if the patient is not diabetic. Severe hypoglycemia should be immediately treated per protocol. A patent IV line may be needed for delivery of emergency drugs. Electrolyte and ammonia levels are relevant data for this patient, and abnormalities in these parameters may be contributing to change in mental status. (Note: Laboratory results [i.e., electrolytes and ammonia levels] may be concurrently available; however, you should train yourself to systematically look at data. Look at electrolytes first because these are more commonly ordered. In some cases, you may actually have to remind the physician to order the ammonia level if the patient with a hepatic disorder is having a change in mental status.) **Focus:** Prioritization

16. **Ans: 1. Advanced practice nurse, MD, 2. Advanced practice nurse, MD, RN, 3. Advanced practice nurse, RN, 4. Advanced practice nurse, MD, RN, 5. Advanced practice nurse, MD, RN, LPN/LVN, 6. MD** Advanced practice nurses could do any of the tasks; however, explaining results of a mammogram may be handled by the supervising physician, especially if complex follow-up is needed (e.g., surgery). Physicians could do any of the tasks except they do not make nursing diagnoses. RNs could do tasks 2, 3, 4, and 5 but usually do not do clinical breast examination, unless specially trained, and do not interpret results of diagnostic tests for patients. LPNs/LVNs could reinforce standard information about screening recommendations. The RN should make the nursing diagnoses, and the LPN/LVN assists in planning and implementing the interventions. **Focus:** Assignment

17. **Ans: 2** Potentially life-threatening hypercalcemia can occur in cancers with destruction of bone. Other laboratory values are pertinent for overall patient management but are less specific to bone cancers. **Focus:** Prioritization

18. **Ans: 2, 4** Debulking of tumor and laminectomy are palliative procedures. These patients can be placed in the same room. The patient with a low neutrophil count and the patient who has had a bone marrow transplantation need protective isolation. **Focus:** Assignment

19. **Ans: 3** The patient is not coping with the recent diagnosis of cancer and prospect of losing his leg. His decision to go hiking may be a form of denial, or possibly a veiled suicide threat. It is also possible that he has decided not to have any treatment; however, you need to make additional assessment about his decision and actions and help him to discuss alternatives and consequences. The other diagnoses may also apply, but if he leaves the hospital there will be no chance to address any other issues. **Focus:** Prioritization

20. **Ans: 2** Tumor lysis syndrome can result in severe electrolyte imbalances and potential kidney failure. The other laboratory values are important to monitor to identify general chemotherapy side effects but are less pertinent to tumor lysis syndrome. **Focus:** Prioritization

21. **Ans: 1, 3, 4, 5** Women age 21 or over should have annual Pap smears, regardless of sexual activity. African-American men should begin prostate-specific antigen testing at age 45. Colonoscopy and annual fecal occult blood testing are recommended for those with average risk starting at age 50. Annual mammograms are recommended for women over the age of 40. Women age 65 or older who have normal results on previous Pap tests may forego additional screenings for cervical cancer. **Focus:** Prioritization

22. **Ans: 2** Hyponatremia is a concern; therefore, fluid restrictions would be ordered. Urinalysis is less pertinent; however, the nurse should monitor for changes in urine specific gravity. The diet may need to include sodium supplements. Fluid bolus is unlikely to be ordered for patients with SIADH; however, IV normal saline or hypertonic saline solutions may be given very cautiously. **Focus:** Prioritization

23. **Ans: 1, 2, 4, 6** Measuring vital signs and reporting on specific parameters, practicing good hand washing, and gathering equipment are within the scope of duties for a UAP. Assessing for symptoms of infections and superinfections is the responsibility of the RN. **Focus:** Delegation

24. **Ans: 2** An LPN/LVN is versed in medication administration and able to teach patients standardized information. The other options require more in-depth assessment, planning, and teaching, which should be performed by the RN. Helping patients with smoking cessation is a Core Measure. **Focus:** Delegation

25. **Ans: 1** Morphine elixir is the therapy of choice because it is thought to reduce anxiety and the subjective sensation of air hunger. It also increases venous capacitance. End-of-life-care should not include

aggressive measures such as intubation or resuscitation. Support and comfort are always welcome, but in this case you should not sit quietly because there is an option that would offer some physical relief for the patient. **Focus:** Prioritization

26. **Ans: 3** Explain that you are not chemotherapy certified so that the charge nurse can quickly rearrange the patient assignments. You can assess the patient, site, and infusion; however, you do not have the expertise to recognize the side effects of the medication or to give specialized care that may be needed. Asking the nurse to stay is not the best solution, because the care of the patient and the effects of the medication continue after the infusion has been completed. Looking up the side effects of the drug is okay for your own information, but you are still not qualified to deal with this situation. In addition, knowing how to properly discontinue the infusion and dispose of the equipment are essential for your own safety and the safety of others. **Focus:** Prioritization

27. **Ans: 2** If the radiation implant has obviously been expelled (i.e., is on the bed linens), use a pair of forceps to place the radiation source in a lead container. The other options would be appropriate after safety of the patient and personnel are ensured. **Focus:** Prioritization, supervision

28. **Ans: 3** You must try to find out what Nurse A is thinking and feeling. If you can discover the underlying issue, there is a better chance that you can help her (e.g., referral to counseling or in-service training). You should try to avoid being too draconian with your staff by insisting that they switch back to the original assignments, or too condescending by lecturing them about patients' rights. Nurses frequently can and do switch patients to help each other out, but the charge nurse should always be informed prior to making the switch. **Focus:** Assignment, supervision

CHAPTER 3: Immunologic Problems, pages 19-22

1. **Ans: 3** Epinephrine is the initial drug of choice for treatment of anaphylaxis. Giving epinephrine rapidly at the onset of an anaphylactic reaction may prevent or reverse cardiovascular collapse as well as airway narrowing caused by bronchospasm and inflammation. Oxygen use is also appropriate, but oxygen would be administered using a nonrebreather mask in order to achieve a fraction of inspired oxygen closer to 100%. Albuterol may also be administered to decrease airway narrowing but would not be the first therapy used for anaphylaxis. IV access will take longer to establish and should not be the first intervention. **Focus:** Prioritization

2. **Ans: 1** Supplying sterile injection supplies to patients who are at risk for HIV infection can be done by staff

members with health assistant education. Assessing for high-risk behaviors, education, and community assessment are RN-level skills. **Focus:** Delegation

3. **Ans: 2** Nystatin should be in contact with the oral and esophageal tissues as long as possible for maximum effect. The other actions are also inappropriate and should be discussed with the student but do not require action as quickly. HIV-positive patients do not require droplet/contact precautions or visitor restrictions to prevent opportunistic infections. Hot or spicy foods are not usually well tolerated by patients with oral or esophageal fungal infections. **Focus:** Prioritization

4. **Ans: 4** Pentamidine can cause fatal hypoglycemia, so the low blood glucose level indicates a need for a change in therapy. The low blood pressure suggests that the pentamidine infusion rate may need to be slowed. The other responses indicate a need for independent nursing actions (such as establishing a new IV site and encouraging oral intake) but are not associated with pentamidine infusion. **Focus:** Prioritization

5. **Ans: 2** Drug therapy for HIV infection requires taking medications very consistently. Failure to take the medications daily can lead to mutations and the emergence of more virulent forms of the virus. Although the other data indicate the need for further assessments or interventions, they will not affect the decision to initiate antiretroviral therapy for this patient. **Focus:** Prioritization

6. **Ans: 1** Patients with severe immunodeficiency may be unable to produce an immune response, so a negative TB skin test result does not completely rule out a TB diagnosis for this patient. The next steps in diagnosis are chest radiography and sputum culture. Teaching about isoniazid and follow-up TB testing may be required, depending on the radiographic findings and sputum culture results. **Focus:** Prioritization

7. **Ans: 2** The collection of data used to evaluate the therapeutic and adverse effects of medications is included in LPN/LVN education and scope of practice. Assessment, planning, and teaching are more complex skills that require RN education. Assistance with hygiene and activities of daily living should be delegated to the UAP. **Focus:** Delegation

8. **Ans: 3** To be most effective, cyclosporine must be mixed and administered in accordance with the manufacturer's instructions, so the RN who is likely to have the most experience with the medication should care for this patient or monitor the new graduate carefully during medication preparation and administration. The coronary care unit float nurse and the nurse who is new to the unit would not have experience with this medication. **Focus:** Assignment

9. **Ans: 4** Both naproxen (a nonsteroidal anti-inflammatory drug [NSAID]) and prednisone (a corticosteroid) can cause gastrointestinal bleeding, and the stool appearance indicates that blood may be present in the stool. The health care provider should be notified so that

actions such as testing a stool specimen for occult blood and administering proton pump inhibitors can be prescribed. The other symptoms are common in patients with RA and will require further assessment or intervention, but do not indicate that the patient is experiencing adverse effects from the medications. **Focus:** Prioritization

10. **Ans: 1**   Nausea and vomiting are common adverse effects of interferon alfa-2a, but continued vomiting should be reported to the physician, because dehydration may occur. The medication may be given by either the subcutaneous or intramuscular route. Flu-like symptoms such as a mild temperature elevation, headache, muscle aches, and anorexia are common after initiation of therapy but tend to decrease over time. **Focus:** Prioritization

11. **Ans: 3**   Patients taking immunosuppressive medications are at increased risk for development of cancer. A nontender swelling or lump may signify that the patient has lymphoma. The other data indicate that the patient is experiencing common side effects of the immunosuppressive medications. **Focus:** Prioritization

12. **Ans: 4**   Viral load testing measures the amount of HIV genetic material in the blood, so a decrease in viral load indicates that the HAART is effective. The CD4 level, total lymphocytes, and complete blood count will also be used to assess the impact of HIV on immune function but will not directly measure the effectiveness of antiretroviral therapy. **Focus:** Prioritization

13. **Ans: 1**   Administration of oral medication is included in LPN/LVN education and scope of practice. Assessment, planning of care, and teaching are more complex RN-level interventions. **Focus:** Delegation

14. **Ans: 2**   Methotrexate is teratogenic and should not be used by patients who are pregnant. The physician will need to discuss the use of contraception during the time the patient is taking methotrexate. The other patient information may require further patient assessment or teaching, but does not indicate that methotrexate may be contraindicated for the patient. **Focus:** Prioritization

15. **Ans: 2**   The varicella (chickenpox) vaccine is a live-virus vaccine and should not be administered to patients who are receiving immunosuppressive medications such as prednisone. The other medical orders are appropriate. Prednisone doses should be tapered gradually when patients have received long-term steroid therapy, but tapering is not necessary for short-term prednisone use. Measurement of C-reactive protein level is not the most specific test for monitoring treatment, but the test is inexpensive and frequently used. High doses of NSAIDs such as ibuprofen are more likely to cause side effects such as gastrointestinal bleeding but are useful in treating the joint pain associated with SLE exacerbations. **Focus:** Prioritization

16. **Ans: 3**   Albuterol is the most rapidly acting of the medications listed. Corticosteroids are helpful in preventing allergic reactions but are not rapidly acting. Cromolyn is used as a prophylactic medication to prevent asthma attacks but not to treat acute attacks. Aminophylline is not a first-line treatment for bronchospasm. **Focus:** Prioritization

17. **Ans: 1**   A high number of patients with SLE develop nephropathy, so an increase in blood urea nitrogen level may indicate a need for a change in therapy or for further diagnostic testing such as a creatinine clearance test or renal biopsy. The other laboratory results are expected in patients with SLE. **Focus:** Prioritization

18. **Ans: 2**   A high incidence of latex allergy in seen in individuals with allergic reactions to these fruits. More information and/or testing is needed to determine whether the new employee has a latex allergy, which might affect his or her ability to provide direct patient care. The other findings are important to include in documenting the employee's health history but do not affect the ability to provide patient care. **Focus:** Prioritization

19. **Ans: 2**   Because protease inhibitors decrease the metabolism of many drugs, including midazolam, serious toxicity can develop when protease inhibitors are given with other medications. Midazolam should not be given to this patient. The other patient data are consistent with the patient's diagnosis of panic attack and do not indicate an urgent need to communicate with the provider. **Focus:** Prioritization

20. **Ans: 4**   A major purpose of HIV testing for asymptomatic patients is to ensure that HIV-positive individuals are aware of their HIV status, take actions to prevent HIV transmission, and effectively treat the HIV infection. According to current national guidelines, the other actions are also appropriate. Rapid HIV testing must be confirmed by another test, usually the Western blot test. Antiretroviral therapy is recommended for all HIV-positive patients. Risk factor information will be used in tracking patient contacts and in teaching the patient how to reduce the risk for transmission to others. **Focus:** Prioritization

CHAPTER 4: Fluid, Electrolyte, and Acid-Base Balance Problems, pages 23-26

1. **Ans: 2**   UAPs can reinforce additional fluid intake once it is part of the care plan. Administering IV fluids, developing plans, and teaching families require additional education and skills that are within the scope of practice of an RN. **Focus:** Delegation, supervision

2. **Ans: 1**   Normally, neck veins are distended when the client is in the supine position. These veins flatten as the client moves to a sitting position. The other three responses are characteristic of the nursing diagnosis of Excess Fluid Volume. **Focus:** Prioritization

3. **Ans: 1, 2, 3, 4** The LPN/LVN scope of practice and educational preparation includes oral care and routine observation. State practice acts vary as to whether LPNs/LVNs are permitted to perform assessment. The client should be reminded to avoid most commercial mouthwashes, which contain alcohol, a drying agent. Initiating a dietary consult is within the purview of the RN or physician. **Focus:** Delegation, supervision

4. **Ans: 4** Bilateral moist crackles indicate fluid-filled alveoli, which interferes with gas exchange. Furosemide is a potent loop diuretic that will help mobilize the fluid in the lungs. The other orders are important, but are not urgent. **Focus:** Prioritization

5. **Ans: 2** Suspect hypokalemia and check the client's potassium level. Common ECG changes with hypokalemia include ST-segment depression, inverted T waves, and prominent U waves. Clients with hypokalemia may also develop heart block. **Focus:** Prioritization

6. **Ans: 1** The client's potassium level is high (normal range is 3.5 to 5 mEq/L). Kayexalate removes potassium from the body through the gastrointestinal system. Spironolactone is a potassium-sparing diuretic that may cause the client's potassium level to go even higher. The beginning nursing student does not have the skill to assess ECG strips. **Focus:** Delegation, supervision

7. **Ans: 3** SIADH causes a relative sodium deficit due to excessive retention of water. **Focus:** Prioritization

8. **Ans: 1** Providing oral care is within the scope of practice of the UAP. Monitoring and assessing clients, as well as administering IV fluids, require the additional education and skills of the RN. **Focus:** Assignment, delegation, supervision

9. **Ans: 2** A positive Chvostek sign (facial twitching of one side of the mouth, nose, and cheek in response to tapping the face just below and in front of the ear) is a neurologic manifestation of hypocalcemia. The LPN/LVN is experienced and possesses the skills to accurately measure vital signs. **Focus:** Prioritization

10. **Ans: 4** Clients with low calcium levels should be encouraged to eat dairy products, seafood, nuts, broccoli, and spinach, which are all good sources of dietary calcium. **Focus:** Prioritization

11. **Ans: 3** A musculoskeletal manifestation of low phosphorus levels is generalized muscle weakness, which may lead to acute muscle breakdown (rhabdomyolysis). Phosphate is necessary for energy production in the form of ATP, and when not produced, leads to generalized muscle weakness. Although the other statements are true, they do not answer the UAP's question. **Focus:** Delegation, supervision

12. **Ans: 4** Although all of these laboratory values are outside of the normal range, the magnesium level is furthest from normal. With a magnesium level this low, the client is at risk for ECG changes and life-threatening ventricular dysrhythmias. **Focus:** Prioritization

13. **Ans: 2** The client with COPD, although ventilator dependent, is in the most stable condition of the clients in this group. Clients with acid-base imbalances often require frequent laboratory assessment and changes in therapy to correct their disorders. In addition, the client with diabetic ketoacidosis is a new admission and will require an in-depth admission assessment. All three of these clients need care from an experienced critical care nurse. **Focus:** Assignment

14. **Ans: 1** The blood gas component responsible for respiratory acidosis is carbon dioxide. Increasing the ventilator rate will blow off more carbon dioxide and decrease the acidosis. Changes in the oxygen setting may improve oxygenation but will not affect respiratory acidosis. **Focus:** Prioritization

15. **Ans: 2, 3** The UAP's training and education includes how to measure vital signs and record intake and output. Performing fingerstick glucose checks and assessing clients requires additional education and skill, as possessed by licensed nurses. Notifying the provider of glucose changes is within the scope of practice for licensed nurses. Some facilities may train experienced UAPs to perform fingerstick glucose checks and change their role descriptions to designate their new skills, but this task is beyond the normal scope of practice of a UAP. **Focus:** Delegation, supervision

16. **Ans: 4** Risk factors for acid-base imbalances in the older adult include chronic kidney disease and pulmonary disease. Occasional antacid use will not cause imbalances, although antacid abuse is a risk factor for metabolic alkalosis. **Focus:** Prioritization

17. **Ans: 1** A decreased respiratory rate indicates respiratory depression, which also puts the client at risk for respiratory acidosis. All of the other findings are important and should be reported to the RN, but the respiratory rate demands urgent attention. **Focus:** Delegation, supervision

18. **Ans: 2** The client is most likely hyperventilating and blowing off carbon dioxide. This decrease in carbon dioxide will lead to an increase in pH and cause respiratory alkalosis. **Focus:** Prioritization, supervision

19. **Ans: 1** Prolonged nausea and vomiting can result in acid deficit that can lead to metabolic alkalosis. The other findings are important and need to be assessed, but are not related to acid-base imbalances. **Focus:** Prioritization, supervision

20. **Ans: 2** Nasogastric suctioning can result in a decrease in acid components and metabolic alkalosis. The client's decrease in rate and depth of ventilation is an attempt to compensate by retaining carbon dioxide. The first response may be true, but it does not address all the components of the question. The third and fourth answers are inaccurate. **Focus:** Supervision, prioritization

21. **Ans: 1, 4, 5** HCTZ is a thiazide diuretic. It should not be taken at night because it will cause the client

to wake up to urinate. This type of diuretic causes a loss of potassium, so you should teach the client about eating foods rich in potassium. Weight gain and increased edema should not occur while the client is taking this drug, so these should be reported to the prescriber. **Focus:** Prioritization

22. **Ans: 2** Potassium is lost when a client is taking HCTZ, and potassium level should be monitored regularly. **Focus:** Prioritization

23. **Ans: 4** To correct hypovolemic shock with dehydration, the client needs IV fluids that are isotonic and will increase intravascular volume, such as normal saline. With D_5W, the body rapidly metabolizes the dextrose and the solution becomes hypotonic. All of the other orders are appropriate for a client with shock. **Focus:** Prioritization

CHAPTER 5: Safety and Infection Control, pages 27-30

1. **Ans: 3** Current Centers for Disease Control and Prevention (CDC) guidelines indicate that rapid implementation of standard, contact, and airborne precautions are needed for any client suspected of having SARS in order to protect other clients and health care workers. If an airborne-agent isolation (negative-pressure) room is not available in the ED, droplet precautions should be initiated until the client can be moved to a negative-pressure room. The other actions should also be taken rapidly but are not as important as preventing transmission of the disease. **Focus:** Prioritization

2. **Ans: 1** Because the respiratory manifestations associated with avian influenza are potentially life-threatening, the nurse's initial action should be to start oxygen therapy. The other interventions should be implemented after addressing the client's respiratory problems. **Focus:** Prioritization

3. **Ans: 3, 2, 4, 1, 5** This sequence will prevent contact of the contaminated gloves and gown with areas (such as your hair) that cannot be easily cleaned after client contact and stop transmission of microorganisms to you and your other clients. The correct method for donning and removal of personal protective equipment (PPE) has been standardized by agencies such as the CDC and the Occupational Safety and Health Administration. **Focus:** Prioritization

4. **Ans: 2, 3, 4** Because herpes zoster (shingles) is spread through airborne means and by direct contact with the lesions, you should wear an N95 respirator or high-efficiency particulate air filter respirator, a gown, and gloves. Surgical face masks filter only large particles and will not provide protection from herpes zoster. Goggles and shoe covers are not needed for airborne or contact precautions. **Focus:** Prioritization

5. **Ans: 2** Varicella (chickenpox) is spread by airborne means and could be rapidly transmitted to other clients in the ED. The child with the rash should be quickly isolated from the other ED clients through placement in a negative-pressure room. Droplet and/or contact precautions should be instituted for the clients with possible pertussis and MRSA infection, but this can be done after isolating the child with possible chickenpox. The client who has been exposed to TB does not place other clients at risk for infection because there are no symptoms of active TB. **Focus:** Prioritization

6. **Ans: 3** According to CDC guidelines, several factors increase the risk for infection for this client: central lines are associated with a higher infection risk, jugular vein lines are more prone to infection, and the line is nontunneled. Peripherally inserted IV lines such as PICC lines and midline catheters are associated with a lower incidence of infection. Implanted ports are placed under the skin and are the least likely central line to be associated with catheter infection. **Focus:** Prioritization

7. **Ans: 3** LPN/LVN education and scope of practice include performing dressing changes and obtaining specimens for wound culture. Teaching, assessment, and planning of care are complex actions that should be carried out by the RN. **Focus:** Delegation

8. **Ans: 4** The client's age, history of antibiotic therapy, and watery stools suggest that he may have *Clostridium difficile* infection. The initial action should be to place him on contact precautions to prevent the spread of *C. difficile* to other clients. The other actions are also needed and should be taken after placing the client on contact precautions. **Focus:** Prioritization

9. **Ans: 2** To prevent contamination of staff or other clients by anthrax, decontamination of the client by removal and disposal of clothing and showering is the initial action in possible anthrax exposure. Assessment of the client for signs of infection should be performed after decontamination. Notification of security personnel (and local and regional law enforcement agencies) is necessary in the case of possible bioterrorism, but this should occur after decontaminating and caring for the client. According to the CDC guidelines, antibiotics should be administered only if there are signs of infection or the contaminating substance tests positive for anthrax. **Focus:** Prioritization

10. **Ans: 3** All hospital personnel who care for the client are responsible for correct implementation of contact precautions. The other actions should be carried out by licensed nurses, whose education covers monitoring of laboratory results, client teaching, and communication with other departments about essential client data. **Focus:** Delegation

11. **Ans: 3** The client's clinical manifestations suggest possible avian influenza ("bird flu"). If the client has

traveled recently in Asia or the Middle East, where outbreaks of bird flu have occurred, you will need to institute airborne and contact precautions immediately. The other actions may also be appropriate but are not the initial action to take for this client, who may transmit the infection to other clients or staff members. **Focus:** Prioritization

12. **Ans: 4**   The UAP can follow agency policy to disinfect items that come in contact with intact skin (e.g., blood pressure cuffs) by cleaning with chemicals such as alcohol. Teaching and assessment for upper respiratory tract symptoms or use of immunosuppressants require more education and a broader scope of practice, and these tasks should be performed by licensed nurses. **Focus:** Delegation

13. **Ans: 1, 2**   A gown and gloves should be used when coming in contact with linens that may be contaminated by the client's wound secretions. The other PPE items are not necessary, because transmission by splashes, droplets, or airborne means will not occur when the bed is changed. **Focus:** Prioritization

14. **Ans: 3**   LPN/LVN scope of practice and education include administration of medications. Assessment of hydration status, client and family education, and assessment of client risk factors for diarrhea should be done by the RN. **Focus:** Delegation

15. **Ans: 2**   Because the hands of health care workers are the most common means of transmission of infection from one client to another, the most effective method of preventing the spread of infection is to make supplies for hand hygiene readily available for staff to use. Wearing a gown to care for clients who are not on contact precautions is not necessary. Although some hospitals have started screening newly-admitted clients for MRSA, this is not considered a priority action according to current national guidelines. Because administration of antibiotics to individuals who are colonized by bacteria may promote development of antibiotic resistance, antibiotic use should be restricted to clients who have clinical manifestations of infection. **Focus:** Prioritization

16. **Ans: 1**   According to the CDC, CAUTIs are the most common health care–acquired infection in the United States. Primary CDC recommendations include avoiding the use of indwelling catheters and the removal of catheters as soon as possible. Although a high fluid intake will also help to reduce the risk for CAUTIs, 1500 mL may be excessive for some clients. The CDC recommends against routine screening for asymptomatic bacteriuria. Antimicrobial catheters are a secondary recommendation and may be appropriate if other measures are not effective in reducing CAUTI incidence. **Focus:** Prioritization

17. **Ans: 3**   Clients with infections that require airborne precautions (such as TB) need to be in private rooms. Clients with infections that require contact precautions (such as those with *C. difficile* and VRE infections)

should ideally be placed in private rooms; however, they can be placed in rooms with other clients with the same diagnosis. Standard precautions are required for the client with toxic shock syndrome. **Focus:** Prioritization

18. **Ans: 2**   Current CDC evidence-based guidelines indicate that droplet precautions for clients with meningococcal meningitis can be discontinued when the client has received antibiotic therapy (with drugs that are effective against *Neisseria meningitidis*) for 24 hours. The other information may indicate that the client's condition is improving but does not indicate that droplet precautions should be discontinued. **Focus:** Prioritization

19. **Ans: 2**   "Red man" syndrome occurs when vancomycin is infused too quickly. Because the client needs the medication to treat the infection, the vancomycin should not be discontinued. Antihistamines may help decrease the flushing, but vancomycin should be administered over at least 60 minutes. Although the client's temperature will be monitored, a temperature elevation is not the most likely cause of the client's flushing. **Focus:** Prioritization

20. **Ans: 4**   Individuals who have contact with infants should be immunized against pertussis in order to avoid infection and to prevent transmission to the infant. The influenza and pneumococcal vaccines can be administered later in the year, prior to the influenza season. The herpes zoster vaccine is important, but does not need to be administered today. **Focus:** Prioritization

21. **Ans: 1, 2, 5**   The ventilator bundle developed by the Institute for Healthcare Improvement includes recommendations for continuous elevation of the head of the bed, daily assessment for extubation readiness, and daily oral care with chlorhexidine solution. Pneumococcal immunization will prevent pneumococcal pneumonia, but it is not designed to prevent VAP. The use of a kinetic bed may also be of benefit to the client, but it is not considered essential in preventing VAP. **Focus:** Prioritization

22. **Ans: 3**   The current Institute for Healthcare Improvement guidelines indicate that chlorhexidine is more effective than the other options at reducing the risk for central line–associated bloodstream infections (CLABSIs). The other solutions provide some decrease in the number of microorganisms on the skin, but are not as effective as chlorhexidine. **Focus:** Prioritization

23. **Ans: 3**   The staff member who is most knowledgeable about the regulations regarding HIV prophylaxis and about obtaining a client's HIV status and/or ordering HIV testing is the occupational health nurse. Performing unauthorized HIV testing or asking the client yourself would be unethical. The charge nurse is not responsible for obtaining this information (unless the charge nurse is also in charge of occupational health). **Focus:** Prioritization

24. **Ans: 1**   The Institute for Safe Medication Practices (ISMP) guidelines indicate that the use of a trailing zero is not appropriate when writing medication orders because the order can easily be mistaken for a larger dose (in this case, 10 mg). The order should be clarified before administration. The other orders are appropriate, based on the client's diagnosis. **Focus:** Prioritization

25. **Ans: 1**   The first priority for an ambulating client who is dizzy is to prevent falls, which could lead to serious injury. The other actions are also appropriate but are not as high a priority. **Focus:** Prioritization

26. **Ans: 1, 4, 3, 2**   The first action after a medication error should be to assess the client for adverse outcomes. You should evaluate this client for symptoms such as bradycardia and excessive salivation. These may indicate cholinergic crisis, a possible effect of excessive doses of anticholinesterase medications such as neostigmine. The physician should be rapidly notified so that treatment with atropine can be ordered to counteract the effects of the neostigmine, if necessary. Determining the circumstances that led to the error will help decrease the risk for future errors and will be needed to complete the medication error report. **Focus:** Prioritization

27. **Ans: 2**   Hospital staff who have been trained in the appropriate application of restraints may reposition the restraints. Evaluation of the continued need for restraints, communication with the provider about the client's status, and teaching of the family require RN-level education and scope of practice. **Focus:** Delegation

28. **Ans: 1**   Leukeran is an antineoplastic drug used to treat cancer. The medication used to treat methotrexate toxicity is leucovorin (Wellcovorin), a reduced form of folic acid. Leukeran and leucovorin are "look-alike, sound-alike" drugs that have been identified by the ISMP as being at high risk for involvement in medication errors. All treatment prescriptions that are communicated by telephone should be reconfirmed with the health care provider; however, the most important order to clarify is the Leukeran order, which is likely an error. **Focus:** Prioritization

CHAPTER 6: Respiratory Problems, pages 31-34

1. **Ans: 1, 2, 4**   The experienced LPN/LVN is capable of gathering data and making observations, including noting breath sounds and performing pulse oximetry. Administering medications, such as those delivered via MDIs, is within the scope of practice of the LPN/LVN. Independently completing the admission assessment, developing the nursing care plan, and evaluating a patient's abilities require additional education and skills within the scope of

practice of the professional RN. **Focus:** Delegation, supervision

2. **Ans: 2**   For patients with chronic emphysema, the stimulus to breathe is a low serum oxygen level (the normal stimulus is a high carbon dioxide level). This patient's oxygen flow is too high and is causing a high serum oxygen level, which results in a decreased respiratory rate. If you do not intervene, the patient is at risk for respiratory arrest. Crackles, barrel chest, and assumption of a sitting position leaning over the nightstand are common in patients with chronic emphysema. **Focus:** Prioritization

3. **Ans: 1**   When the oxygen flow rate is higher than 4 L/min, the mucous membranes can be dried out. The best treatment is to add humidification to the oxygen delivery system. Applying water-soluble jelly to the nares can also help decrease mucosal irritation. None of the other options will treat the problem. **Focus:** Prioritization

4. **Ans: 3**   When tracheostomy care is performed, a sterile field is set up and sterile technique is used. Standard precautions such as washing hands must also be maintained but are not enough when performing tracheostomy care. The presence of a tracheostomy tube provides direct access to the lungs for organisms, so sterile technique is used to prevent infection. All of the other steps are correct and appropriate. **Focus:** Delegation, supervision

5. **Ans: 2, 3, 4, 5**   The correct position for a patient with an anterior nosebleed is upright and leaning forward to prevent blood from entering the stomach and to avoid aspiration. All of the other instructions are appropriate according to best practice for emergency care of a patient with an anterior nosebleed. **Focus:** Delegation, supervision, assignment

6. **Ans: 3**   The UAP can remind patients about actions that have already been taught by the nurse and are part of the patient's plan of care. Discussing and teaching require additional education and training. These actions are within the scope of practice of the RN. The RN can delegate medication administration to an LPN/LVN. **Focus:** Delegation, supervision

7. **Ans: 1, 2**   The new RN is at an early point in her orientation. The most appropriate patients to assign to her are those in stable condition who require routine care. The patient with the lobectomy will require the care of an experienced nurse, who will perform frequent assessments and monitoring for postoperative complications. The patient admitted with newly-diagnosed esophageal cancer will also benefit from care by an experienced nurse. This patient may have questions and needs a comprehensive admission assessment. As the new nurse advances through her orientation, you will want to work with him or her in providing care for these patients with more complex needs. The newly-diagnosed diabetic patient will need much teaching as well as careful monitoring. **Focus:** Assignment, delegation, supervision

8. **Ans: 1, 2, 4, 5**   Bedding should be washed in hot water to destroy dust mites. All of the other points are accurate and appropriate to a teaching plan for a patient with a new diagnosis of asthma. **Focus:** Prioritization

9. **Ans: 1, 3, 2, 5, 4, 6**   Before each use, the cap is removed and the inhaler is shaken according to the instructions in the package insert. Next the patient should breathe out completely. As the patient begins to breathe in deeply through the mouth, the canister should be pressed down to release 1 puff (dose) of the medication. The patient should continue to breathe in slowly over 3 to 5 seconds and then hold the breath for at least 10 seconds to allow the medication to reach deep into the lungs. The patient should wait at least 1 minute between puffs from the inhaler. **Focus:** Prioritization

10. **Ans: 1**   Assisting patients with positioning and activities of daily living (ADLs) is within the educational preparation and scope of practice of UAPs. Teaching, instructing, and assessing patients all require additional education and skills and are more appropriate to the scope of practice of licensed nurses. **Focus:** Delegation, supervision

11. **Ans: 1**   Experienced LPNs/LVNs can use observation of patients to gather data regarding how well patients perform interventions that have already been taught. Assisting patients with ADLs is more appropriately delegated to UAPs. Planning and consulting require additional education and skills, appropriate to the RN's scope of practice. **Focus:** Delegation, supervision

12. **Ans: 4**   A patient who did not have the pneumonia vaccination or flu shot is at increased risk for developing pneumonia or influenza. An elevated temperature indicates some form of infection, which may be respiratory in origin. All of the other vital sign values are slightly elevated but are not a cause for immediate concern. **Focus:** Delegation, supervision

13. **Ans: 2**   The UAP's training includes how to monitor and record intake and output. After the nurse has taught the patient about the importance of adequate nutritional intake for energy, the UAP can remind and encourage the patient to take in adequate nutrition. Instructing patients and planning activities require more education and skill, and are appropriate to the RN's scope of practice. Monitoring the patient's cardiovascular response to activity is a complex process requiring additional education, training, and skill, and falls within the RN's scope of practice. **Focus:** Delegation, supervision

14. **Ans: 2**   Continuous bubbling indicates an air leak that must be identified. With the physician's order, you can apply a padded clamp to the drainage tubing close to the occlusive dressing. If the bubbling stops, the air leak may be at the chest tube insertion, which will require you to notify the physician. If the air bubbling does not stop when you apply the padded clamp, the air leak is between the clamp and the drainage system, and you must assess the system carefully to locate the leak. Chest tube drainage of 10 to 15 mL/hr is acceptable. Chest tube dressings are not changed daily but may be reinforced. The patient's reports of pain need to be assessed and treated. This is important but is not as urgent as investigating a chest tube leak. **Focus:** Delegation, supervision

15. **Ans: 4**   The patient with asthma did not achieve relief from shortness of breath after using the bronchodilator and is at risk for respiratory complications. This patient's needs are urgent. The other patients need to be assessed as soon as possible, but none of their situations is urgent. In COPD patients, pulse oximetry oxygen saturations of more than 90% are acceptable. **Focus:** Prioritization

16. **Ans: 3**   UAPs can remind the patient to perform actions that are already part of the plan of care. Assisting the patient into the best position to facilitate coughing requires specialized knowledge and understanding that is beyond the scope of practice of the basic UAP. However, an experienced UAP could assist the patient with positioning after the UAP and the patient had been taught the proper technique. UAPs would still be under the supervision of the RN. Teaching patients about adequate fluid intake and techniques that facilitate coughing requires additional education and skill, and is within the scope of practice of the RN. **Focus:** Delegation, supervision

17. **Ans: 3**   Many surgical patients are taught about coughing, deep breathing, and the use of incentive spirometry preoperatively. To care for the patient with TB in isolation, the nurse must be fitted for a high-efficiency particulate air (HEPA) respirator mask. The bronchoscopy patient needs specialized and careful assessment and monitoring after the procedure, and the ventilator-dependent patient needs a nurse who is familiar with ventilator care. Both of these patients need experienced nurses. **Focus:** Assignment

18. **Ans: 2**   Patients taking isoniazid must continue taking the drug for 6 months. The other three statements are accurate and indicate an understanding of TB. Family members should be tested because of their repeated exposure to the patient. Covering the nose and mouth when sneezing or coughing, and placing tissues in plastic bags, help prevent transmission of the causative organism. The dietary changes are recommended for patients with TB. **Focus:** Prioritization

19. **Ans: 1**   Patients who have recently experienced trauma are at risk for deep vein thrombosis and pulmonary embolus. None of the other findings are risk factors for pulmonary embolus. Prolonged immobilization is also a risk factor for deep vein thrombosis and pulmonary embolus, but this period of bed rest was very short. **Focus:** Prioritization

Answer Key

20. **Ans: 4**   An LPN/LVN who has been trained to auscultate lung sounds can gather data by routine assessment and observation, under supervision of an RN. Independently evaluating patients, assessing for symptoms of respiratory failure, and monitoring and interpreting laboratory values require additional education and skill, appropriate to the scope of practice of the RN. **Focus:** Delegation, supervision

21. **Ans: 1, 2, 3, 5**   While a patient is receiving anticoagulation therapy, it is important to avoid trauma to the rectal tissue, which could cause bleeding (e.g., avoid rectal thermometers and enemas). All of the other instructions are appropriate to the care of a patient receiving anticoagulants. **Focus:** Delegation, supervision

22. **Ans: 1**   A nonrebreather mask can deliver nearly 100% oxygen. When the patient's oxygenation status does not improve adequately in response to delivery of oxygen at this high concentration, refractory hypoxemia is present. Usually at this stage, the patient is working very hard to breathe and may go into respiratory arrest unless health care providers intervene by providing intubation and mechanical ventilation to decrease the patient's work of breathing. **Focus:** Prioritization

23. **Ans: 3**   The endotracheal tube should be marked at the level where it touches the incisor tooth or nares. This mark is used to verify that the tube has not shifted. The other three actions are appropriate after endotracheal tube placement. The priority at this time is to verify that the tube has been correctly placed. **Focus:** Delegation, supervision, prioritization

24. **Ans: 2**   The UAP's educational preparation includes measuring vital signs, and an experienced UAP would know how to check oxygen saturation by pulse oximetry. Assessing and observing the patient, as well as checking ventilator settings, require the additional education and skills of the RN. **Focus:** Delegation, supervision

25. **Ans: 4**   Infections are always a threat for the patient receiving mechanical ventilation. The endotracheal tube bypasses the body's normal air-filtering mechanisms and provides a direct access route for bacteria or viruses to the lower parts of the respiratory system. **Focus:** Prioritization

26. **Ans: 3**   Confusion in a patient this age is unusual and may be an indication of intracerebral bleeding associated with enoxaparin use. The right leg symptoms are consistent with a resolving deep vein thrombosis; the patient may need teaching about keeping the right leg elevated above the heart to reduce swelling and pain. The presence of ecchymoses may point to a need to do more patient teaching about avoiding injury while taking anticoagulants but does not indicate that the physician needs to be called. **Focus:** Prioritization

27. **Ans: 2**   Manual ventilation of the patient will allow you to deliver an FiO_2 of 100% to the patient while you attempt to determine the cause of the high-pressure alarm. The patient may need reassurance, suctioning, and/or insertion of an oral airway, but the first step should be assessing the reason for the high-pressure alarm and resolving the hypoxemia. **Focus:** Prioritization

28. **Ans: 4**   The patient's history and symptoms suggest the development of ARDS, which will require intubation and mechanical ventilation. The maximum oxygen delivery with a nasal cannula is an FiO_2 of 44%. This is achieved with the oxygen flow at 6 L/min, so increasing the flow to 10 L/min will not be helpful. Helping the patient to cough and deep breathe will not improve the lung stiffness that is causing his respiratory distress. Morphine sulfate will only decrease the respiratory drive and further contribute to his hypoxemia. **Focus:** Prioritization

29. **Ans: 3**   Removal of large quantities of fluid from the pleural space can cause fluid to shift from the circulation into the pleural space, causing hypotension and tachycardia. The patient may need to receive IV fluids to correct this. The other data indicate that the patient needs ongoing monitoring and/or interventions but would not be unusual findings for a patient with this diagnosis or after this procedure. **Focus:** Prioritization

30. **Ans: 3**   Research indicates that nursing actions such as maintaining the head of the bed at 30 to 45 degrees decrease the incidence of VAP. These actions are part of the standard of care for patients who require mechanical ventilation. The other actions are also appropriate for this patient but will not decrease the incidence of VAP. **Focus:** Prioritization

CHAPTER 7: Cardiovascular Problems, pages 35-40

1. **Ans: 2**   Cardiac troponin levels are elevated 3 hours after the onset of ACS (unstable angina or myocardial infarction [MI]) and are very specific to cardiac muscle injury or infarction. Although levels of creatine kinase MB and myoglobin also increase with MI, the increases occur later and/or are not as specific to myocardial damage as troponin levels. Elevated C-reactive protein levels are a risk factor for coronary artery disease but are not useful in detecting acute injury or infarction. **Focus:** Prioritization

2. **Ans: 4**   Chest pain in a client undergoing a stress test indicates myocardial ischemia and is an indication to stop the testing to avoid ongoing ischemia, injury, or infarction. Moderate elevations in blood pressure and heart rate and slight decreases in oxygen saturation are a normal response to exercise and are expected during stress testing. **Focus:** Prioritization

3. **Ans: 1, 4, 6**   Attaching cardiac monitor leads, obtaining an ECG, and administering oral medications

are within the scope of practice for LPN/LVNs. An experienced ED LPN/LVN would be familiar with these activities. Although anticoagulants and narcotics may be administered by LPNs/LVNs to stable clients, these are high-alert medications that should be given by the RN to this unstable client. Obtaining a pertinent medical history requires RN-level education and scope of practice. **Focus:** Delegation

4. **Ans: 4** Research indicates that reducing sodium intake will lower blood pressure. Lifestyle management is appropriate initial therapy for this client with stage 1 hypertension and no cardiovascular disease or risk factors. Antihypertensive medications would not be prescribed unless lifestyle changes were attempted for several months without a decrease in blood pressure. This client's assessment data indicate that she is not overweight and does not drink alcohol excessively, so discussing changes in these risk factors would not be appropriate. **Focus:** Prioritization

5. **Ans: 3** A persistent and irritating cough (caused by accumulation of bradykinin) is a possible adverse effect of angiotensin-converting enzyme (ACE) inhibitors such as enalapril and is a common reason for changing to another medication category such as the angiotensin II receptor blockers. The other assessment data indicate a need for more client teaching and ongoing monitoring but would not require a change in therapy. **Focus:** Prioritization

6. **Ans: 1, 2** The client's major modifiable risk factor is her ongoing smoking. The family history is significant, and she should be aware that this increases her cardiovascular risk. The goal when treating hypertension with medications is reduction of blood pressure to under 140/90 mm Hg. There is no indication that stress is a risk factor for this client. The client's work involves moderate physical activity; although leisure exercise may further decrease her cardiac risk, this is not an immediate need for this client. **Focus:** Prioritization

7. **Ans: 2** An RN who worked on a medical-surgical unit would be familiar with left ventricular failure, the administration of IV medications, and ongoing monitoring for therapeutic and adverse effects of furosemide. The other clients need to be cared for by RNs who are more familiar with the care of clients who have ACS and with collaborative treatments such as coronary angioplasty and coronary artery stenting. **Focus:** Assignment

8. **Ans: 4** Because continuous chest pain lasting for more than 12 hours indicates that reversible myocardial injury has progressed to irreversible myocardial necrosis, fibrinolytic drugs are not recommended for clients with chest pain that has lasted for more than 12 hours. The other information is also important to communicate but would not impact the decision about alteplase use. **Focus:** Prioritization

9. **Ans: 1** Administration of nitroglycerin and appropriate client monitoring for therapeutic and adverse effects are included in LPN/LVN education and scope of practice. Monitoring of blood pressure, pulse, and oxygen saturation should be delegated to the UAP. Client teaching requires RN-level education and scope of practice. **Focus:** Delegation

10. **Ans: 3** The priority for a client with unstable angina or MI is treatment of pain. It is important to remember to assess vital signs before administering sublingual nitroglycerin. The other activities also should be accomplished rapidly but are not as high a priority. **Focus:** Prioritization

11. **Ans: 3** The best option in this situation is to educate the client about the purpose of the docusate (to counteract the negative effects of immobility and narcotic use on peristalsis). Charting the medication as "refused" or telling the client that he should take the docusate simply because it was prescribed are possible actions but are not as appropriate as client education. It is unethical to administer a medication to a client who is unwilling to take it, unless someone else has health care power of attorney and has authorized use of the medication. **Focus:** Prioritization

12. **Ans: 4** The goal in pain management for the client with an acute MI is to completely eliminate the pain. Even pain rated at a level of 1 out of 10 should be treated with additional morphine sulfate (although possibly a lower dose). The other data indicate a need for ongoing assessment for the possible adverse effects of hypotension, respiratory depression, and tachycardia but do not require further action at this time. **Focus:** Prioritization

13. **Ans: 2** For behavior to change, the client must be aware of the need to make changes. This response acknowledges the client's statement and asks for further clarification. This will give you more information about the client's feelings, current diet, and activity levels and may increase the willingness to learn. The other responses (although possibly accurate) indicate an intention to teach whether the client is ready or not and are not likely to lead to changes in lifestyle. **Focus:** Prioritization

14. **Ans: 3** Hyperkalemia is a common adverse effect of both ACE inhibitors and potassium-sparing diuretics. The other laboratory values may be affected by these medications but are not as likely or as potentially life threatening. **Focus:** Prioritization

15. **Ans: 2** Since proton pump inhibitors such as omeprazole affect the metabolism of clopidogrel and decrease its effectiveness, the health care provider may want to discontinue the omeprazole in this client with unstable angina. The other medications should also be verified, but current national guidelines for clients with unstable angina indicate that providers should consider avoiding proton pump inhibitors in those who require clopidogrel. **Focus:** Prioritization

16. **Ans: 1** Because TEE is performed after the throat is numbed using a topical anesthetic and possibly after IV sedation, it is important that the client be placed on NPO status for several hours before the test. The other actions also will need to be accomplished before the TEE but do not need to be implemented immediately. **Focus:** Prioritization

17. **Ans: 4** The most common complication after coronary arteriography is hemorrhage, and the earliest indication of hemorrhage is an increase in heart rate. The other data may also indicate a need for ongoing assessment, but the increase in heart rate is of most concern. **Focus:** Prioritization

18. **Ans: 1** Measurement of ankle and brachial blood pressures for ankle-brachial index calculation is within the UAP's scope of practice. Calculating the ankle-brachial index and any referrals or discussion with the client are the responsibility of the supervising RN. The other clients require more complex assessments or client teaching, which should be done by an experienced RN. **Focus:** Delegation

19. **Ans: 2** The new RN's education and hospital orientation would have included safe administration of IV medications. The preceptor will be responsible for the supervision of the new graduate in assessments and client care. The other clients require more complex assessment or client teaching by an RN with experience in caring for clients with these diagnoses. **Focus:** Assignment

20. **Ans: 3** Premature ventricular contractions occurring in the setting of acute myocardial injury or infarction can lead to ventricular tachycardia and/or ventricular fibrillation (cardiac arrest), so rapid treatment is necessary. The other clients also have dysrhythmias that will require further assessment, but these are not as immediately life threatening as the premature ventricular contractions in the setting of MI. **Focus:** Prioritization

21. **Ans: 1** Research indicates that rapid defibrillation improves the success of resuscitation in cardiac arrest. If defibrillation is unsuccessful in converting the client's rhythm into a perfusing rhythm, CPR should be initiated. Administration of medications and intubation are later interventions. Determining which of these interventions will be used first depends on other factors, such as whether IV access is available. **Focus:** Prioritization

22. **Ans: 3** Research indicates that mortality is decreased when clients with heart failure use beta-blocking medications such as carvedilol. When beta-blocker therapy is started for clients with heart failure, heart failure symptoms may initially become worse for a few weeks, so increased fatigue, activity intolerance, weight gain, and edema are not indicative of a need to discontinue the medication at this time. However, the slow heart rate does require further follow-up, because bradycardia may progress to

more serious dysrhythmias such as heart block. **Focus:** Prioritization

23. **Ans: 2** The client's symptoms indicate acute hypoxia, so immediate further assessments (such as assessment of oxygen saturation, neurologic status, and breath sounds) are indicated. The other clients also should be assessed soon, because they are likely to require nursing actions such as medication administration and teaching, but they are not as acutely ill as the dyspneic client. **Focus:** Prioritization

24. **Ans: 2** LPN/LVN education and scope of practice include data collection such as listening to lung sounds and checking for peripheral edema when caring for stable clients. Weighing the residents should be delegated to a UAP. Reviewing medications with residents and planning appropriate activity levels are nursing actions that require RN-level education and scope of practice. **Focus:** Delegation

25. **Ans: 3** The client's visual disturbances may be a sign of digoxin toxicity. The nurse should notify the health care provider and obtain an order to measure the digoxin level. An irregularly irregular pulse is expected with atrial fibrillation; there are no contraindications to taking digoxin with food; and crackles that clear with coughing are indicative of atelectasis, not worsening of heart failure. **Focus:** Prioritization

26. **Ans: 2, 4, 3, 1** The primary goal is to decrease the cardiac ischemia that may be causing the client's tachycardia. This would be most rapidly accomplished by decreasing the workload of the heart and administering supplemental oxygen. Changes in blood pressure indicate the impact of the tachycardia on cardiac output and tissue perfusion. Finally, the physician should be notified about the client's response to activity, because changes in therapy may be indicated. **Focus:** Prioritization

27. **Ans: 3** The client's history and symptoms indicate that acute arterial occlusion has occurred. Because it is important to return blood flow to the foot rapidly, the physician should be notified immediately so that interventions such as balloon angioplasty or surgery can be initiated. Changing the position of the foot and improving blood oxygen saturation will not improve oxygen delivery to the foot. Telling the client that embolization is a common complication of endocarditis will not reassure a client who is experiencing acute pain. **Focus:** Prioritization

28. **Ans: 4** Assisting with hygiene is included in the role and education of UAP. Assessments and teaching are appropriate activities for licensed nursing staff members. **Focus:** Delegation

29. **Ans: 1** Elevated blood pressure in the immediate postoperative period puts stress on the graft suture line and could lead to graft rupture and/or hemorrhage, so it is important to lower blood pressure quickly. The other data also indicate the need for ongoing assessments and possible interventions but do

not pose an immediate threat to the client's hemodynamic stability. **Focus:** Prioritization

30. **Ans: 3** Development of plans for client care or teaching requires RN-level education and is the responsibility of the RN. Wound care, medication administration, assisting with ambulation, and reinforcing previously-taught information are activities that can be delegated to other nursing personnel under the supervision of the RN. **Focus:** Delegation

31. **Ans: 4** Anticoagulant medications are high-alert medications and require special safeguards, such as double-checking of medications by two nurses before administration. Although the other medications require the usual medication safety procedures, double-checking is not needed. **Focus:** Prioritization

32. **Ans: 2** Research indicates that B-type natriuretic peptide levels increase in clients with poor left ventricular function and symptomatic heart failure and can be used to differentiate heart failure from other causes of dyspnea and fatigue such as pneumonia. The other values should also be monitored, but do not indicate whether the client has heart failure. **Focus:** Prioritization

CHAPTER 8: Hematologic Problems, pages 41-44

1. **Ans: 4** Centers for Disease Control and Prevention (CDC) guidelines for the prevention of surgical site infections indicate that surgery should be postponed when there is evidence of a pre-existing infection such as an elevation in white blood cell count. The other values are slightly abnormal, but would not be likely to cause postoperative problems for knee arthroscopy. **Focus:** Prioritization

2. **Ans: 3** Normal saline, an isotonic solution, should be used when priming the IV line to avoid causing hemolysis of red blood cells (RBCs). Ideally, blood products should be infused as soon as possible after they are obtained; however, a 20-minute delay would not be unsafe. Large-bore IV catheters are preferable for blood administration; if a smaller catheter must be used, normal saline may be used to dilute the RBCs. Although the new RN should avoid increasing patient anxiety by indicating that a serious transfusion reaction may occur, this action is not as high a concern as using an inappropriate fluid for priming the IV tubing. **Focus:** Prioritization

3. **Ans: 2** Hypoxia and deoxygenation of the RBCs are the most common cause of sickling, so administration of oxygen is the priority intervention here. Pain control and hydration are also important interventions for this patient and should be accomplished rapidly. Vaccination may help prevent future sickling episodes by decreasing the risk of infection, but it will not help with the current sickling crisis. **Focus:** Prioritization

4. **Ans: 1** An experienced UAP will have been taught how to obtain a stool specimen for the Hemoccult slide test, because this is a common screening test for hospitalized patients. Having the patient sign an informed consent form should be done by the physician who will be performing the colonoscopy. Administering medications and checking for allergies are within the scope of practice of licensed nursing staff. **Focus:** Delegation

5. **Ans: 3** A nurse who works in the PACU will be familiar with the monitoring needed for a patient who has just returned from a procedure such as a colonoscopy, which requires conscious sedation. Care of the other patients requires staff with more experience with various types of hematologic disorders and would be better to assign to nursing personnel who regularly work on the medical-surgical unit. **Focus:** Assignment

6. **Ans: 1** Patients with pancytopenia are at higher risk for infection. The patient with digoxin toxicity presents the least risk of infecting the new patient. Viral pneumonia, shingles, and cellulitis are infectious processes. **Focus:** Prioritization

7. **Ans: 3** Because aspirin will decrease platelet aggregation, patients with thrombocytopenia should not use aspirin routinely. Patient teaching about this should be included in the care plan. Bruising is consistent with the patient's admission problem of thrombocytopenia. Soft, dark brown stools indicate that there is no frank blood in the bowel movements. Although the patient's decreased appetite requires further assessment by the nurse, this is a common complication of chemotherapy. **Focus:** Prioritization

8. **Ans: 2** When a hemophiliac patient is at high risk for bleeding, the priority intervention is to maximize the availability of clotting factors. The other orders also should be implemented rapidly but do not have as high a priority as administering clotting factors. **Focus:** Prioritization

9. **Ans: 1** Patients taking warfarin are advised to avoid making sudden dietary changes, because changing the oral intake of foods high in vitamin K (such as green leafy vegetables and some fruits) will have an impact on the effectiveness of the medication. The other statements suggest that further teaching may be indicated, but more assessment for teaching needs is required first. **Focus:** Prioritization

10. **Ans: 3** Because the decrease in oxygen saturation will have the greatest immediate effect on all body systems, improvement in oxygenation should be the priority goal of care. The other data also indicate the need for rapid intervention, but improvement of oxygenation is the most urgent need. **Focus:** Prioritization

11. **Ans: 3** More assessment about what the patient means is needed before any interventions can be planned or implemented. All of the other statements indicate an assumption that the patient is afraid of

dying of Hodgkin disease, which may not be the case. **Focus:** Prioritization PCC

12. **Ans: 4**   Any temperature elevation in a neutropenic patient may indicate the presence of a life-threatening infection, so actions such as drawing blood for culture and administering antibiotics should be initiated quickly. The other patients need to be assessed as soon as possible but are not critically ill. **Focus:** Prioritization

13. **Ans: 2**   UAP education covers routine nursing skills such as assessment of vital signs. Evaluation, baseline assessment of patient abilities, and nutrition planning are activities appropriate to RN practice. **Focus:** Delegation

14. **Ans: 3**   The patient's symptoms indicate that a transfusion reaction may be occurring, so the first action should be to stop the transfusion. Chills are an indication of a febrile reaction, so warming the patient may not be appropriate. Checking the patient's temperature and administering oxygen are also appropriate actions if a transfusion reaction is suspected; however, stopping the transfusion is the priority. **Focus:** Prioritization

15. **Ans: 1**   LPNs/LVNs should be assigned to care for stable patients. Subcutaneous administration of epoetin is within the LPN/LVN scope of practice. Blood transfusions should be administered by RNs, because evaluation for and management of transfusion reactions require RN-level education and scope of practice. The other patients will require teaching about phlebotomy and bone marrow aspiration that should be implemented by the RN. **Focus:** Assignment

16. **Ans: 4**   The leg numbness may indicate spinal cord compression, which should be evaluated and treated immediately by the health care provider to prevent further loss of function. Chronic bone pain, hyperuricemia, and the presence of Bence Jones proteins in the urine all are typical of multiple myeloma and do require assessment and/or treatment; the loss of motor or sensory function is an emergency. **Focus:** Prioritization

17. **Ans: 2**   Because the spleen has an important role in the phagocytosis of microorganisms, the patient is at higher risk for severe infection after a splenectomy. Medical therapy, such as antibiotic administration, is usually indicated for any symptoms of infection. The other information also indicates the need for more assessment and intervention, but prevention and treatment of infection are the highest priorities for this patient. **Focus:** Prioritization

18. **Ans: 3**   The infusion of IV fluids is a common intervention that can be implemented by RNs who do not have experience in caring for patients who are severely immunosuppressed. Administering cyclosporine, assessing for subtle indications of infection, and patient teaching are more complex tasks that should be done by RN staff members who have experience caring for immunosuppressed patients. **Focus:** Delegation

19. **Ans: 3**   Because many aspects of nursing care need to be modified to prevent infection when a patient has a low absolute neutrophil count, care should be provided by the staff member with the most experience with neutropenic patients. The other staff members have the education required to care for this patient but are not as clinically experienced. When LPN/LVN staff members are given acute care patient assignments, they must work under the supervision of an RN. The LPN/LVN in this case would report to the RN assigned to the patient. **Focus:** Assignment

20. **Ans: 4**   A patient with neutropenia is at increased risk for infection, so the LTC charge nurse needs to know about the neutropenia to make decisions about the patient's room assignment and to plan care. The other information also will impact planning for patient care, but the charge nurse needs the information about neutropenia before the patient is transferred. **Focus:** Prioritization

21. **Ans: 1**   Fatal hyperkalemia may be caused by tumor lysis syndrome, a potentially serious consequence of chemotherapy in acute leukemia. The other symptoms also indicate a need for further assessment or interventions but are not as critical as the elevated potassium level. **Focus:** Prioritization

22. **Ans: 2**   A nontender lump in this area (or near any lymph node) may indicate that the patient has developed lymphoma, a possible adverse effect of immunosuppressive therapy. The patient should receive further evaluation immediately. The other symptoms may also indicate side effects of cyclosporine (gingival hyperplasia, nausea, paresthesia), but do not indicate the need for immediate action. **Focus:** Prioritization

23. **Ans: 4**   Skin care is included in UAP education and job description. Assessment and patient teaching are more complex tasks that should be delegated to RNs. Because the patient's clothes need to be carefully chosen to prevent irritation or damage to the skin, the RN should assist the patient with this. **Focus:** Delegation

24. **Ans: 1**   The newly-admitted patient should be assessed first, because the baseline assessment and plan of care need to be completed. The other patients also need assessments or interventions but do not need immediate nursing care. **Focus:** Prioritization

CHAPTER 9: Neurologic Problems, pages 45-48

1. **Ans: 1**   The priority for interdisciplinary care for the client experiencing a migraine headache is pain management. All of the other nursing diagnoses are accurate, but none of them is urgent like the issue of pain, which is often incapacitating. **Focus:** Prioritization

2. **Ans: 1, 2, 3, 4, 5**   Medications such as estrogen supplements may actually trigger a migraine head-

ache attack. All of the other statements are accurate. **Focus:** Prioritization

3. **Ans: 3** Measurement of vital signs is within the education and scope of practice of UAPs. The nurse should perform neurologic checks and document the seizure. Clients with seizures should not be restrained; however, the nurse may guide the client's movements if necessary. **Focus:** Delegation, supervision

4. **Ans: 2** The LPN/LVN can set up the equipment for oxygen and suctioning. The RN should perform the complete initial assessment. Controversy exists as to whether padded side rails actually provide safety, and their use may embarrass the client and family. Tongue blades should not be at the bedside and should never be inserted into the client's mouth after a seizure begins. **Focus:** Delegation, supervision

5. **Ans: 4** A client with a seizure disorder should not take over-the-counter medications without consulting with the health care provider first. The other three statements are appropriate teaching points for clients with seizure disorders and their families. **Focus:** Delegation, supervision

6. **Ans: 3** The UAP should help the client with morning care as needed, but the goal is to keep this client as independent and mobile as possible. The client should be encouraged to perform as much morning care as possible. Assisting the client in ambulating, reminding the client not to look at his feet (to prevent falls), and encouraging the client to feed himself are all appropriate to the goal of maintaining independence. **Focus:** Delegation, supervision

7. **Ans: 1** Exercises are used to strengthen the back, relieve pressure on compressed nerves, and protect the back from reinjury. Ice, heat, and firm mattresses are appropriate interventions for back pain. People with chronic back pain should avoid wearing high-heeled shoes at all times. **Focus:** Prioritization

8. **Ans: 2** These signs and symptoms are characteristic of autonomic dysreflexia, a neurologic emergency that must be promptly treated to prevent a hypertensive stroke. The cause of this syndrome is noxious stimuli, most often a distended bladder or constipation, so checking for poor catheter drainage, bladder distention, and fecal impaction is the first action that should be taken. Adjusting the room temperature may be helpful, because too cool a temperature in the room may contribute to the problem. Acetaminophen will not decrease the autonomic dysreflexia that is causing the client's headache. Notifying the physician may be necessary if nursing actions do not resolve symptoms. **Focus:** Prioritization

9. **Ans: 2** The new RN graduate who is on orientation to the unit should be assigned to care for clients with stable, noncomplex conditions, such as the client with stroke. The task of helping the client with Parkinson disease to bathe is best delegated to the UAP. The client being transferred to the nursing home and the newly-admitted client with SCI should be assigned to experienced nurses. **Focus:** Assignment

10. **Ans: 4** The first priority for the client with an SCI is assessing respiratory patterns and ensuring an adequate airway. A client with a high cervical injury is at risk for respiratory compromise, because spinal nerves C3 through C5 innervate the phrenic nerve, which controls the diaphragm. The other assessments are also necessary but are not as high a priority. **Focus:** Prioritization

11. **Ans: 2** The UAP's training and education covers measuring and recording vital signs. The UAP may help with turning and repositioning the client and may remind the client to cough and deep breathe, but he or she does not teach the client how to perform these actions. Assessing and monitoring clients require additional education and are appropriate to the scope of practice of professional nurses. **Focus:** Delegation, supervision

12. **Ans: 1, 2, 4, 5** All of the strategies except straight catheterization may stimulate voiding in clients with an SCI. Intermittent bladder catheterization can be used to empty the client's bladder, but it will not stimulate voiding. **Focus:** Prioritization

13. **Ans: 1, 3, 4** Checking and observing for signs of pressure or infection is within the scope of practice of the LPN/LVN. The LPN/LVN also has the appropriate skills for cleaning the halo insertion sites with hydrogen peroxide. Neurologic examination and care plan development require additional education and skill appropriate to the professional RN. **Focus:** Delegation, supervision

14. **Ans: 3** The client's statement indicates impaired individual resilience in adjusting to the limitations of the injury and the need for additional counseling, teaching, and support. The other three nursing diagnoses may be appropriate for a client with SCI but are not related to the client's statement. **Focus:** Prioritization

15. **Ans: 2** The traveling nurse is relatively new to neurologic nursing and should be assigned clients whose condition is stable and not complex, such as the client with chronic ALS. The newly-diagnosed client with MS will need a lot of teaching and support. The client with respiratory distress will need frequent assessments and may need to be transferred to the intensive care unit. The client with a C4-level SCI is at risk for respiratory arrest. All three of these clients should be assigned to nurses experienced in neurologic nursing care. **Focus:** Assignment

16. **Ans: 4** At this time, based on the client's statement, the priority is Bathing Self-Care Deficit related to fatigue after physical therapy. The other three nursing diagnoses are appropriate to a patent with MS but are not related to the client's statement. **Focus:** Prioritization

17. **Ans: 4** The priority intervention for a client with GBS is maintaining adequate respiratory function.

Clients with GBS are at risk for respiratory failure, which requires urgent intervention. The other findings are important and should be reported to the nurse, but they are not life threatening. **Focus:** Prioritization, delegation, supervision

18. **Ans: 2**   The changes that the UAP is reporting are characteristic of myasthenic crisis, which often follows some type of infection. The client is at risk for inadequate respiratory function. In addition to notifying the physician, the nurse should carefully monitor the client's respiratory status. The client may need intubation and mechanical ventilation. **Focus:** Prioritization

19. **Ans: 3**   Alteplase is a clot buster. In a client who has experienced hemorrhagic stroke, there is already bleeding into the brain. A drug such as alteplase can worsen the bleeding. The other statements about the use of alteplase are accurate but are not pertinent to this client's diagnosis. **Focus:** Prioritization

20. **Ans: 1**   Clients with right cerebral hemisphere stroke often manifest neglect syndrome. They lean to the left and, when asked, respond that they believe they are sitting up straight. They often neglect the left side of their bodies and ignore food on the left side of their food trays. The nurse needs to remind the student of this phenomenon and discuss the appropriate interventions. **Focus:** Delegation, supervision

21. **Ans: 1, 2, 3, 5**   An experienced UAP would know how to reposition the client, reapply compression boots, and feed a client, and would remind the client to perform activities the client has been taught to perform. Assessing for redness and swelling (signs of deep venous thrombosis) requires additional education and skill, appropriate to the professional nurse. **Focus:** Delegation, supervision

22. **Ans: 1**   Positioning the client in a sitting position decreases the risk of aspiration. The UAP is not trained to assess gag or swallowing reflexes. The client should not be rushed during feeding. A client who needs suctioning performed between bites of food is not handling secretions and is at risk for aspiration. Such a client should be assessed further before feeding. **Focus:** Delegation, supervision

23. **Ans: 2**   Bacterial meningitis is a medical emergency, and antibiotics are administered even before the diagnosis is confirmed (after specimens have been collected for culture). The other interventions will also help to reduce central nervous system stimulation and irritation and should be implemented as soon as possible, but are not as important as starting antibiotic therapy. **Focus:** Prioritization

24. **Ans: 1**   Meningococcal meningitis is spread through contact with respiratory secretions, so use of a mask and gown is required to prevent transmission of the infection to staff members or other clients. The other actions may not be appropriate but do not require intervention as rapidly. The presence of a family member at the bedside may decrease client confusion and agitation. Clients with hyperthermia frequently report feeling chilled, but warming the client is not an appropriate intervention. Checking the pupils' response to light is appropriate but is not needed every 30 minutes and is uncomfortable for a client with photophobia. **Focus:** Prioritization

25. **Ans: 1, 2**   Any nursing staff member who is involved in caring for the client should observe for the onset and duration of any seizures (although a more detailed assessment of seizure activity should be done by the RN). Administration of medications is included in LPN/LVN education and scope of practice. Teaching, discharge planning, and assessment for adverse effects of new medications are complex activities that require RN-level education and scope of practice. **Focus:** Delegation

26. **Ans: 1**   The priority action during a generalized tonic-clonic seizure is to protect the airway by turning the client to one side. Administering lorazepam should be the next action, because it will act rapidly to control the seizure. Although oxygen may be useful during the postictal phase, the hypoxemia during tonic-clonic seizures is caused by apnea, which cannot be corrected by oxygen administration. Checking level of consciousness is not appropriate during the seizure, because generalized tonic-clonic seizures are associated with a loss of consciousness. **Focus:** Prioritization

27. **Ans: 2**   Leukopenia is a serious adverse effect of phenytoin therapy and would require discontinuation of the medication. The other data indicate a need for further assessment and/or client teaching but will not require a change in medical treatment for the seizures. **Focus:** Prioritization

28. **Ans: 4**   Urinary tract infections (UTIs) are a frequent complication in clients with MS because of the effect of the disease on bladder function, and UTIs may lead to sepsis in these clients. The elevated temperature and flank pain suggest that this client may have pyelonephritis. The physician should be notified immediately so that IV antibiotic therapy can be started quickly. The other clients should be assessed as soon as possible, but their needs are not as urgent as those of this client. **Focus:** Prioritization

29. **Ans: 1, 3, 5**   UAP education and scope of practice include taking pulse and blood pressure measurements. In addition, UAPs can reinforce previous teaching or skills taught by the RN or personnel in other disciplines, such as speech or physical therapists. Evaluating client response to medications and developing and individualizing the plan of care require RN-level education and scope of practice. **Focus:** Delegation

30. **Ans: 1**   LPN/LVN education and team leader responsibilities include checking for the therapeutic and adverse effects of medications. Changes in the

residents' memory would be communicated to the RN supervisor, who is responsible for overseeing the plan of care for each resident. Assessing for changes in score on the Mini-Mental State Examination and developing the plan of care are RN responsibilities. Assisting residents with personal care and hygiene would be delegated to UAPs working at the long-term care facility. **Focus:** Delegation

31. **Ans: 2** The husband's statement about lack of sleep and anxiety about whether his wife is receiving the correct medications are behaviors that support this diagnosis. There is no evidence that the client's cardiac output is decreased. The husband's statements about how he monitors the client and his concern with medication administration indicate that the risk for ineffective family therapeutic regimen management and falls are not priority diagnoses at this time. **Focus:** Prioritization

32. **Ans: 1** The inability to recognize family members is a new neurologic deficit for this client and indicates a possible increase in intracranial pressure (ICP). This change should be communicated to the health care provider immediately so that treatment can be initiated. The continuing headache also indicates that the ICP may be elevated but is not a new problem. The glucose elevation and weight gain are common adverse effects of dexamethasone that may require treatment but are not emergencies. **Focus:** Prioritization

33. **Ans: 2** The client's history and assessment data indicate that he may have a chronic subdural hematoma. The priority goal is to obtain a rapid diagnosis and send the client to surgery to have the hematoma evacuated. The other interventions also should be implemented as soon as possible, but the initial nursing activities should be directed toward diagnosis and treatment of any intracranial lesion. **Focus:** Prioritization

34. **Ans: 3** Of the clients listed, the client with bacterial meningitis is in the most stable condition. An RN from the medical unit would be familiar with administering IV antibiotics. The other clients require assessments and care from RNs more experienced in caring for clients with neurologic diagnoses. **Focus:** Assignment

CHAPTER 10: Visual and Auditory Problems, pages 49-52

1. **Ans: 3** If the client is wearing contact lenses, the lenses may be causing the symptoms, and removing them will prevent further eye irritation or damage. Policies on giving telephone advice vary among institutions, and knowledge of your facility policy is essential. The other options may be appropriate, but you should gather additional information before suggesting anything else. **Focus:** Prioritization

2. **Ans: 3** Most accidental eye injuries (90%) could be prevented by wearing protective eyewear for sports and hazardous work. Other options should be considered in the overall prevention of injuries, but these have less impact. **Focus:** Prioritization

3. **Ans: 1, 3, 5, 6** Providing postoperative and preoperative instructions, making home health referrals, and assessing for needs related to loss of vision should be done by an experienced nurse who can give specific details and specialized information about follow-up eye care and adjustment to loss. The principles of applying an eye pad and shield and teaching the administration of eyedrops are basic procedures that should be familiar to all nurses. **Focus:** Assignment

4. **Ans: 6, 2, 5, 4, 3, 1** Have the client sit with the head tilted back. Pulling down the lower conjunctival sac creates a small pocket for the drops. Stabilizing the hand prevents accidentally poking the client's eye. Having the client look up prevents the drops from falling on the cornea and stimulating the blink reflex. When the client gently moves the eye, the medication is distributed. Pressing on the lacrimal duct prevents systemic absorption. **Focus:** Prioritization

5. **Ans: 2, 3, 4, 7** Administering medications, reviewing and demonstrating standard procedures, and performing standardized assessments with predictable outcomes in noncomplex cases are within the scope of the LPN/LVN. Assessing for systemic manifestations and behaviors, risk factors, and nutritional factors is the responsibility of the RN. **Focus:** Delegation

6. **Ans: 2** Try to find out how much and how frequently she has been taking the drops by mouth. This information will be needed if you call the ophthalmologist for an order or if you call Poison Control. A good follow-up question is to try to find out why she is taking the drops by mouth. She may be very confused, or there may have been an error of omission in client education by all health care team members who were involved in the initial prescription. **Focus:** Prioritization

7. **Ans: 1** Warm compresses will usually provide relief. If the problem persists, eyelid scrubs and antibiotic drops would be appropriate. The ophthalmologist could be consulted, but other providers such as the family physician or the nurse practitioner could give a prescription for antibiotics. **Focus:** Prioritization

8. **Ans: 4** A curtainlike shadow is a symptom of retinal detachment, which is an emergency situation. A change in color vision is a symptom of cataract. Crusty drainage is associated with conjunctivitis. Increased lacrimation is associated with many eye irritants, such as allergies, contact lenses, or foreign bodies. **Focus:** Prioritization

9. **Ans: 2, 5** Assisting the client with ambulating in the hall and obtaining supplies are within the scope of practice of the UAP. Counseling for emotional problems, orienting the client to the room, and encouraging independence require formative evaluation to gauge readiness, and these activities should be the responsibility of

the RN. Storing items and rearranging furniture are inappropriate actions, because the client needs be able to consistently locate objects in the immediate environment. **Focus:** Delegation

10. **Ans: 4**   Pain may signal hemorrhage, infection, or increased ocular pressure. A scratchy sensation and loss of depth perception with the patch in place are not uncommon. Adequate vision may not return for 24 hours. **Focus:** Prioritization

11. **Ans: 3, 4, 5, 6**   The client's symptoms are suggestive of angle-closure glaucoma. Immediate inventions include instillation of miotics, which open the trabecular network and facilitate aqueous outflow, and intravenous or oral administration of hyperosmotic agents to move fluid from the intracellular space to the extracellular space. Applying cool compresses and providing a dark, quiet space are appropriate comfort measures. Photodynamic therapy is a treatment for age-related macular degeneration. Use of mydriatics is contraindicated because dilation of the pupil will further block the outflow. **Focus:** Prioritization

12. **Ans: 4**   All beta-adrenergic blockers are contraindicated in bradycardia. Alpha-adrenergic agents can cause tachycardia and hypertension. Carbonic anhydrase inhibitors should not be given to clients with rheumatoid arthritis who are taking high dosages of aspirin. **Focus:** Prioritization

13. **Ans: 2**   Asking the nurse to explain the documentation is a way of assessing her knowledge of documentation, how the client's complaint contributes to what should be assessed, and her understanding of the use of abbreviations. The nurse may have a good reason for charting "N/A," but you should explain how a reader could misunderstand. For example, "visual acuity N/A" could be interpreted as the nurse making a clinical judgment that assessing vision was not important for this client. The documentation is not acceptable, because the client's chief complaint indicates that vision should be tested if at all possible. Redoing the assessment yourself does not help the nurse to correct mistakes. Contacting the educator for assistance is an option that is based on your assessment of her rationale. **Focus:** Supervision, prioritization

14. **Ans: 1, 2, 3**   Irrigating the ear, giving medication, and reminding the client about postoperative instructions that were given by an RN are within the scope of practice of the LPN/LVN. Counseling clients and families and assessing for meningitis signs in a client with labyrinthitis are the responsibilities of the RN. **Focus:** Delegation

15. **Ans: 1, 2, 3, 4**   Medications such as aspirin or diuretics (and many others) can cause tinnitus (ringing in the ears). Loud noises, impacted earwax or foreign bodies in the ear canal, or ear infections can also cause tinnitus. Asking about frequency of hygiene is less relevant than asking about the method the client uses to clean the ears. For example, the insertion of cotton-tipped swabs may be contributing to the impaction of earwax. **Focus:** Prioritization

16. **Ans: 2**   This client has a hearing loss, and it seems likely that a referral for a hearing aid or rehabilitation program will allow her to participate in her baseline social habits. The other diagnoses are pertinent if the hearing loss continues to interfere with her quality of life. **Focus:** Prioritization

17. **Ans: 3**   A bulging red or blue tympanic membrane is a possible sign of otitis media or perforation. The other signs are considered normal anatomy. **Focus:** Prioritization

18. **Ans: 3**   The client reporting vertigo without hearing loss should be further assessed for nonvestibular causes, such as cardiovascular or metabolic. The other descriptions are more commonly associated with inner ear or labyrinthine causes. **Focus:** Prioritization

19. **Ans: 1. MD, 2. UAP, 3. LPN/LVN or RN, 4. MD, 5. RN, 6. Physical therapist**   The physician is responsible for determining the medical diagnosis and for explaining the outcomes and risks of surgical procedures. A physical therapist evaluates movement and the need for adaptive equipment and teaches ambulation techniques; however, the UAP (under supervision) is able to help clients with routine ambulation and position changes. The LPN/LVN and RN are qualified to give medications. The RN should assess the client to identify situations associated with vertigo. **Focus:** Assignment

20. **Ans: 3**   Heavy lifting should be strictly avoided for at least 3 weeks after stapedectomy. Water in the ear and air travel should be avoided for at least 1 week. Coughing and sneezing should be performed with the mouth open to prevent increased pressure in the ear. **Focus:** Prioritization

21. **Ans: 1, 5, 2, 7, 3, 4, 6**   Use an otoscope to assess the ear first and then fill the syringe with warm fluid. Angle the syringe to allow the fluid to flow along the side of the ear canal, not directly at the eardrum. Flush with continuous pressure, rather than a pumping action. You should see fluid return with cerumen. If not, then wait at least 10 minutes and repeat. Tipping the head allows gravity drainage of fluid left in the ear canal. **Focus:** Prioritization

CHAPTER 11: Musculoskeletal Problems, pages 53-56

1. **Ans: 4**   Assisting with activities of daily living (ADLs) is within the scope of the UAP's practice. The other three interventions require additional educational preparation and are within the scope of practice of licensed nurses. **Focus:** Delegation, supervision

2. **Ans: 1, 2, 3, 5**   The purpose of the teaching is to help the patient prevent falls. The hip protector can prevent hip fractures if the patient falls. Throw rugs and obstacles in the home increase the risk of falls. Patients who are tired are also more likely to fall. Exercise helps to strengthen muscles and improve coordination. **Focus:** Prioritization

3. **Ans: 2**   Platybasia (basilar skull invagination) causes brainstem manifestations that threaten life. Patients with Paget disease are usually short and often have bowing of the long bones that results in asymmetrical knees or elbow deformities. The skull is typically soft, thick, and enlarged. **Focus:** Prioritization

4. **Ans: 3**   Applying heat, not ice, is the appropriate measure to help reduce the patient's pain. Ibuprofen is useful to manage mild to moderate pain. Exercise prescribed by the PT would be nonimpact in nature and provide strengthening for the patient. A diet rich in calcium promotes bone health. **Focus:** Delegation, supervision

5. **Ans: 4**   The PACU nurse is very familiar with the assessment skills necessary to monitor a patient who just underwent surgery. For the other patients, nurses familiar with musculoskeletal system–related nursing care are needed to provide teaching and assessment, and prepare a report to the long-term care facility. **Focus:** Assignment

6. **Ans: 1**   An elevated temperature indicates infection and inflammation. This patient needs IV antibiotic therapy. The other vital sign values are normal or high normal. **Focus:** Delegation, supervision

7. **Ans: Clear, Concise, Correct, Complete**   Implementing the Four Cs of communication helps the nurse ensure that the UAP understands what is being said; that the UAP does not confuse the nurse's directions; that the directions comply with policies, procedures, job descriptions, and the law; and that the UAP has all the information necessary to complete the tasks assigned. **Focus:** Delegation, supervision

8. **Ans: 3**   Helping with ADLs is within the scope of practice of UAPs. Placing a splint for the first time is appropriate to the scope of practice of PTs. Assessing and testing for paresthesia are not within the scope of practice of UAPs. **Focus:** Delegation, supervision

9. **Ans: 3**   When a patient with CTS has a splint to immobilize the wrist, the wrist is placed either in the neutral position or in slight extension. The other interventions are correct and are within the scope of practice of a UAP. UAPs may remind patients about elements of their care plans such as avoiding heavy lifting. **Focus:** Delegation, supervision

10. **Ans: 1**   Postoperative pain and numbness occur for a longer period of time with endoscopic carpal tunnel release than with an open procedure. Patients often need assistance postoperatively, even after they are discharged. The dressing from the endoscopic procedure is usually very small, and there should not be a lot of drainage. **Focus:** Prioritization

11. **Ans: 1, 2, 3, 5**   Postoperatively, patients undergoing open carpal tunnel release surgery experience pain and numbness, and their discomfort may last for weeks to months. All of the other directions are appropriate for the postoperative care of this patient. It is important to monitor for drainage, tightness, and neurovascular changes. Raising the hand and wrist above the heart reduces the swelling from surgery, and this is often done for several days. **Focus:** Assignment, delegation, supervision

12. **Ans: 2**   Hand movements, including heavy lifting, may be restricted for 4 to 6 weeks after surgery. Patients experience discomfort for weeks to months after surgery. The surgery is not always a cure; in some cases, CTS may recur months to years after surgery. **Focus:** Prioritization

13. **Ans: 1**   Ibuprofen can cause abdominal discomfort or pain and ulceration of the gastrointestinal tract. In such cases, it should be taken with meals or milk. Removal of throw rugs helps prevent falls. Range-of-motion exercises and rest are important strategies for coping with osteoporosis. **Focus:** Prioritization

14. **Ans: 2**   Fat embolism syndrome is a serious complication that often results from fractures of long bones. Its earliest manifestation is altered mental status caused by a low arterial oxygen level. The nurse would want to know about and treat the pain, but it is not life threatening. The nurse would also want to know about the blood pressure and the patient's voiding; however, this information is not urgent to report. **Focus:** Prioritization, delegation, supervision

15. **Ans: 3**   The patient with the tight cast is at risk for circulation impairment and peripheral nerve damage. Although all of the other patients' concerns are important and the nurse will want to see them as soon as possible, none of their complaints is urgent. **Focus:** Prioritization

16. **Ans: 3**   When the weights are resting on the floor, they are not exerting pulling force to provide reduction and alignment or to prevent muscle spasm. The weights should always hang freely. Attending to the weights may reduce the patient's pain and spasm. With skeletal pins, a small amount of clear fluid drainage is expected. It is important to inspect the traction system after a patient changes position, because position changes may alter the traction. **Focus:** Delegation, supervision, prioritization

17. **Ans: 1**   Moving from a lying position first to a sitting position and then to a standing position allows the patient to establish balance before standing. Administering pain medication before the patient begins exercising decreases pain with exercise. Explanations about the purpose of the exercise program and proper use of crutches are appropriate interventions with this patient. **Focus:** Delegation, supervision

18. **Ans: 2** Monitoring for sufficient tissue perfusion is the priority at this time. Phantom pain is a concern but is more common in patients with above-the-knee amputations. Early ambulation is a goal, but at this time the patient is more likely to be engaged in muscle-strengthening exercises. Elevating the residual limb on a pillow is controversial, because it may promote knee flexion contracture. **Focus:** Delegation, supervision

19. **Ans: 1** Three theories are being researched with regard to phantom limb pain. The peripheral nervous system theory holds that sensations remain as a result of the severing of peripheral nerves during the amputation. The central nervous system theory states that phantom limb pain results from a loss of inhibitory signals that were generated through afferent impulses from the amputated limb. The psychological theory helps predict and explain phantom limb pain because stress, anxiety, and depression often trigger or worsen a pain episode. **Focus:** Prioritization

20. **Ans: 4** The patient is indicating an interest in learning about prostheses. The experienced nurse can initiate discussion and begin educating the patient. Certainly the health care provider can also discuss prostheses with the patient, but the patient's wish to learn should receive a quick response. The nurse can then notify the health care provider about the patient's request. **Focus:** Delegation, supervision

21. **Ans: 1** Pressure and pain may be due to increased compartment pressure and can indicate the serious complication of acute compartment syndrome. This situation is urgent. If it is not treated, cyanosis, tingling, numbness, paresis, and severe pain can occur. **Focus:** Prioritization

22. **Ans: 1** Doses of fluoxetine, a drug used to treat depression, that are greater than 20 mg should be given in two divided doses, not once a day. The other three orders are appropriate for a patient who underwent amputation 4 days earlier. **Focus:** Prioritization

CHAPTER 12: Gastrointestinal and Nutritional Problems, pages 57-60

1. **Ans: 2** The UAP can reinforce dietary and fluid restrictions after the RN has explained the information to the client. It is also possible that the UAP can administer the enema; however, special training is required, and policies may vary among institutions. Medication administration should be performed by licensed personnel. **Focus:** Delegation

2. **Ans: 4** A client with a fractured femur is at risk for fat embolism, so a fat emulsion should be used with caution. Vomiting may be a problem if the emulsion is infused too rapidly. TPN is commonly used in clients with GI obstruction, severe anorexia nervosa, and chronic diarrhea or vomiting. **Focus:** Prioritization

3. **Ans: 7, 3, 5, 2, 1, 4, 6** Always check the order before administering TPN; generally, each bag is individually prepared by the pharmacist. The solution should not be cloudy or turbid. Prepare the equipment by priming the tubing and threading the pump. To prevent infection, scrub the hub and use aseptic technique when inserting the connector into the injection cap and connecting the tubing to the central line. Set the pump at the prescribed rate. **Focus:** Prioritization

4. **Ans: 4** A boardlike abdomen with shoulder pain is a symptom of a perforation, which is the most lethal complication of peptic ulcer disease. A burning sensation is a typical complaint and can be controlled with medications. Projectile vomiting can signal an obstruction. Coffee-ground emesis is typical of slower bleeding, and the client will require diagnostic testing. **Focus:** Prioritization

5. **Ans: 2** Body dysmorphic disorder is a preoccupation with an imagined physical defect. Corrective surgery can exacerbate this disorder when the client continues to feel dissatisfied with the results. The other findings are criterion indicators for this treatment. **Focus:** Prioritization

6. **Ans: 4** Fluctuating level of consciousness and mood swings are associated more with acute delirium, which could be caused by many things, such as electrolyte imbalances, sepsis, or medications. Information about the client's baseline behavior is essential; however, based on your knowledge of pathophysiology, you know that flat affect and rambling and repetitive speech, memory impairments, and disorientation to time are behaviors typically associated with chronic dementia. Lack of motivation and early morning awakening are associated with depression. **Focus:** Prioritization

7. **Ans: 3** Reminding the client to follow through on advice given by the nurse is an appropriate task for the UAP. The RN should take responsibility for teaching rationale, discussing strategies for the treatment plan, and assessing client concerns. **Focus:** Delegation

8. **Ans: 1** The primary concern is the potential for airway complications. Elevating the head, at least 30 degrees, decreases the chance for aspiration and facilitates respiratory effort. The other options are also correct, but will occur later in the postoperative period. **Focus:** Prioritization

9. **Ans: 4** Nausea and vomiting are common after chemotherapy. Administration of antiemetics and fluid monitoring can be done by an LPN/LVN. The RN should perform the preoperative teaching for the glossectomy client. Clients returning from surgery need extensive assessment. The client with anorexia is showing signs of hypokalemia and is at risk for cardiac dysrhythmias. **Focus:** Assignment

10. **Ans: 3** The LPN/LVN can assist in the planning of interventions, but the RN should take ultimate

responsibility for planning. The LPN/LVN can delegate and assign tasks to UAPs; however, if the RN is in charge, it is better if UAPs are not receiving instructions from multiple people. Obtaining equipment should be delegated to a UAP. A physical therapist should be contacted to set up specialized equipment. **Focus:** Delegation

11. **Ans: 4**   Showing the student how to insert the suppository meets both the immediate client need and the student's learning need. The instructor can address the student's fears and long-term learning needs once he or she is aware of the incident. It is preferable that students express fears and learning needs. The other options will discourage the student's future disclosure of clinical limitations and need for additional training. **Focus:** Supervision, assignment

12. **Ans: 7, 3, 1, 5, 2, 8, 4, 6**   Putting on a pair of clean gloves protects the hands from colostomy secretions. The water should be warm (cold water can cause cramping) and the container should be hung at shoulder height (hanging the container too high or too low will alter the rate of flow). Lubricating the stoma and gently inserting the tubing tip will allow the water to flow into the stoma. A slow and steady flow prevents cramps and spillage. Providing adequate time allows for complete evacuation. Walking stimulates the bowel. Careful attention to the skin prevents breakdown. **Focus:** Prioritization

13. **Ans: 3**   Disconnecting the tube from suction is an appropriate task to delegate. Suction should be reconnected by the nurse, so that correct pressure is checked. If the UAP is permitted to reconnect the tube, the RN is still responsible for checking that the pressure setting is correct. During removal of the tube, there is a potential for aspiration, so the nurse should perform this task. If the tube is dislodged, the nurse should recheck placement before it is secured. **Focus:** Delegation

14. **Ans: 3**   The goal of bowel training is to establish a pattern that mimics normal defecation, and many people have the urge to defecate after a meal. If this is not successful, a suppository can be used to stimulate the urge. The use of incontinence briefs is embarrassing for the client, and they must be changed frequently to prevent skin breakdown. Routine use of rectal tubes is not recommended because of the potential for damage to the mucosa and sphincter tone. **Focus:** Prioritization

15. **Ans: 1**   The immediate problem is controlling the diarrhea. Addressing this problem is a step toward correcting the nutritional imbalance and decreasing the diarrheal cramping. Self-care and compliance with the treatment plan are important long-term goals that can be addressed when the client is feeling better physically. **Focus:** Prioritization

16. **Ans: 3, 4, 1, 2, 6, 5**   Immediate decontamination is appropriate, because time can affect viral load. The

occupational health nurse will direct the UAP in filing the correct forms, getting the appropriate laboratory tests, obtaining appropriate prophylaxis, and following up on results. **Focus:** Prioritization, supervision

17. **Ans: 2, 5, 3, 4, 1, 6**   Stay calm and stay with the client. Any increase in intra-abdominal pressure will worsen the evisceration; placement of the client in a semi-Fowler position with knees flexed will decrease the strain on the wound site. (Note: If shock develops, the client's head should be lowered.) Continuously monitor vital signs, particularly for a decrease in blood pressure or increase in pulse rate, while your colleague gathers supplies and notifies the physician. Covering the site protects tissue. Ultimately, the client will need emergency surgery. **Focus:** Prioritization

18. **Ans: 3**   Right upper quadrant pain is a sign of hemorrhage or bile leak. The ability to void should return within 6 hours postoperatively. Right shoulder pain is related to unabsorbed carbon dioxide and will be resolved by placing the client in Sims position. Output that does not equal input after surgery for the first several hours is expected. **Focus:** Prioritization

19. **Ans: 1**   The UAP should use infection control precautions for the protection of self, employees, and other clients. Monitoring is an RN responsibility. UAPs can report valuable information; however, they are not responsible for detecting signs and symptoms that can be subtle or hard to detect, such as skin changes. While playing games with the client may be ideal, it is rarely possible on a medical-surgical unit. **Focus:** Delegation

20. **Ans: 1**   There is a potential for sudden rupture of fragile blood vessels with massive hemorrhage from straining that increases thoracic or abdominal pressure. The client could have fluid accumulation in the abdomen (ascites) that can be mild and hard to detect or severe enough to cause orthopnea. Dependent peripheral edema can also be observed but is less urgent. **Focus:** Prioritization

21. **Ans: 2**   Assisting with procedures for clients in stable condition with predictable outcomes is within the educational preparation of the LPN/LVN. Teaching the client about self-care or pathophysiology and evaluating the outcome of interventions are responsibilities of the RN. **Focus:** Delegation

22. **Ans: 1**   Distention and rigidity can signal hemorrhage or peritonitis. The physician may also decide that these symptoms require a medication to stimulate peristalsis. Absence of bowel sounds is expected within the first 24 to 48 hours. Nausea and vomiting are not uncommon and are usually self-limiting, and an "as needed" (PRN) order for an antiemetic is usually part of the routine postoperative orders. The reason for displacement of the NG tube should be assessed and the tube secured as necessary. **Focus:** Prioritization

Answer Key

23. **Ans: 2, 3**   Both clients will need frequent pain assessments and medications. Clients with copious diarrhea or vomiting will frequently need enteric isolation. Cancer clients receiving chemotherapy are at risk for immunosuppression and are likely to need protective isolation. **Focus:** Assignment

24. **Ans: 4**   Diverticulitis can cause chronic or severe bleeding, so if there is no obvious blood in the stool, the stool may be tested for occult blood. A barium enema is not usually ordered because of the danger of perforation. Laxatives and ambulation increase intestinal motility and are to be avoided in the initial phase of treatment. If a barium enema, PRN laxative, or ambulation is ordered, question the orders before delegating these interventions. **Focus:** Delegation

25. **Ans: 3**   The UAP can take vital signs and report all of the values to the RN. In this case, all of the values are needed in order to detect trends. In other cases, you may decide to give parameters for reporting. The RN should assess skin temperature and pain, and closely monitor the urine because quantity is an indicator of perfusion and red/pink urine can signal damage to the urinary system, transfusion reaction, or rhabdomyolysis. **Focus:** Delegation

26. **Ans: 6, 2, 3, 5, 4, 1**   A pair of clean gloves should be put on before touching the skin or pouch. The stoma should be assessed for a healthy pink color. Washing, rinsing, and drying the skin and applying a skin barrier help to protect the skin. A good fit prevents gastric contents from spilling onto the skin. **Focus:** Prioritization

27. **Ans: 1**   Refeeding syndrome occurs when aggressive and rapid feeding results in fluid retention and heart failure. Electrolytes, especially phosphorus, should be monitored, and the client should be observed for signs of fluid overload. Changes in bowel sounds, nausea, and distention may occur but are also appropriate for any client with nutritional issues or for clients receiving enteral feedings. Observing for purging and water ingestion would be appropriate for a client with an eating disorder. Change in stool patterns may occur, but are not related to refeeding syndrome. **Focus:** Prioritization

28. **Ans: 3**   All of these measures should be performed for total care of the client; however weighing the client every day is considered the single best indicator of fluid volume. **Focus:** Prioritization

29. **Ans: 3**   Substance abuse may exclude a person from the transplant list, so the nurse should conduct additional assessment about this comment. The comment about difficulty in taking prescription medications should also be investigated because a true inability to follow the treatment regimen would also exclude the client from the list. **Focus:** Prioritization

30. **Ans: 3**   T-tubes should not be irrigated, aspirated, or clamped without a specific order from the physician.

All of the other actions are appropriate in the care of this client. **Focus:** Supervision

CHAPTER 13: Diabetes Mellitus, pages 61-64

1. **Ans: 3**   The higher the blood glucose level is over time, the more glycosylated the hemoglobin becomes. The $HgbA_{1c}$ level is a good indicator of the average blood glucose level over the previous 120 days. Fasting glucose and oral glucose tolerance tests are important diagnostic tools. Fingerstick blood glucose monitoring provides information that allows adjustment of the patient's therapeutic regimen. **Focus:** Prioritization

2. **Ans: 4**   The UAP's role includes reminding patients about interventions that are already part of the plan of care. Arranging for a consult with the dietitian is appropriate for the unit clerk. Teaching and assessing require additional education and should be carried out by licensed nurses. **Focus:** Delegation, supervision, assignment

3. **Ans: 1, 2, 5**   Sensory alterations are the major cause of foot complications in diabetic patients, and patients should be taught to examine their feet on a daily basis. Properly-fitted shoes protect the patient from foot complications. Broken skin increases the risk of infection. Cotton socks are recommended to absorb moisture. Patients, family, or health care providers may trim toenails. **Focus:** Prioritization

4. **Ans: 3**   Profuse perspiration is a symptom of hypoglycemia, a complication of diabetes that requires urgent treatment. A glucose level of 185 mg/dL will need coverage with sliding-scale insulin, but this is not urgent. Numbness and tingling, as well as bunions, are related to the chronic nature of diabetes and are not urgent problems. **Focus:** Prioritization

5. **Ans: 1**   Checking the bath water temperature is part of assisting with activities of daily living and is within the education and scope of practice of the UAP. Discussing community resources, teaching, and assessing require a higher level of education and are appropriate to the scope of practice of licensed nurses. **Focus:** Delegation

6. **Ans: 1, 2, 5**   When a diabetic patient is ill, glucose levels become elevated, and administration of insulin may be necessary. Teaching or reviewing the components of proper foot care is always a good idea with a diabetic patient. Bed rest is not necessary, and glucose level may be better controlled when a patient is more active. The Atkins diet recommends decreasing the consumption of carbohydrates and is not a good diet for diabetic patients. **Focus:** Prioritization

7. **Ans: 4**   When a diabetic patient is ill or has surgery, glucose levels become elevated, and administration of insulin may be necessary. This is a temporary change that resolves with recovery from the illness or surgery. Option 3 is correct but does not explain

why the patient may currently need insulin. The patient does not have type 1 diabetes, and finger-stick glucose checks are usually prescribed for before meals and at bedtime. **Focus:** Prioritization

8. **Ans: 1** The onset of action for rapid-acting insulin is within minutes, so it should be given only when the patient has food and is ready to eat. Because of this, rapid-acting insulin is sometimes called "see food" insulin. Options 2, 3, and 4 are incorrect. Long-acting insulins mimic the action of the pancreas. Regular insulin is the only insulin that can be given IV. **Focus:** Assignment, supervision

9. **Ans: 1, 3, 5** Giving the patient extra sweetener, recording oral intake, and checking blood pressure are all within the scope of practice of the UAP. Assessing shoe fit and patient teaching are not within the UAP's scope of practice. **Focus:** Assignment

10. **Ans: 2** Rapid, deep respirations (Kussmaul respirations) are symptomatic of diabetic ketoacidosis (DKA). Hammer toe, as well as numbness and tingling, are chronic complications associated with diabetes. Decreased sensitivity and swelling (lipohypertrophy) occurs at a site of repeated insulin injections, and treatment involves teaching the patient to rotate injection sites. **Focus:** Prioritization

11. **Ans: 1** The nurse should not leave the patient. The scope of the unit clerk's job includes calling and paging physicians. LPNs/LVNs generally do not administer IV push medication. IV fluid administration is not within the scope of practice of UAPs. Patients with DKA already have a high glucose level and do not need orange juice. **Focus:** Delegation, supervision

12. **Ans: 2** The new nurse is still on orientation to the unit. Appropriate patient assignments at this time include patients whose conditions are stable and not complex. **Focus:** Assignment

13. **Ans: 2** The signs and symptoms the patient is exhibiting are consistent with hyperglycemia. The RN should not give the patient additional glucose. All of the other interventions are appropriate for this patient. The RN should also notify the provider at this time. **Focus:** Prioritization

14. **Ans: 3** The UAP's scope of practice includes checking vital signs and assisting with morning care. UAPs with special training can check the patient's glucose level before meals. It is generally not within the UAP's scope of practice to administer medications, but this is within the scope of practice of the LPN/LVN. **Focus:** Assignment

15. **Ans: 4** Before orange juice or insulin is given, the patient's blood glucose level should be checked. Checking blood pressure is a good idea but is not the first action the nurse should take. **Focus:** Prioritization

16. **Ans: 4** The low morning fasting blood glucose level indicates possible nocturnal hypoglycemia. Research indicates that it is important to avoid hypoglycemic episodes in pediatric patients because of the risk for permanent neurologic damage and adverse developmental outcomes. Although a lower hemoglobin A_{1c} might be desirable, the upper limit for hemoglobin A_{1c} levels ranges from 7.5% to 8.5% in pediatric patients. The parents' questions about diet and the child's activity level should also be addressed, but the most urgent consideration is education about the need to avoid hypoglycemia. **Focus:** Prioritization

17. **Ans: 2, 4, 5** National guidelines published by the American Diabetes Association (ADA) indicate that administration of emergency treatment for hypoglycemia, obtaining blood glucose readings, and reminding children are appropriate tasks for non–health care professional personnel such as teachers, paraprofessionals, and unlicensed health care personnel. Assessments and education require more specialized education and scope of practice and should be done by the school nurse. **Focus:** Delegation

18. **Ans: 2** Alcohol has the potential for causing alcohol-induced hypoglycemia. It is important to know when the patient drinks alcohol and to teach the patient to ingest it shortly after meals to prevent this complication. The other questions are important, but not urgent. The lipid profile question is important because alcohol can raise plasma triglycerides but is not as urgent as the potential for hypoglycemia. **Focus:** Prioritization

19. **Ans: 1, 3, 5** Guidelines for exercise are based on blood glucose and urine ketone levels. Patients should test blood glucose before, during, and after exercise to be sure that it is safe. When ketones are present in urine, the patient should not exercise because they indicate that current insulin levels are not adequate. Vigorous exercise is permitted in patients with type 1 diabetes if glucose levels are between 100 and 250 mg/dL. Warm-up and cool-down should be included in exercise to gradually increase and decrease the heart rate. **Focus:** Prioritization

20. **Ans: 4** An unexpected rise in blood glucose is associated with increased mortality and morbidity after surgical procedures. Current ADA guidelines recommend insulin protocols to maintain blood glucose levels between 140 and 180 mg/dL. Also, unexpected rises in blood glucose values may indicate wound infection. **Focus:** Delegation, supervision, prioritization

21. **Ans: 2** Urine ketone testing should be done whenever the patient's blood glucose is greater than 240 mg/dL. All of the other teaching points are appropriate "sick day rules." For dehydration, teaching should also include that if the patient's blood glucose is lower than her target range, she should drink fluids containing sugar. **Focus:** Supervision, delegation

22. **Ans: 1, 3** HHS often occurs in older adults with type 2 diabetes. Risk factors include taking diuretics and inadequate fluid intake. Weight loss (not weight gain) would be a symptom. While the patient's blood

Answer Key

pressure is high, this is not a risk factor. A urine output of 50 to 75 mL/hr is adequate. **Focus:** Prioritization

23. **Ans: 1**   While it is important to rotate injection sites for insulin, it is preferred that the injection sites be rotated within one anatomic site (e.g., the abdomen) to prevent day-to-day changes in the absorption rate of the insulin. All of the other teaching points are appropriate. **Focus:** Supervision, prioritization

24. **Ans: 3**   Repaglinide is a meglitinide analog drug. These drugs are short-acting agents used to prevent postmeal blood glucose elevation. They should be given within 1 to 30 minutes before meals and cause hypoglycemia shortly after dosing when a meal is delayed or omitted. **Focus:** Supervision, delegation, prioritization

25. **Ans: 1, 4, 5**   The manifestations listed in option 1 are correct. The symptoms should be treated with carbohydrate, but 10 to 15 g (not 4 to 8 g). Glucose should be retested at 15 minutes; 30 minutes is too long to wait. Options 4 and 5 are correct. **Focus:** Prioritization

CHAPTER 14: Other Endocrine Problems, pages 65-68

1. **Ans: 3**   Exophthalmos (abnormal protrusion of the eyes) is characteristic of patients with hyperthyroidism due to Graves disease. Periorbital edema, bradycardia, and hoarse voice are all characteristics of patients with hypothyroidism. **Focus:** Prioritization

2. **Ans: 1**   The cardiac problems associated with hyperthyroidism include tachycardia, increased systolic blood pressure, and decreased diastolic blood pressure. Patients with hyperthyroidism also may have increased body temperature related to increased metabolic rate. Respiratory changes are usually not symptomatic of this condition. **Focus:** Delegation, supervision

3. **Ans: 2**   Monitoring vital signs and recording their values are within the education and scope of practice of UAPs. An experienced UAP should have been taught how to monitor the apical pulse. However, a nurse should observe the UAP to be sure that the UAP has mastered this skill. Instructing and teaching patients, as well as performing venipuncture to obtain laboratory samples, are more suited to the education and scope of practice of licensed nurses. In some facilities, an experienced UAP may perform venipuncture, but only after special training. **Focus:** Delegation, supervision, assignment

4. **Ans: 3**   Although patients with hypothyroidism often have cardiac problems that include bradycardia, a heart rate of 48 beats/min may have significant implications for cardiac output and hemodynamic stability. Patients with Graves disease usually have a rapid heart rate, but 94 beats/min is within normal limits. The diabetic patient may need sliding-scale insulin dosing. This is important but not urgent. Patients with Cushing disease frequently have dependent edema. **Focus:** Prioritization

5. **Ans: 1**   Patients with hypofunction of the adrenal gland often have hypotension and should be instructed to change positions slowly. Once a patient has been so instructed, it is appropriate for the UAP to remind the patient of those instructions. Assessing, teaching, and planning nursing care require more education and should be done by licensed nurses. **Focus:** Delegation, supervision

6. **Ans: 4**   The presence of crackles in the patient's lungs indicate excess fluid volume due to excess water and sodium reabsorption and may be a symptom of pulmonary edema, which must be treated rapidly. Striae (stretch marks), weight gain, and dependent edema are common findings in patients with Cushing disease. These findings should be monitored but do not require urgent action. **Focus:** Prioritization

7. **Ans: 4**   Monitoring vital signs is within the education and scope of practice for UAPs. The nurse should be sure to instruct the UAP that blood pressure measurements are to be taken with the cuff on the same arm each time. Revising the care plan and instructing and assessing patients are beyond the scope of UAPs and fall within the purview of licensed nurses. **Focus:** Assignment

8. **Ans: 2**   Palpating the abdomen can cause the sudden release of catecholamines and severe hypertension. **Focus:** Delegation, supervision

9. **Ans: 1**   Rapid weight gain and edema are signs of excessive drug therapy, and the dosage of the drug would need to be adjusted. Hypertension, hyponatremia, hyperkalemia, and hyperglycemia are common in patients with adrenal hypofunction. **Focus:** Prioritization

10. **Ans: 1**   The presence of glucose in nasal drainage indicates that the fluid is cerebrospinal fluid (CSF) and suggests a CSF leak. Packing is normally inserted in the nares after the surgical incision is closed. Urine output of 40 to 50 mL/hr is adequate, and patients may experience thirst postoperatively. When patients are thirsty, nursing staff should encourage fluid intake. **Focus:** Prioritization

11. **Ans: 2**   The 83-year-old has no complicating factors at the moment. Providing care for patients in stable and uncomplicated condition falls within the LPN/LVN's educational preparation and scope of practice, with the care always being provided under the supervision and direction of an RN. The nurse should assess the patient who has just undergone surgery and the newly-admitted patient. The patient who is preparing for discharge after myocardial infarction may need some complex teaching. **Focus:** Delegation, supervision, assignment

12. **Ans: 1**   The parathyroid glands are located on the back of the thyroid gland. The parathyroids are important in maintaining calcium and phosphorus balance. The nurse should be attentive to all patient laboratory values, but calcium and phosphorus levels

are important to monitor after thyroidectomy because abnormal values could be the result of removal of the parathyroid glands during the procedure. **Focus:** Prioritization

13. **Ans: 4**   A patient with permanent diabetes insipidus requires lifelong vasopressin therapy. All of the other statements are appropriate to the home care of this patient. **Focus:** Prioritization

14. **Ans: 1, 2, 4, 5**   A patient with Cushing disease experiences body changes affecting body image and is at risk for bruising, infection, and hypertension. Such a patient usually gains weight. **Focus:** Prioritization

15. **Ans: 1**   A patient with Addison disease is at risk for anemia. The nurse should expect this patient's sodium level to decrease, and potassium and calcium levels to increase. **Focus:** Prioritization

16. **Ans: 1**   Vitiligo, or patchy areas of pigment loss with increased pigmentation at the edges, is seen with primary hypofunction of the adrenal glands and is caused by autoimmune destruction of melanocytes in the skin. The other findings are signs of pituitary hypofunction. **Focus:** Prioritization

17. **Ans: 4**   The thyroid gland should always be palpated gently because vigorous palpation can stimulate a thyroid storm in a patient who may have hyperthyroidism. You should stand either behind or in front of the patient and use both hands to palpate the thyroid. Having the patient swallow can help with locating the thyroid gland. **Focus:** Supervision, delegation

18. **Ans: 2**   The patient with Cushing disease usually has paper-thin skin that is easily injured. The UAPs should use a lift or a draw sheet to carefully move the patient and prevent injury to the skin. All of the other actions are appropriate to moving this patient up in bed. **Focus:** Delegation, supervision

19. **Ans: 3**   This patient's potassium level is very high, placing the patient at risk for cardiac dysrhythmias that could be life threatening. The other patients need to be seen also, but are not as urgent as this patient. **Focus:** Prioritization

20. **Ans: 1, 2, 3, 6**   Weighing patients, recording intake and output, and checking vital signs are all within the scope of practice for a UAP. An experienced UAP would have been trained to perform fingerstick glucose monitoring also. Administering medications and monitoring for cardiac dysrhythmias are within the scope of practice of licensed nurses. **Focus:** Delegation

21. **Ans: 2**   A key cardiovascular feature seen in patients with Cushing disease is capillary fragility, which results in bruising and petechiae. Bleeding disorders are not a sign of Cushing disease, and although these patients have delicate skin, this is not the cause of the bruising. You may want to investigate whether the patient fell, but these patients have bruising and petechiae despite falls. **Focus:** Supervision, prioritization

22. **Ans: 3**   Diuretics and hydration help reduce serum calcium for patients who are not surgery candidates.

Furosemide increases kidney excretion of calcium when combined with IV saline in large volumes. **Focus:** Prioritization

23. **Ans: 1, 2, 6**   Assessment, auscultation, and reminding patients about information that has been taught to them are within the scope of practice of the LPN/LVN. Certainly the LPN/LVN could check the patient's vital signs, but this would be more appropriately delegated to the UAP. Creating nursing care plans falls within the scope of practice of the RN. The use of sedation is discouraged for patients with hypothyroidism because it may make respiratory problems more difficult. If sedation is used, dosage is reduced and it is not given around the clock. **Focus:** Delegation, supervision

24. **Ans: 1**   When caring for a patient with hyperthyroidism, even after a partial thyroidectomy, a temperature elevation of 1° must be reported immediately because it may indicate an impending thyroid crisis. The other changes should be monitored, but none is urgent. **Focus:** Prioritization

25. **Ans: 2**   These assessment findings are classic initial manifestations for growth hormone excess. **Focus:** Prioritization

CHAPTER 15: Integumentary Problems, pages 69-72

1. **Ans: 3**   An LPN/LVN who is experienced in working with postoperative clients will know how to monitor for pain, bleeding, or swelling and will notify the supervising RN. Client teaching requires more education and a broader scope of practice and is appropriate for RN staff members. **Focus:** Delegation

2. **Ans: 4**   LPN/LVN education and scope of practice includes sterile and nonsterile wound care. LPNs/LVNs do function as wound care nurses in some LTC facilities, but the choice of dressing type and assessment for risk factors are more complex skills that are appropriate to the RN level of practice. Assisting the client to change position is a task included in UAP education and would be more appropriate to delegate to the UAP. **Focus:** Delegation

3. **Ans: 2**   Facial burns are frequently associated with airway inflammation and swelling, so this client requires the most immediate assessment. The other clients also require rapid assessment or interventions, but not as urgently as the client with facial burns. **Focus:** Prioritization

4. **Ans: 3, 4, 2, 1, 5**   Pain medication should be administered before changing the dressing, because changing dressings for partial-thickness burns is painful, especially if the dressing change involves removal of eschar. The wound should be débrided before obtaining wound specimens for culture to avoid including bacteria that are skin contaminants rather than causes

of the wound infection. Culture specimens should be obtained prior to the application of antibacterial creams. The antibacterial cream should then be applied to the area after débridement to gain the maximum effect. Finally, the wound should be covered with a sterile dressing. **Focus:** Prioritization

5. **Ans: 3**   A nurse from the oncology unit would be familiar with dressing changes and sterile technique. The charge RN in the burn unit would work closely with the float RN to provide partners to assist in providing care and to answer any questions. Admission assessment and development of the initial care plan, discharge teaching, and splint positioning in burn clients all require expertise in caring for clients with burns. These clients should be assigned to RNs who regularly work on the burn unit. **Focus:** Assignment

6. **Ans: 4**   Irregular borders and a black or variegated color are characteristics associated with malignant skin lesions. Striae and toenail thickening or yellowing are common in elderly individuals. Silver scaling is associated with psoriasis, which may need treatment but is not as urgent a concern as the appearance of the mole. **Focus:** Prioritization

7. **Ans: 1**   A blue color or cyanosis may indicate that the client has significant problems with circulation or ventilation. More detailed assessments are needed immediately. The other data may also indicate health problems in major body systems, but potential respiratory or circulatory abnormalities are the priority. **Focus:** Prioritization

8. **Ans: 1**   Because isotretinoin is associated with a high incidence of birth defects, it is important that the client stop using the medication at least a month before attempting to become pregnant. Nausea and poor night vision are possible adverse effects of isotretinoin that would require further assessment but are not as urgent as discussing the fetal risks associated with this medication. The client's concern about whether treatment is effective should be addressed, but this is a lower-priority intervention. **Focus:** Prioritization

9. **Ans: 3**   Scheduling a follow-up appointment for the client is within the legal scope of practice and training for the medical assistant role. Client teaching, assessment for positive skin reactions to the test, and monitoring for serious allergic reactions are appropriate to the education and practice role of licensed nursing staff. **Focus:** Delegation

10. **Ans: 1**   Systemic use of tetracycline is associated with severe photosensitivity reactions to ultraviolet light. All individuals should be taught about the potential risks of overexposure to sunlight or other ultraviolet light, but the client taking tetracycline is at the most immediate risk for severe adverse effects. **Focus:** Prioritization

11. **Ans: 3**   Although it is not appropriate for UAPs to plan or implement initial client or family teaching, reinforcement of previous teaching is an important function of UAPs (who are likely to be in the home on a daily basis). Teaching about medication use, nutritional assessment and planning, and evaluation for improvement are included in the RN scope of practice. **Focus:** Delegation

12. **Ans: 1**   Medication administration is included in LPN/LVN education and scope of practice. Bathing and cleaning clients require the least education and would be better delegated to a UAP. Assessment and evaluation of outcomes of care are more complex skills best performed by RNs. **Focus:** Delegation

13. **Ans: 2**   The highest priority diagnoses for this client are Acute Pain and Imbalanced Nutrition. The Acute Pain diagnosis takes precedence, because the client's acute oral pain will need to be controlled to increase the ability to eat and to improve nutrition. Disturbed Body Image and Social Isolation are major concerns for the client but are not as high a priority as the need for pain control and improved nutrition. **Focus:** Prioritization

14. **Ans: 4**   Wheals are frequently associated with allergic reactions, so asking about exposure to new medications is the most appropriate question for this client. The other questions would be useful in assessing the skin health history but do not directly relate to the client's symptoms. **Focus:** Prioritization

15. **Ans: 2**   With chemical injuries, it is important to remove the chemical from contact with the skin to prevent ongoing damage. The other actions also should be accomplished rapidly; however, rinsing the chemical off is the priority for this client. **Focus:** Prioritization

16. **Ans: 3**   This client's vital signs indicate that the life-threatening complications of sepsis and septic shock may be developing. The other clients also need rapid assessment and/or nursing interventions, but their symptoms do not indicate that they need care as urgently as the febrile and hypotensive client. **Focus:** Prioritization

17. **Ans: 4**   Because aspirin affects platelet aggregation, the client is at increased risk for postprocedure bleeding, and the surgeon may need to reschedule the procedure. The other information is also pertinent but will not affect the scheduling of the procedure. **Focus:** Prioritization

18. **Ans: 3**   A new graduate would be familiar with the procedure for a sterile dressing change, especially after working for 3 weeks on the unit. Clients whose care requires more complex skills such as admission assessments, preprocedure teaching, and discharge teaching should be assigned to more experienced RN staff members. **Focus:** Assignment

19. **Ans: 3**   Epigastric pain may indicate that the client is developing peptic ulcers, which require collaborative interventions such as the use of antacids, histamine$_2$ receptor blockers (e.g., famotidine [Pepcid]), or

proton pump inhibitors (e.g., esomeprazole [Nexium]). The elevation in blood glucose level, increased appetite, and slight elevation in blood pressure may be related to prednisone use but are not clinically significant when steroids are used for limited periods and do not require treatment. **Focus:** Prioritization

20. **Ans: 2** Dairy products inhibit the absorption of doxycycline, so this action would decrease the effectiveness of the antibiotic. The other activities are not appropriate but would not cause as much potential harm as the administration of doxycycline with milk. Anaerobic bacteria would not be likely to grow in a superficial wound. The herpes zoster vaccine is recommended for clients who are 60 years or older. Pressure garments may be used after graft wounds heal and during the rehabilitation period after a burn injury, but this should be discussed when the client is ready for rehabilitation, not when the client is admitted. **Focus:** Prioritization

CHAPTER 16: Renal and Urinary Problems, pages 73-76

1. **Ans: 4** Providing the equipment that the patient needs to collect the urine sample is within the scope of practice of a UAP. Teaching, planning, and assessing all require additional education and skill, which is appropriate to the scope of practice of professional nurses. **Focus:** Delegation, supervision

2. **Ans: 3** The presence of 100,000 bacterial colonies per milliliter of urine or the presence of many white blood cells (WBCs) and red blood cells (RBCs) indicates a urinary tract infection. The WBC count is within normal limits and the hematocrit is a little low, which may need follow-up. Neither of these results indicates infection. **Focus:** Prioritization

3. **Ans: 1** The patient with cystitis who is taking oral antibiotics is in stable condition with predictable outcomes, and caring for this patient is therefore appropriate to the scope of practice of an LPN/LVN under the supervision of an RN. The patient with a new order for lithotripsy will need teaching about the procedure, which should be accomplished by the RN. The patient in need of bladder training will need the RN to plan this intervention. The patient with flank pain needs careful and skilled assessment by the RN. **Focus:** Assignment

4. **Ans: 2** Prostate disease increases the risk of UTIs in men because of urinary retention. The wife's UTI should not affect the patient. The times of the catheter usage and kidney stone removal are too distant to cause this UTI. **Focus:** Prioritization

5. **Ans: 4** A cystoscopy is needed to accurately diagnose interstitial cystitis. Urinalysis may show WBCs and RBCs, but no bacteria. The patient will probably need a urinalysis upon admission, but daily samples do not need to be obtained. Intake and output may be assessed, but results will not contribute to the diagnosis. Cystitis does not usually affect urine electrolyte levels. **Focus:** Prioritization

6. **Ans: 3** For uncomplicated cystitis, a 3-day course of antibiotics is an effective treatment, and research has shown that patients are more likely to adhere to shorter antibiotic courses. Seven-day courses of antibiotics are appropriate for complicated cystitis, and 10- to 14-day courses are prescribed for uncomplicated pyelonephritis. This patient is being discharged and should not be at risk for a nosocomial infection. **Focus:** Prioritization, supervision

7. **Ans: 4** Women should avoid irritating substances such as bubble bath, nylon underwear, and scented toilet tissue to prevent UTIs. Adequate fluid intake, consumption of cranberry juice, and regular voiding are all good strategies for preventing UTIs. **Focus:** Delegation, supervision, prioritization

8. **Ans: 3** A patient with urge incontinence can be taught to control the bladder as long as the patient is alert, aware, and able to resist the urge to urinate by starting a schedule for voiding, then increasing the intervals between voids. Patients with functional incontinence related to mental status changes or loss of cognitive function will not be able to follow a bladder-training program. A better treatment for a patient with stress incontinence is exercises such as pelvic floor (Kegel) exercises to strengthen the pelvic floor muscles. **Focus:** Prioritization

9. **Ans: 1** Oxybutynin is an anticholinergic agent, and these drugs often cause an extremely dry mouth. The maximum dosage is 20 mg/day. Oxybutynin should be taken between meals, because food interferes with absorption of the drug. **Focus:** Prioritization

10. **Ans: 4** Teaching about bladder emptying, self-catheterization, and medications requires additional knowledge and training and is appropriate to the scope of practice of the RN. The LPN/LVN can reinforce information that has already been taught to the patient. **Focus:** Delegation, supervision

11. **Ans: 1** When patients with urolithiasis pass stones, they can be in excruciating pain for up to 24 to 36 hours. All of the other nursing diagnoses for this patient are accurate; however, at this time, pain is the most urgent concern for the patient. **Focus:** Prioritization

12. **Ans: 3** Bruising is to be expected after lithotripsy. It may be quite extensive and take several weeks to resolve. All of the other statements are accurate for a patient after lithotripsy. **Focus:** Prioritization

13. **Ans: 3, 4** Both these patients will need frequent assessments and medications. The patient receiving chemotherapy and the patient who has just undergone surgery should not be exposed to any patient with infection. **Focus:** Assignment

14. **Ans: 4** Administering oral medications appropriately is covered in the educational program for LPNs/LVNs

and is within their scope of practice. Teaching and assessing the patient require additional education and skill and are appropriate to the scope of practice of RNs. **Focus:** Delegation, supervision

15. **Ans: 1, 5, 3, 2, 7, 4, 6, 8**   Before checking postvoid residual, you should ask the patient to void, and then position him. Next you should open the catheterization kit and put on sterile gloves, position the patient's penis, clean the meatus, then lubricate and insert the catheter. All urine must be drained from the bladder to assess the amount of postvoid residual the patient has. Finally, the catheter is removed, the penis cleaned, and the urine measured. **Focus:** Prioritization

16. **Ans: 1**   The underlying pathophysiology of nephrotic syndrome involves increased glomerular permeability, which allows larger molecules to pass through the membrane into the urine and be removed from the blood. This process causes massive loss of protein, edema formation, and decreased serum albumin levels. Key features include hypertension and renal insufficiency (decreased urine output) related to concurrent renal vein thrombosis, which may be a cause or an effect of nephrotic syndrome. Flank pain is seen in patients with acute pyelonephritis. **Focus:** Prioritization

17. **Ans: 2**   Chemotherapy has limited effectiveness against renal cell carcinoma. This form of cancer is usually treated surgically by nephrectomy. **Focus:** Supervision, prioritization

18. **Ans: 1, 2, 3, 5**   A patient with only one kidney should avoid all contact sports and high-risk activities to protect the remaining kidney from injury and preserve kidney function. All of the other points are key to preventing renal trauma. **Focus:** Prioritization

19. **Ans: 1, 2, 4, 6**   Administering oral medications is appropriate to the scope of practice for an LPN/LVN or RN. Assessing breath sounds requires additional education and skill development and is most appropriately within the scope of practice of an RN, but it may be part of the observations of an experienced and competent LPN/LVN. All other actions are within the educational preparation and scope of practice of an experienced UAP. **Focus:** Delegation, supervision

20. **Ans: 1**   During the oliguric phase of acute kidney failure, a patient's urine output is greatly reduced. Fluid boluses and diuretics do not work well. This phase usually lasts from 8 to 15 days. Although there are frequent omissions in recording intake and output, this is probably not the cause of the patient's decreased urine output. Retention of sodium and water is the rationale for giving furosemide, not the reason that it is ineffective. Nitrogenous wastes build up as a result of the kidneys' inability to perform their elimination function. **Focus:** Prioritization, supervision

21. **Ans: 2**   A nurse from the surgical ICU will be thoroughly familiar with the care of patients who have just undergone surgery. The patient scheduled for lithotripsy may need education about the procedure.

The newly-admitted patient needs an in-depth admission assessment, and the patient with chronic kidney failure needs teaching about peritoneal dialysis. All of these interventions would best be accomplished by an experienced nurse with expertise in the care of patients with kidney problems. **Focus:** Assignment

22. **Ans: 1**   Gentamicin can be a highly nephrotoxic substance. You would monitor creatinine and blood urea nitrogen levels for elevations indicating possible nephrotoxicity. All of the other measures are important but are not specific to gentamicin therapy. **Focus:** Prioritization

23. **Ans: 2**   Patients with acute kidney failure usually go through a diuretic phase 2 to 6 weeks after the onset of the oliguric phase. The diuresis can result in an output of up to 10 L/day of dilute urine. During this phase it is important to monitor for electrolyte and fluid imbalances. This is followed by the recovery phase. A patient with acute kidney failure caused by hypovolemia would receive IV fluids to correct the problem; however, this would not necessarily lead to the onset of diuresis. **Focus:** Supervision

24. **Ans: 1**   CAVH is a continuous renal replacement therapy that is prescribed for patients with kidney failure who are critically ill and do not tolerate the rapid shifts in fluids and electrolytes that are associated with hemodialysis. A teaching plan is not urgent at this time. A patient must have a mean arterial pressure (MAP) of at least 60 mm Hg or more for CAVH to be of use. The physician should be notified about this patient's MAP; it is a priority, but not the highest priority. When a patient urgently needs a procedure, morning care does not take priority and may be deferred until later in the day. **Focus:** Prioritization

25. **Ans: 4**   A patient with dehydration due to deficient ADH would have diluted urine with a decreased urine specific gravity. Normal urine specific gravity ranges from 1.003 to 1.030. A specific gravity of 1.035 would indicate urine that is concentrated. **Focus:** Prioritization

26. **Ans: 1**   The risk for contrast-induced kidney failure is greatest in patients who are older or dehydrated. If possible, arrange for the patient to have this procedure early in the day to prevent dehydration. The purpose of this procedure is to assess kidney function and identify anomalies. The administration of drugs that affect the gag reflex is not done during this procedure. **Focus:** Supervision, prioritization

CHAPTER 17: Reproductive Problems, pages 77-80

1. **Ans: 3**   A palpable bladder and restlessness are indicators of urinary retention, which would require action (such as insertion of a catheter) to empty the bladder. The other data would be consistent with the client's diagnosis of BPH. More detailed assessment may be indicated, but no immediate action is required. **Focus:** Prioritization

2. **Ans: 4** Irregularly shaped and nontender lumps are consistent with a diagnosis of breast cancer, so this client needs immediate referral for diagnostic tests such as mammography or ultrasound. The other information is not unusual and does not indicate the need for immediate action. **Focus:** Prioritization

3. **Ans: 1** An LPN/LVN working in a PACU would be expected to check dressings for bleeding and alert RN staff members if bleeding occurs. The other tasks are more appropriate for nursing staff with RN-level education and licensure. **Focus:** Delegation

4. **Ans: 2** Positioning the client's arm is a task within the scope of practice for UAP working on a surgical unit. Client teaching and assessment are RN-level skills. The RN should reinforce dressings as necessary, because this requires assessment of the surgical site and possible communication with the surgeon. **Focus:** Delegation

5. **Ans: 4** The bladder spasms may indicate that blood clots are obstructing the catheter, which would indicate the need for irrigation of the catheter with 30 to 50 mL of normal saline using a piston syringe. The other data would all be normal after a TURP, but the client may need some teaching about the usual post-TURP symptoms and care. **Focus:** Prioritization

6. **Ans: 4** Because tamsulosin blocks alpha receptors in the peripheral arterial system, the most significant side effects are orthostatic hypotension and dizziness. To avoid falls, it is important that the client change positions slowly. The other information is also accurate and may be included in client teaching but is not as important as decreasing the risk for falls. **Focus:** Prioritization

7. **Ans: 2** Hemorrhage is a major complication after TURP and should be reported to the surgeon immediately. The other assessment data also indicate a need for nursing action, but not as urgently. **Focus:** Prioritization

8. **Ans: 1** Reinforcement of previous teaching is an expected role of the LPN/LVN. Planning and implementing client initial teaching and documentation of a client's discharge assessment should be performed by experienced RN staff members. **Focus:** Delegation

9. **Ans: 4** It is important to assess oxygenation, because the client's calf tenderness and shortness of breath suggest a possible deep vein thrombosis and pulmonary embolus, serious complications of TURP. The other activities are appropriate but are not as high a priority as ensuring that oxygenation is adequate. **Focus:** Prioritization

10. **Ans: 1** This client has symptoms of testicular torsion, an emergency that needs immediate assessment and intervention, because it can lead to testicular ischemia and necrosis within a few hours. The other clients also have symptoms of acute problems (primary syphilis, acute bacterial prostatitis, and prostatic hyperplasia and urinary retention), which also need

rapid assessment and intervention, but these are not as urgent as the possible testicular torsion. **Focus:** Prioritization

11. **Ans: 2, 1, 3, 4** Bladder spasms after a TURP are usually caused by the presence of clots that obstruct the catheter, so irrigation should be the first action taken. Administration of analgesics may help to reduce spasm. Administration of a bolus of IV fluids is commonly used in the immediate postoperative period to help maintain fluid intake and increase urinary flow. Oral fluid intake should be encouraged once you are sure that the client is not nauseated and has adequate bowel tone. **Focus:** Prioritization

12. **Ans: 3** Sildenafil is a potent vasodilator and has caused cardiac arrest in clients who were also taking nitrates such as nitroglycerin. The other client data indicate the need for further assessment and/or teaching, but it is essential for the client who uses nitrates to avoid concurrent use of sildenafil. **Focus:** Prioritization

13. **Ans: 2** Administration of narcotics and the associated client monitoring are included in LPN/LVN education and scope of practice. Assessments and teaching are more complex skills that require RN-level education and are best accomplished by an RN with experience in caring for clients with this diagnosis. **Focus:** Delegation

14. **Ans: 3** An RN from the ED would be experienced in assessment and management of pain. Because of their diagnoses and treatments, the other clients should be assigned to RNs who are experienced in caring for clients with cancer. **Focus:** Assignment

15. **Ans: 4, 3, 2, 1** The bilateral orchiectomy client needs immediate assessment, because confusion may be an indicator of serious postoperative complications such as hemorrhage, infection, or pulmonary embolism. The client who had a perineal prostatectomy should be assessed next, because pain medication may be needed to allow him to perform essential postoperative activities such as deep breathing, coughing, and ambulating. The vaginal hysterectomy client's anxiety needs further assessment next. Although the breast implant client has questions about care of the drains at the surgical site, there is nothing in the report indicating that these need to be addressed immediately. **Focus:** Prioritization

16. **Ans: 3** Although infection occurs only rarely as a complication of transrectal prostate biopsy, it is important that the client receive teaching about checking his temperature and calling the physician if there is any fever or other signs of systemic infection. The client should understand that the test results will not be available immediately but that he will be notified about the results. Transient rectal bleeding may occur after the biopsy, but bleeding that lasts for more than a few hours indicates that there may have been rectal trauma. **Focus:** Prioritization

17. **Ans: 4** Cramping or aching abdominal pain is common after dilation and curettage; however, sharp, continuous pain may indicate uterine perforation, which would require rapid intervention by the surgeon. The other data indicate a need for ongoing assessment or interventions. Transient blood pressure elevation may occur due to the stress response after surgery. Bleeding following the procedure is expected but should decrease over the first 2 hours. And although the oxygen saturation is not at an unsafe level, interventions to improve the saturation should be carried out. **Focus:** Prioritization

18. **Ans: 2, 4, 5** Assisting with catheter care, ambulation, and hygiene are included in home health aide education and would be expected activities for this staff member. Client assessments are the responsibility of RN members of the home health care team. **Focus:** Delegation

19. **Ans: 1** Because the most likely source of the bacteria causing the toxic shock syndrome is the client's tampon, it is essential to remove it first. The other actions should be implemented in the following order: obtain blood culture samples (best done before initiating antibiotic therapy to ensure accurate culture and sensitivity results), infuse nafcillin (rapid initiation of antibiotic therapy will decrease bacterial release of toxins), and administer acetaminophen (fever reduction may be necessary, but treating the infection has the highest priority). **Focus:** Prioritization

20. **Ans: 2** Right calf swelling and tenderness indicate the possible presence of deep vein thrombosis. This will change the plan of care, because the client should be placed on bed rest, whereas the usual plan is to ambulate the client as soon as possible after surgery. The other data indicate the need for common postoperative nursing actions such as having the client cough, assessing her pain, and increasing her fluid intake. **Focus:** Prioritization

21. **Ans: 3** Clients with intracavitary implants are kept in bed during the treatment to avoid dislodgement of the implant. The other actions may also require you to intervene by providing guidance to the student. Minimal time should be spent close to clients who are receiving internal irradiation. Asking the client about her reaction to losing childbearing abilities may be inappropriate at this time. Clients are frequently placed on low-residue diets to decrease bowel distention while implants are in place. **Focus:** Prioritization

22. **Ans: 1** The client has symptoms of a urinary tract infection. Inserting a straight catheter will enable you to obtain an uncontaminated urine specimen for culture and sensitivity testing before the antibiotic is started. In addition, the client is probably not emptying her bladder fully because of the painful urination. The antibiotic therapy should be initiated as rapidly as possible once the urine specimen is obtained. Administration of acetaminophen is the lowest priority, because

the client's temperature is not dangerously elevated. **Focus:** Prioritization

23. **Ans: 2** After an A & P repair, it is essential that the bladder be empty to avoid putting pressure on the suture lines. The abdominal firmness and tenderness indicate that the client's bladder is distended. The physician should be notified and an order for catheterization obtained. The other data also indicate a need for further assessment of her cardiac status and actions such as having the client cough and deep breathe, but these are not such immediate concerns. **Focus:** Prioritization

24. **Ans: 3** The client should be positioned in a semi-Fowler position to minimize the risk of abscess development higher in the abdomen. The other actions also require correction, but not as rapidly. Tampon use is not contraindicated after an episode of PID, although some sources recommend not using tampons during the acute infection. Heat application to the abdomen and pelvis is used for pain relief. Intercourse is safe a few weeks after effective treatment for PID. **Focus:** Prioritization

25. **Ans: 3** Centers for Disease Control and Prevention guidelines indicate that the HPV immunization should not be given during pregnancy. Ideally, the immunization series should start at age 11 or 12 for females and males, but it may be started up through age 26. HPV immunization is most effective in preventing HPV infection and cervical cancer when it is started before the individual is sexually active and prior to any HPV infection, but these are not contraindications for vaccination. **Focus:** Prioritization

26. **Ans: 2** The initial action should be to ensure that the abdominal contents remain moist by covering the wound and loops of intestine with dressings soaked with sterile normal saline. Since national guidelines addressing the use of Rapid Response Teams (RRTs) indicate that the role of the RRT is immediate assessment and stabilization of the client, the nurse's next action should be to activate the RRT. The surgeon should be notified once further assessments of the client (i.e., pulse and blood pressure) are obtained. Wound cultures may be obtained, but protection of the wound, further assessment of the client, then notification of the surgeon so that other actions can be taken are the priority. **Focus:** Prioritization

27. **Ans: 3** LPN/LVN education includes vital sign monitoring; an experienced LPN/LVN would recognize and report significant changes in vital signs to the RN. The paracentesis tray could be obtained by a UAP. Client admission assessment and teaching require RN-level education and experience, although part of the data gathering may be done by an LPN/LVN. **Focus:** Delegation

28. **Ans: 4** The current national guidelines, supported by nonrandomized screening trials and observational data, call for first-degree relatives of clients with the *BRCA* gene to be screened with both annual mammography

and magnetic resonance imaging (MRI). Although annual mammography, breast self-examination, and clinical breast examination by a health care provider may help to detect cancer, the best option for this client is annual mammography and MRI. **Focus:** Prioritization

CHAPTER 18: Problems in Pregnancy and Childbearing, pages 81-84

1. **Ans: 4**   The incidence of congenital anomalies is three times higher in the offspring of diabetic women. Good glycemic control during preconception and early pregnancy significantly reduces this risk and would be the highest priority message to this patient at this point. The other responses are correct but are not of greatest importance at this time. **Focus:** Prioritization

2. **Ans: 1**   The UAP can check the blood pressure of this patient and report it to the RN. The RN would include this information in her full assessment of the patient, who may be showing signs of preeclampsia. The other tasks listed require nursing assessment, analysis, and planning, and should be performed by the RN. Provision of accurate and supportive education about breast-feeding and breast pumping supports the Perinatal Core Measure of increasing the percentage of women who exclusively breast-feed. **Focus:** Delegation

3. **Ans: 2**   A multiparous patient in active labor with an urge to have a bowel movement will probably give birth imminently. She needs to be the first assessed, the provider must be notified immediately, and she must be moved to a safe location for the birth. She should not be allowed up to the bathroom at this time. The other patients all have needs requiring prompt assessment, but the imminent birth takes priority. Vaginal bleeding after intercourse could be due to cervical irritation or a vaginal infection, or could have a more serious cause such as placenta previa. This patient should be the second one assessed. **Focus:** Prioritization

4. **Ans: 1, 3, 4**   Magnesium sulfate toxicity can cause fatal cardiovascular events and/or respiratory depression or arrest, so monitoring of respiratory rate is of utmost importance. The drug is excreted by the kidneys, and therefore monitoring for adequate urine output is essential. Deep tendon reflexes disappear when serum magnesium is reaching a toxic level. Vaginal bleeding is not associated with magnesium sulfate use. Calf pain can be a sign of a deep vein thrombosis, but is not associated with magnesium sulfate therapy. **Focus:** Prioritization

5. **Ans: 2**   It is recommended to avoid artificial nipples and pacifiers while establishing breast feeding unless medically indicated. Improper latch and position are common causes of nipple soreness and can be corrected with assessment and assistance to the mother. This practice supports the Perinatal Core Measure of increasing the percentage of newborns who are fed breast milk only. **Focus:** Prioritization

6. **Ans: 2**   The positive group B streptococci result requires immediate action. The provider must be notified and orders obtained for prompt antibiotic prophylaxis during labor to reduce the risk of mother-to-newborn transmission of group B streptococci. The other data are not as significant in the care of the patient at this moment. Intrapartum-appropriate antibiotic treatment of the mother with group B streptococci supports the Perinatal Core Measure of reducing health care–acquired bloodstream infections in newborns. **Focus:** Prioritization

7. **Ans: 1**   An RN in a prenatal clinic can safely give telephone advice regarding nausea, vomiting, and pedal edema, which can be considered normal in pregnancy. The RN would assess the complaint, give the patient evidence-based advice, and define the circumstances under which the patient should call back. Vaginal itching at 20 weeks could be a yeast infection. Depending on clinic protocols, the RN could, after phone assessment, safely recommend an over-the-counter medication or arrange an office visit for the patient. Leaking vaginal fluid at 34 weeks requires immediate attention, however, because it could indicate premature rupture of membranes with the risk of premature birth. **Focus:** Prioritization

8. **Ans: 4**   The RN must follow through on the findings of a nonreassuring fetal heart rate. Where patient safety is concerned, the nurse is obligated to pursue an appropriate response. Documenting the conversation with the provider and discussing it with a colleague are appropriate, but something must be done to address the immediate safety concern and possible need for intervention at this time. The RN must persist until the safety concern has been addressed appropriately. **Focus:** Prioritization

9. **Ans: 1**   The cause of variable fetal heart decelerations is compression of the umbilical cord, which can often be corrected by a change in maternal position. **Focus:** Prioritization

10. **Ans: 1, 3, 5**   Late fetal heart rate decelerations can be an ominous sign of fetal hypoxemia, especially if repetitive and accompanied by decreased variability. Notification of the provider is indicated. Turning off the oxytocin and administering oxygen to the mother are recommended nursing interventions to improve fetal oxygenation. An increase in the IV rate can improve hydration, correct hypovolemia, and increase blood flow to the uterus. Putting the woman in a lateral position can increase blood flow to the uterus and increase oxygenation to the fetus. Promptly addressing fetal heart rate changes may allow intrauterine resuscitation and may decrease the need for cesarean section if those measures are effective. This supports the Perinatal Core Measure of reducing of cesarean section rates. **Focus:** Prioritization

11. **Ans: 3**   The care of a vegetarian woman who is pregnant should begin with assessment of her diet,

because vegetarian practices vary widely. The RN must first assess exactly what the woman's diet consists of and then determine any deficiencies. The reason for the diet is less important than what the diet actually contains. It is probable that the woman will need a vitamin B_{12} supplement, but the assessment comes first. Vegetarian diets can be completely adequate in protein, and therefore protein supplementation is not routinely recommended. **Focus:** Prioritization

12. **Ans: 1, 3, 5** The UAP could provide an abdominal binder, measure the vital signs of the patient, and assist her to ambulate. The RN would be responsible for evaluating the normality of the vital sign values. The UAP should be given parameter limits for vital signs and told to report values outside these limits to the RN. Assisting in breast feeding for a first-time mother is a very important nursing function, because the RN needs to give consistent, evidence-based advice to enhance success at breast feeding. A common complaint of postpartum patients is inconsistent help with and advice on breast feeding. The RN should also be the one to check the amount of lochia, because the evaluation requires nursing judgment. The use of the professionally educated RN to provide evidence-based and consistent information and assistance with breast feeding supports the Perinatal Core Measure of increasing the percentage of newborns who are fed breast milk only. **Focus:** Delegation

13. **Ans: 1** Fundal pressure should never be applied in a case of shoulder dystocia, because it may worsen the problem by impacting the fetal shoulder even more firmly into the symphysis pubis. This issue of patient safety would require the supervising RN to intervene immediately. The other responses are appropriate actions in a case of shoulder dystocia. **Focus:** Assignment

14. **Ans: 1, 3, 4** It is recommended that a newborn be placed on the back in a crib with a firm mattress with no toys and a minimum of blankets as a safety measure for prevention of sudden infant death syndrome. A newborn discharged before 72 hours of life should be seen by an RN or MD within 2 days of discharge. Breast-feeding women should breast-feed at all feedings, especially in these early weeks of establishing breast feeding. This supports the Perinatal Core Measure of increasing the percentage of newborns who are fed breast milk only. A more appropriate response would be for the father to help with household chores to allow breast feeding to be established successfully. A flu shot in flu season is a recommended intervention for a new mother. **Focus:** Prioritization

15. **Ans: 1, 4** Patient 1 is in the latent phase of labor with her first child; she typically will cope well at this point and will have many hours before labor becomes more active. Patient 4 would most likely be managed expectantly at this point and require observation and assessment for labor or signs of infection. Patient 2 can be expected to deliver soon and so requires intensive nursing care. Patient 3 is in the first hour of recovery and therefore requires frequent assessments, newborn assessments, and help with initiation of breast feeding if this is her chosen feeding method. Breast feeding in the first hour of life supports the Perinatal Core Measure of increasing the percentage of newborns who are fed breast milk only. Patient 5 could be in premature labor and require administration of tocolytic medications to stop contractions or preparation for a preterm delivery if dilation is advanced. **Focus:** Assignment

16. **Ans: 3** Fundal massage would be the priority nursing action because it helps the uterus to contract firmly and thus reduces bleeding. The first two Answer choices are appropriate nursing actions, but do nothing to stop the immediate bleeding. Putting the baby to the breast does release oxytocin, which causes uterine contraction, but it will be slower to do so than fundal massage. **Focus:** Prioritization

17. **Ans: 2, 4, 5** Staying with the parents at this moment and offering physical and emotional support is appropriate. It is also appropriate to prepare the infant in a way that demonstrates care and respect for the baby and to offer the parents the opportunity to view and/or hold the infant as they desire. The RN must ask the parents if there are cultural or religious rituals they would like for their child to ensure that they feel their infant has been treated properly with respect to their religion or culture. Autopsy should be discussed, but not at the very moments after birth. The infant should not be placed on the maternal abdomen until the nurse assesses the parents' wishes of when and how to view the infant. **Focus:** Prioritization

18. **Ans: 3** Slight redness in the left calf could be suggestive of thrombophlebitis and requires further investigation. The other findings are within normal limits. **Focus:** Prioritization

19. **Ans: 2, 4** Insertion of a Foley catheter is indicated because the woman will usually be unable to void due to the effect of the anesthetic in the bladder area. Positioning the patient on her side enhances blood flow and helps to prevent hypotension. Changing maternal position encourages progress in labor. In management of the second stage of labor when epidural anesthesia is used, laboring down as opposed to immediately pushing without the urge to push is advocated. It is not recommended to routinely discontinue an epidural anesthetic at complete dilation. A continuous epidural infusion provides pain relief throughout labor and birth. Use of evidence-based practices with a laboring woman supports the Perinatal Core Measure of reducing the percentage of women who are delivered by cesarean section. **Focus:** Prioritization

20. **Ans: 2, 3** The patient may be experiencing supine hypotension caused by the pressure of the uterus on

the vena cava and the effects of epidural medication. Maternal hypotension can cause uteroplacental insufficiency leading to fetal hypoxia. Placing the woman in lateral position can relieve the pressure on the vena cava. The anesthesiologist should be notified and may need to treat the patient with ephedrine to correct the hypotension. IV fluids are increased per protocol when supine hypotension occurs. The correction of common problems in labor supports the Perinatal Core Measure of reducing the percentage of women who are delivered by cesarean section. **Focus:** Prioritization

21. **Ans: 3** The RN remains an important part of the labor and birth in this scenario. Even with a good support team present, the RN needs to observe and assess the patient's comfort and safety as part of essential nursing care during labor. The RN's expertise allows the RN to make helpful suggestions to the support people and patient. The patient should be encouraged to utilize positions and activities that are most comfortable to her. It is appropriate to let the patient and support people know of all pain control options, but it would not be appropriate to continually offer pain medication to a patient who has chosen natural childbirth. Expert nursing care in labor supports the Perinatal Core Measure of reducing the percentage of women who are delivered by cesarean section. **Focus:** Prioritization

22. **Ans: 3** Painless vaginal bleeding can be a symptom of placenta previa. A digital vaginal examination is contraindicated until ultrasound can be performed to rule out placenta previa. If a digital examination is performed when placenta previa is present, it can cause increased bleeding. The other statements reflect appropriate assessment of an incoming patient with vaginal bleeding. **Focus:** Assignment

23. **Ans: 1** Administration of antiviral medications to the pregnant woman and the newborn, cesarean birth, and avoidance of breast feeding have reduced the incidence of perinatal transmission of HIV from approximately 26% to 1% to 2%. Pregnancy is not known to accelerate HIV disease in the mother. The most important nursing action is to engage the mother in prenatal care and educate her as to the great benefits of medication for HIV during pregnancy. **Focus:** Prioritization

24. **Ans: 3** When a patient discloses fear of hurting herself or her baby, the RN must have the woman immediately evaluated before allowing her to leave. Merely informing the patient about community resources is not sufficient. The "baby blues" are typically milder and occur 1 to 2 weeks postpartum. Once the woman has been evaluated, the provider can prescribe antidepressants that can be safely used while breastfeeding. **Focus:** Prioritization

25. **Ans: 2** There is no evidence that exercise should be avoided in the first trimester of pregnancy in a healthy woman without medical or obstetric complications. The American College of Obstetricians and Gynecologists recommends 30 minutes or more of exercise on most if not all days of the week for pregnant women. Exercise in which injury is more likely to occur should be avoided. **Focus:** Prioritization

26. **Ans: 4** A newborn baby should feed 8 to 12 times in 24 hours. The other findings are normal for an infant of this age. The baby should void 6 to 8 times a day after the fourth day of life. Helpful guidance at this point may help parents understand infant feeding and help support the Perinatal Core Measure of increasing the percentage of infants who are fed breast milk only. **Focus:** Prioritization

27. **Ans: 4** The yellow eye discharge could be a conjunctivitis related to an infection acquired during birth or afterward. The other findings are normal variants on a newborn of this age. A newborn may normally experience a weight loss of 5% to 10% in the first days of life. **Focus:** Prioritization

28. **Ans: 1, 2** During phototherapy, the infant's eyes must be protected and the temperature carefully monitored to avoid both hypothermia and hyperthermia. Breastfeeding should be continued to avoid dehydration and to increase passage of meconium, which helps to excrete bilirubin. Ointments or lotions should not be applied to the skin during phototherapy as they may cause burns. Encouraging continued breast feeding and teaching the family the benefits of breast feeding in this scenario supports the Perinatal Core Measure of increasing the percentage of infants who are fed breast milk only. **Focus:** Assignment

CHAPTER 19: Pediatric Problems, pages 85-90

1. **Ans: 3** Pain rating scales using faces (depicting smiling, neutral, frowning, crying, etc.) are appropriate for young children who may have difficulty describing pain or understanding the correlation of pain to numerical or verbal descriptors. The other tools require abstract reasoning abilities to make analogies and the use of advanced vocabulary. **Focus:** Prioritization

2. **Ans: 2** The set of circumstances is least complicated for the child with the fracture, and this would be the best patient for a new and relatively inexperienced nurse. The child is likely to have a good response to pain medication, and with gentle encouragement and pain management the anxiety will resolve. The other three children have more complex social and psychological issues related to pain management. **Focus:** Delegation

3. **Ans: 3** National guidelines indicate that rapid treatment of infection in neutropenic patients is essential to prevent complications such as overwhelming sepsis and secondary infections; therefore, the child with

fever and a low neutrophil count is the priority. A potassium level of 3.3 mEq/L is borderline low and should be monitored. Nosebleeds are common, and the patient and parents should be taught to apply direct pressure to the nose, have the child sit upright, and not disturb the clot. Severe spontaneous hemorrhage is not expected until the platelet count drops below 20,000 mm³. Children can withstand low hemoglobin levels. The nurse should help the patient and parents regulate activity to prevent excessive fatigue. **Focus:** Prioritization

4. **Ans: 4**   Help the mother to understand that the child may be angry about being left in the hospital or about her inability to prevent the illness and protect the child. Reminding the child about the food and the purpose of the food does not address the strong emotions underlying the outburst. Allowing the mother and child time alone is a possibility, but the assumption would be that the mother understands the child's behavior and is prepared to deal with the behavior in a constructive manner. Asking the mother to leave the child suggests that the mother is a source of stress. **Focus:** Prioritization

5. **Ans: 4**   Helping the patient to eat is within the scope of responsibilities for a UAP. Assessing ability and willingness to drink and checking for extent of mucosal ulceration is the responsibility of an RN. Plain water or saline rinses are preferable if the child cannot gargle or spit out fluids. The RN should assess and administer oral preparations as needed. **Focus:** Delegation

6. **Ans: 3**   LPN/LVN scope of practice includes care of patients with chronic and stable health problems, such as the patient with chronic graft-versus-host disease. Chemotherapy medications are considered high-alert medications and should be given by RNs who have received additional education in chemotherapy administration. Platelets and other blood products should be given by RNs. The 6-year-old patient has a history and clinical manifestations consistent with neutropenia and sepsis and should be assessed by an RN as quickly as possible. **Focus:** Assignment

7. **Ans: 1**   Patients who are neutropenic should be placed in positive-airflow rooms; placement of the child in a negative-airflow room will increase the likelihood of infection for this patient. Although private rooms are preferred for patients who need droplet precautions, such as patients with RSV infection, they can be placed in rooms with other patients who are infected with the same microorganism. The use of an N95 respirator is not necessary for pertussis, and goggles are not needed for changing the linens of patients infected with *C. difficile;* however, these precautions do not increase risk to the patients. **Focus:** Prioritization

8. **Ans: 1, 3, 4**   Because all patient care staff members should be familiar with the various types of isolation, a UAP will be able to stock the room and post the precautions on the patient's door. Reminding visitors about previously taught information is also a task that can be done by a UAP, although the RN is responsible for the initial teaching. Patient teaching and discussion of the reasons for the protective isolation fall within the RN-level scope of practice. **Focus:** Delegation

9. **Ans: 2**   The incidence of once-common infectious diseases such as measles, chickenpox, and mumps has been most effectively reduced by the immunization of all school-age children. The other actions are also helpful but will not have as great an impact as immunization. **Focus:** Prioritization

10. **Ans: 1**   The administration of varicella-zoster immune globulin can prevent the development of varicella in immunosuppressed patients and will typically be prescribed. Acyclovir therapy and hospitalization may be required if the child develops a varicella-zoster virus infection. Contact and airborne precautions will be implemented to prevent the spread of infection to other children if the child develops varicella. **Focus:** Prioritization

11. **Ans: 2**   Because patients with rubeola require implementation of airborne precautions, which include placement in a negative-airflow room, this child cannot be admitted to the pediatric unit. The other circumstances may require actions such as staff reassignments but would not prevent the admission of a patient with rubeola. **Focus:** Prioritization

12. **Ans: 3**   National guidelines indicate that airway clearance techniques are critical for patients with cystic fibrosis; CPT should take priority over the other activities. Although allowing more independent decision making is important for adolescents, the physiologic need for improved respiratory function takes precedence at this time. A private room may be desirable for the patient but is not necessary. With increased shortness of breath, it will be more important that the patient have frequent respiratory treatments than 8 hours of sleep. **Focus:** Prioritization

13. **Ans: 1**   Frequent swallowing after tonsillectomy may indicate bleeding. You should inspect the back of the throat for evidence of bleeding. The other assessment results are expected in a 3-year-old after surgery. **Focus:** Prioritization

14. **Ans: 3**   Tracheal deviation suggests tension pneumothorax, a possible complication of positive-pressure ventilation. The nurse will need to communicate rapidly with the health care provider and assist with actions such as chest tube insertion. The heart rate, crackles, and oxygen saturation will be reported to the health care provider, but are expected in RDS and do not require immediate intervention. **Focus:** Prioritization

15. **Ans: 2**   Research indicates that the administration of synthetic surfactant improves respiratory status and decreases the incidence of pneumothorax in premature infants with RDS. The other medications may be

used if respiratory distress persists, but the first medication administered will be the surfactant. **Focus:** Prioritization

16. **Ans: 4** Circumoral cyanosis indicates a drop in the partial pressure of oxygen that may precipitate seizures and loss of consciousness. The nurse should rapidly place the child in a knee-chest position, administer oxygen, and take steps to calm the child. The other assessment data are expected in a child with congenital heart defects such as tetralogy of Fallot. **Focus:** Prioritization

17. **Ans: 3** Crackles throughout both lungs indicate that the child has severe left ventricular failure as a complication of endocarditis. Hypoxemia is likely, so the child needs rapid assessment of oxygen saturation, initiation of supplemental oxygen delivery, and administration of medications such as diuretics. The other children should also be assessed as quickly as possible, but they are not experiencing life-threatening complications of their medical diagnoses. **Focus:** Prioritization

18. **Ans: 1** This patient requires the least complex assessments and interventions of the four patients. Safe administration of oral medications such as digoxin would have been included in the orientation of the new RN graduate. The conditions of the other patients are more complex, and they require assessments and/or interventions (such as teaching) that should be carried out by an RN with more experience. **Focus:** Assignment

19. **Ans: 4** Children who receive aspirin therapy are at risk for the development of Reye syndrome if they contract viral illnesses such as varicella or influenza, so the lack of immunization is the greatest concern for this child. Peeling skin on the fingers and toes and irritability are consistent with Kawasaki disease, but do not require any change in therapy. Since Kawasaki disease is not a communicable disease, day care need not be avoided. **Focus:** Prioritization

20. **Ans: 2** The joint pain that occurs in sickle cell crisis is caused by obstruction of blood flow by the red blood cells. Cold packs will further decrease blood flow to the patient's knees and increase sickling. The appropriate therapy for this patient is application of moist heat to the joints to cause vasodilation and improve circulation. Genetic counseling may be provided to patients with sickle cell disease but is not appropriate to suggest to a 10-year-old. Although infection control is important in preventing and treating sickle cell crisis, there is no need to restrict all visitors or to check the patient's temperature every 2 hours. **Focus:** Prioritization

21. **Ans: 1** Because decreased responsiveness in a 1-year-old with a clotting disorder may indicate intracerebral bleeding, this patient should be assessed immediately. The other patients also require assessments or interventions but are not at immediate risk for life-threatening or disabling complications. **Focus:** Prioritization

22. **Ans: 2** The low hemoglobin level suggests that the child may have active bleeding, and rapid actions such as diagnostic testing and transfusions are indicated. The other laboratory data are expected in a child with idiopathic thrombocytopenic purpura. **Focus:** Prioritization

23. **Ans: 3** Methotrexate is a high-alert drug, and extra precautions, such as double-checking with another nurse, should be taken when administering this medication. Although many pediatric units have a policy requiring that all medication administration to children be double-checked, the other medications listed are not on the high-alert list published by the Institute for Safe Medication Practices. **Focus:** Prioritization

24. **Ans: 2** National guidelines indicate that medication dosing for pediatric patients should be based on the child's weight. The weight for the 6-year-old is not provided. For phenytoin, the dose for children is prescribed as 5 mg/kg in 2 or 3 divided doses; 300 mg is a typical maintenance dose for an adult, but would be an unusual dose for a 6-year-old. All telephone orders should be verified; however, the dosages for the other three prescriptions are appropriately based on the child's weight. **Focus:** Prioritization

25. **Ans: 2** Pupil dilation may indicate increased intracranial pressure and should be reported immediately to the surgeon. The other data are not unusual in a 3-year-old after surgery, although they indicate the need for ongoing assessments or interventions. **Focus:** Prioritization

26. **Ans: 4** The elevated temperature indicates possible infection and should be reported immediately to the physician so that treatment can be started. The other data are typical in an infant with this defect. **Focus:** Prioritization

27. **Ans: 2** Despite the fact that the child is screaming, the mother must continue to irrigate the eyes for at least 20 minutes. Another adult, if present, should call the Poison Control Center and 911. **Focus:** Prioritization

28. **Ans: 3** Vegetable or insect matter will swell if water is used for irrigation. Tightly wedged objects such as beads are difficult to flush. If perforation is suspected or if the object is not easily removed, the nurse should not attempt irrigation or instillation. **Focus:** Prioritization

29. **Ans: 2** The shift report indicates that the patient still has a disturbed body image; however, she is actively working on gaining weight and improving self-esteem, and has appropriate knowledge that she can use to maintain her health. **Focus:** Prioritization

30. **Ans: 2** Passage of brown stool indicates resolution of the intussusception, so surgery may not be necessary. The other findings are part of the clinical presentation of this disorder. **Focus:** Prioritization

31. **Ans: 4** Even though the caller reports that the child is "breathing okay," additional questions about possible airway obstruction are the priority (i.e., coughing, gagging, choking, drooling, refusing to eat or drink). Gastrointestinal symptoms should be assessed but are less urgent. The type of foreign body, in the absence of symptoms, may dictate a wait-and-see approach, in which case the parent would be directed to check the stools for passage of the foreign body. **Focus:** Prioritization

32. **Ans: 1** Hand washing is the most important aspect to emphasize. Addressing fecal incontinence and sharing of personal items may be recommended when the disease is in an infectious stage. Immunizations are recommended, but this would be emphasized to parents rather than day-care providers. **Focus:** Prioritization

33. **Ans: 3** Oral sedation agents such as the benzodiazepines are considered high-alert medications when ordered for children, and extra precautions should be taken before administration. Many facilities require that all medications administered to pediatric patients be double-checked before administration, but the lorazepam is the most important to double-check with another nurse. **Focus:** Prioritization

34. **Ans: 3** Theories about bed-wetting relate it to immature bladder and deep sleep patterns. Although it is true that most children stop bed-wetting by the time they start school, this does not answer the mother's question. Many boys wet the bed until after the age of 5. The fourth response is not accurate, because often bed-wetting is not within the control of a 5-year-old child. **Focus:** Prioritization

35. **Ans: 1** Reminding the child about something that has already been taught is within the scope of practice for a UAP. An LPN/LVN could administer the oral medication. Teaching and discussion of other strategies for dealing with bed-wetting require additional education and are more appropriate to the scope of practice of the professional RN. **Focus:** Delegation

36. **Ans: 4** Because *Chlamydia trachomatis* infection is the most prevalent sexually transmitted disease in the United States, national research-based guidelines state that *Chlamydia* screening is strongly recommended for all sexually active females age 25 or younger. Screening for the other STDs may also be considered, but is recommended only if other risk factors or evidence of disease is present. **Focus:** Prioritization

37. **Ans: 2** The UAP can help with the removal of outer clothing, which allows the heat to dissipate from the child's skin. Assessments, advising, and explaining require RN-level education and scope of practice. **Focus:** Delegation

38. **Ans: 1** Iron is a toxic substance that can lead to massive hemorrhage, coma, shock, and hepatic failure. Deferoxamine is an antidote that can be used for severe cases of iron poisoning. The other information needs additional investigation but will not change the immediate diagnostic testing or treatment plan. **Focus:** Prioritization

39. **Ans: 3** Parental refusal is an absolute contraindication; therefore, the provider must be notified. Tetanus status can be addressed later. The RN can reestablish the IV access and provide information about conscious sedation; if the parent is still not satisfied, the provider can give more information. **Focus:** Prioritization

40. **Ans: 2** An impaled object may be providing a tamponade effect, and removal can precipitate sudden hemodynamic decompensation. Additional history, including a more definitive description of the blood loss, depth of penetration, and medical history, should be obtained. Other information, such as the dirt on the stick or history of diabetes, is important in the overall treatment plan but can be addressed later. **Focus:** Prioritization

41. **Ans: 1, 3, 4, 5** Children have proportionately larger heads that predispose them to head injuries. Hypoxemia is more likely because of their higher oxygen demand. Liver and spleen injuries are more likely because the thoracic cage of children offers less protection. Hypothermia is more likely because of children's thinner skin and proportionately larger body surface area. They have strong hearts; therefore pulse rate will increase to compensate, but other arrhythmias are less likely to occur. Children have relatively flexible bones compared with those of adults. The most likely spinal injury in children is injury to the cervical area. **Focus:** Prioritization

CHAPTER 20: Emergencies and Disasters, pages 91-94

1. **Ans: 3** Triage requires at least one experienced RN. Pairing an experienced RN with an inexperienced RN provides opportunities for mentoring. Advanced practice nurses are qualified to perform triage; however, their services are usually required in other areas of the ED. An LPN/LVN is not qualified to perform the initial client assessment or decision making. Pairing an experienced RN with an experienced UAP is the second best option, because the UAP can measure vital signs and assist in transporting. **Focus:** Assignment

2. **Ans: 2, 1, 4, 3** An irritable infant with fever and petechiae should be further assessed for other signs of meningitis. The client with the head wound needs additional history taking and assessment for intracranial pressure. The client with moderate abdominal pain is in discomfort, but her condition is not unstable at this point. For the ankle injury, medical evaluation could be delayed up to 24 to 48 hours if necessary, but the client should receive the appropriate first aid. **Focus:** Prioritization

3. **Ans: 3** A brief neurologic assessment to determine level of consciousness and pupil reaction is part of the primary survey. Measuring vital signs, assessing the abdomen, and checking pulse oximetry readings are considered part of the secondary survey. **Focus:** Prioritization

4. **Ans: 3** The priority goal is to increase myocardial oxygenation. The other actions are also appropriate and should be performed immediately after administering oxygen. **Focus:** Prioritization

5. **Ans: 1, 3, 4, 5, 6** Strangulated intestinal obstruction is a surgical emergency. The NG tube is for decompression of the intestine. Abdominal radiography is the most useful diagnostic aid. IV fluids are needed to maintain fluid and electrolyte balance and allow IV delivery of medication. IV broad-spectrum antibiotics are usually ordered. Pain medications are likely to be withheld during the initial period to prevent masking of peritonitis or perforation. In addition, morphine slows gastric motility. A barium enema examination is not ordered if perforation is suspected. **Focus:** Prioritization

6. **Ans: 4** The homeless person has symptoms of heat stroke, a medical emergency that increases the risk for brain damage. The elderly client is at risk for heat syncope and should be educated to rest in a cool area and avoid future similar situations. The runner is having heat cramps, which can be managed with rest and fluids. The housewife is experiencing heat exhaustion, and management includes administration of fluids (IV or oral) and cooling measures. **Focus:** Prioritization

7. **Ans: 2, 4, 1, 3, 5** Establish unresponsiveness first. (The client may have fallen and sustained a minor injury.) If the client is unresponsive, get help and activate the code team. Performing the chin lift or jaw thrust maneuver opens the airway. The nurse is then responsible for starting CPR. (Use a pocket mask or bag-valve mask.) CPR should not be interrupted until the client recovers or it is determined that all heroic efforts have been exhausted. A crash cart should be at the site when the code team arrives; however, basic CPR can be effectively performed until the team is present. **Focus:** Prioritization

8. **Ans: 1** UAPs are trained in basic cardiac life support and can perform chest compressions. The use of the bag-valve mask requires practice, and usually a respiratory therapist will perform this function. The nurse or the respiratory therapist should provide assistance as needed during intubation. The defibrillator pads are clearly marked; however, placement should be done by the RN or physician because of the potential for skin damage and electrical arcing. **Focus:** Delegation

9. **Ans: 3** The client is hyperventilating secondary to anxiety, and breathing into a paper bag will allow rebreathing of carbon dioxide. Also, encouraging slow breathing will help. Other treatments such as oxygen administration and medication may be needed if other causes are identified. **Focus:** Prioritization

10. **Ans: 3** The fast-track clinic deals with clients in relatively stable condition. The triage, trauma, and pediatric medicine areas should be staffed with experienced nurses who know the hospital routines and policies and can rapidly locate equipment. **Focus:** Assignment

11. **Ans: 3** An LPN/LVN is able to listen and provide emotional support for clients. The other tasks are the responsibility of an RN or, if available, a sexual assault nurse examiner who has received training in assessing, collecting, and safeguarding evidence, and caring for assault victims. **Focus:** Delegation

12. **Ans: 3, 2, 4, 1, 5** The client should be removed from the cold environment first, then the rewarming process can be initiated. It will be painful, so pain medication should be given before immersing the feet in warm water. A loose, sterile, bulky bandage should be applied to the area after warming to protect the feet. The client should be monitored for compartment syndrome every hour after initial treatment. **Focus:** Prioritization

13. **Ans: 1, 2, 4, 5** The only correct intervention is to gently cleanse the digits with normal saline, wrap them in sterile gauze moistened with saline, and place them in a plastic bag or container. The container is then placed on ice. **Focus:** Supervision, knowledge

14. **Ans: 1** Safety is a priority for this client, and she should not return to a place where violence could recur. The other options are important for the long-term management of this case. **Focus:** Prioritization

15. **Ans: 2** First try to express your concerns to the physician. The ED can be very hectic, and the ED staff should work as a team and watch out for each other as well as the clients. If the physician refuses to consider your concerns, then you may have to contact the nursing supervisor or write an incident report. This client has the signs of peritonitis. If the client dies or suffers a poor outcome, you are as liable as the physician if you fail to intervene. **Focus:** Prioritization

16. **Ans: 4** The client has symptoms of alcohol abuse and there is a risk for Wernicke-Korsakoff syndrome, which is caused by a thiamine deficiency. Multiple drug abuse is not uncommon; however, the primary concern with an opiate overdose is respiratory depression, and the client does not show any respiratory distress or alterations in respiratory pattern. Additional information or the results of the blood alcohol testing are part of the total treatment plan but should not delay the immediate treatment. **Focus:** Prioritization

17. **Ans: 3** Postmortem care requires some turning, cleaning, lifting, and so on, and the UAP is able to assist with these duties. The RN should take responsibility for the other tasks to help the family begin the grieving process. In cases of questionable death, belongings may be retained for evidence, so the chain of custody would have to be maintained. **Focus:** Delegation

Answer Key

18. **Ans: 5, 3, 4, 2, 1** Checking exhaled carbon dioxide levels is the most accurate way of immediately verifying placement. Auscultating and confirming equal bilateral breath sounds should be performed in rapid succession. If the sounds are not equal or if the sounds are heard over the midepigastric area, tube placement must be corrected immediately. Securing the tube can be performed after these assessments are performed. Finally, radiographic study will verify and document correct placement. **Focus:** Prioritization

19. **Ans: 1** The client demonstrates neurologic hyperreactivity and is on the verge of a seizure. Client safety is the priority. The client needs medications such as chlordiazepoxide (Librium) to decrease neurologic irritability and phenytoin (Dilantin) for seizures. Thiamine and haloperidol (Haldol) may also be ordered to address the other problems. The other diagnoses are pertinent but less urgent. **Focus:** Prioritization

20. **Ans: 2** The stinger will continue to release venom into the skin, so prompt removal of the stinger is advised. Cool compresses and antihistamines can follow. The caller should be further advised about symptoms that require 911 assistance. **Focus:** Prioritization

21. **Ans: 1** Cats' mouths contain a virulent organism, *Pasteurella multocida,* that can lead to septic arthritis or bacteremia. Appropriate first aid would include rigorous washing of the wound site with soap and water to combat infection. There is also a risk for tendon damage due to deep puncture wounds, but this is usually evaluated by an orthopedic surgeon after initial emergency care is started. A tetanus shot can be given before discharge. **Focus:** Prioritization

22. **Ans: 4, 5, 2, 3, 1, 6** The client with a pulsating mass has an abdominal aneurysm that may rupture, and he may decompensate suddenly. The woman with lower left quadrant pain is at risk for ectopic pregnancy, which is a life-threatening condition. The 11-year-old boy needs evaluation to rule out appendicitis. The woman with vomiting needs evaluation for gallbladder problems, which appear to be worsening. The 35-year-old man has food poisoning, which is usually self-limiting. The woman with midepigastric pain may have an ulcer, but follow-up diagnostic testing and teaching of lifestyle modification can be scheduled with the primary care provider. **Focus:** Prioritization

23. **Ans: 4** At least one representative from each group should be included, because all employees are potential targets for violence in the ED. **Focus:** Assignment

24. **Ans: 1** A deviated trachea is a symptom of tension pneumothorax, which will result in respiratory arrest if not corrected. All of the other symptoms need to be addressed, but are of lower priority. **Focus:** Prioritization

25. **Ans: 3, 2, 4, 1, 5, 6, 7** For a trauma client with multiple injuries, many interventions will occur simultaneously as team members assist in the resuscitation.

Assessing for spontaneous respirations, performing techniques to open the airway such as chin lift or jaw thrust, and applying oxygen may occur simultaneously. However, in the nursing process, recall that first you must assess, then you intervene. Opening the airway must precede the administration of oxygen because, if the airway is closed, the oxygen cannot enter the air passages. Starting IV lines for fluid resuscitation is part of supporting circulation. (Emergency medical service personnel will usually establish at least one IV line in the field.) UAPs can be directed to measure vital signs and remove clothing. Insertion of a Foley catheter is necessary for close monitoring of output. **Focus:** Prioritization

26. **Ans: 2** Decontamination in a specified area is the priority. Performing assessments delays decontamination and does not protect the total environment. These clients do not need to don personal protective equipment (PPE); however, personnel should don PPE before assisting with decontamination or assessing the clients. The clients must undergo decontamination before entering cold or clean areas. **Focus:** Prioritization

27. **Ans: 1** In preparing for disasters, the RN should be aware of the emergency response plan. The plan gives guidance that includes the roles of team members, responsibilities, and mechanisms of reporting. Signs and symptoms of exposure to many agents will mimic common complaints, such as flulike symptoms. Discussions with colleagues and supervisors may help the individual nurse to sort through ethical dilemmas related to potential danger to self. **Focus:** Prioritization

28. **Ans: 3, 4, 2, 5, 1** The first priority is to protect personnel, unaffected clients, bystanders, and the facility. Personal protective gear should be donned before victims are assessed or treated. Decontamination of victims in a separate area is followed by triage and treatment. The incident should be reported according to protocol as information about the number of people involved, history, and signs and symptoms becomes available. **Focus:** Prioritization

29. **Ans: 4** Any of these people may need or benefit from psychiatric counseling. Obviously, there will be variations in previous coping skills and support systems; however, a person who experienced a threat to his or her own life is at the greatest risk for psychiatric problems following a disaster incident. **Focus:** Prioritization

30. **Ans: 2, 3, 4, 5, 7** These would be appropriate for disaster triage. The other items are important and would be addressed when the staff has time and resources to collect the additional information. (Note: During nondisaster situations, it would be appropriate to include all items.) **Focus:** Prioritization

31. **Ans: 6, 2, 4, 3, 5, 1** Treat the 12-year-old with asthma first by initiating an albuterol treatment. This action is quick to initiate, and the child or parent can

be instructed to hold the apparatus while you attend to other clients. The firefighter is in greater respiratory distress than the 12-year-old; however, managing a strong combative client is difficult and time consuming (i.e., the 12-year-old could die if you spend too much time trying to control the firefighter). Attend to the teenager with a crush injury next. Anxiety and tachycardia may be caused by pain or stress; however, the swelling suggests hemorrhage. Next attend to the woman with burns on the forearms by providing dressings and pain management. The child with burns over more than 70% of the anterior body should be given comfort measures; however, the prognosis is very poor. The prognosis for the client in cardiac arrest is also very poor, because CPR efforts have been prolonged. **Focus:** Prioritization

CHAPTER 21: Psychiatric–Mental Health Problems, pages 95-98

1. **Ans: 3** The case manager has a relationship with the patient, knows the specific details of agreements made with the patient, and is the most capable of helping him to decrease anxiety and preoccupation with physical symptoms. In general, presenting reality does not have an impact on patients with hypochondriasis. Encouraging expression of feelings and giving in to the patient's wishes contribute to secondary gains of maintaining the sick role. **Focus:** Prioritization

2. **Ans: 4** Patients with conversion disorders are experiencing symptoms, even though there is no identifiable organic cause; therefore, they should be assisted in learning ways to cope and live with the disability. Encouraging the expression of feelings is okay, but it is premature to expect the patient to link the fight to her blindness. It is likely that the sudden onset of blindness will quickly resolve, and the patient may also be physically able to see, but presenting facts would not be helpful at this time. **Focus:** Prioritization

3. **Ans: 2** Teenagers, in general, are self-conscious in the presence of members of the opposite sex, and teens with anorexia are overly concerned with their appearance; therefore, it would be better to assign this patient to a mature female staff member. An experienced LVN, regardless of gender pairing, is able to set boundaries and to assist patients with chronic health problems. An experienced RN should be assigned to new admissions, particularly if there are acute safety issues. An RN with medical-surgical experience would be well acquainted with care issues related to dementia. **Focus:** Assignment

4. **Ans: 3** Jane is experiencing a panic level of anxiety and initially she needs very simple and direct instructions. Instruct her to look at you first, to make a connection and to get her attention, then you can continue with your instructions. Telling her to calm down is not useful at this point, and she may or may not be able to articulate why she is trying to go back into the house. Regardless of her reason, she cannot be allowed to run back into the house. Directing her to go to your house is kind and therapeutic, but it may be difficult to remove her from the scene until her anxiety is more under control. **Focus:** Prioritization

5. **Ans: 3** This patient has trouble with interpersonal interactions, so consistent caregivers who use psychosocial interventions have the best chance of being able to develop a relationship with this difficult individual. Rotating the assignment sheet to give the staff a break and using float staff are frequent strategies that are employed, but these are not necessarily the best for the patient. Taking the patient yourself may seem like the easiest solution, but in the long run strengthening and supporting the staff are better strategies than trying to do all of the hard tasks yourself. **Focus:** Assignment

6. **Ans: 4** You can acknowledge the patient's fears without agreeing or disagreeing with his accusation toward Dr. Smith, and by directing him to talk to the nursing staff you are giving him emotional support and an action that he can use to decrease his anxiety. Telling the patient that no one has died and that the staff will ensure safety is presenting reality; however, he believes that someone has been killed and that Dr. Smith is responsible, so you are opening up opportunities for an argument. Asking him to explain his rationale for his beliefs encourages him to elaborate on his delusion. **Focus:** Prioritization, knowledge

7. **Ans: 1** Assess the content of command hallucinations, because the patient may be getting a command to harm self or others. Ideas of reference occur when an ordinary thing or event (e.g., a song on the radio) has personal significance (e.g., belief that the lyrics were written for him or her). Ideas of reference could escalate into aggression, especially if delusions of persecution are present, so the nurse would check on this patient next. Clang association is a meaningless rhyming of words, and neologisms are new words created by patients. These communication patterns create frustration for staff and patients, but there is no need for immediate intervention. **Focus:** Prioritization

8. **Ans: 3** All of these symptoms signal an increase of anxiety; however, physically aggressive behavior signals a danger to others and to self. Verbal intervention is still possible, but the pacing and fist pounding are a step above the other symptoms. **Focus:** Prioritization

9. **Ans: 2** The patient has a strong family history of completed suicide, which is an increased risk factor. The patient may believe that other family members have successfully used suicide to solve their problems. A long history of depression suggests that the problem is chronic; assess for treatment history, risk factors, and coping strategies. Having a feeling of responsibility toward others and feeling fear are protective factors that can be utilized in the treatment plan. **Focus:** Prioritization

10. **Ans: 3** Before someone enters an alcohol rehabilitation program, there should be a medically-supervised detoxification. This patient has walked in off the street; therefore, you must determine whether he is at risk for withdrawal symptoms. The other questions are relevant and are likely to be included in the interview. **Focus:** Prioritization

11. **Ans: 1** The mental health assistant can initiate this simple cooling measure with minimal instruction. Neuroleptic malignant syndrome is a rare but potentially fatal reaction to antipsychotic medication. Symptoms include fever, altered mental status, muscle rigidity, and autonomic instability. The RN should continuously monitor vital signs, although taking vital signs can be delegated. UAPs in the ICU and emergency department (ED) will be familiar with how to attach ECG leads, but mental health assistants will rarely have occasion to use this equipment; therefore, the RN should perform this task. Making arrangements to transfer the patient takes time, and treatment must begin while arrangements are being made. **Focus:** Delegation

12. **Ans: 4** Although the patient is ruminating about suicide, major depression usually leaves the patient with minimal energy to act. The danger for suicide will increase as the medication and therapy begin to help. A new nurse is more likely to be manipulated by a borderline patient. Psychotic patients can seem very threatening to new nurses. Depression, dementia, and delirium have some behavior and symptom overlap; this patient is best assigned to an experienced nurse until delirium is treated or ruled out. **Focus:** Assignment

13. **Ans: 3** Medical-surgical UAPs frequently assist patients to ambulate and can redirect the patient if he wanders off. Performing one-to-one suicide watch requires experience, because the observer may have to immediately intervene while calling out for help. Assisting the occupational therapist or medication nurse may be possible, but the medical-surgical UAP is unlikely to be familiar with the behavioral interventions required in these situations. **Focus:** Assignment

14. **Ans: 2** The restraints must be tied to a stationary portion of the bed. Physicians are usually much less familiar with how the beds function. Quick-release knots are for safety in case the restraints need to be quickly removed. Distal pulses should be checked. The physician or RN is usually responsible for explaining the restraint procedure; however, restraining a patient is rarely a planned event, and the caregiver who has the best relationship with the patient may be the best spokesperson. **Focus:** Supervision

15. **Ans: 2** First try to determine how the nurses found out about the patient's admission. This is a serious Health Insurance Portability and Accountability Act (HIPAA) violation, and information disclosure must be immediately stopped. Unfortunately for these RNs, administration will have to be notified, but as a professional courtesy it would be better if they went directly to the supervisor and admitted the error, rather than you calling the supervisor and reporting them. **Focus:** Prioritization, supervision

16. **Ans: 2** Switching the assignments at shift change or mid-shift creates delays for everyone, so politely ask her to continue for the day. However, her request is not unreasonable; dealing with depressed patients can be very tiring, so consider her request for future assignments. While many patients benefit by having the same caregiver, a chronically-depressed patient might benefit from stimulation by various caregivers. Explaining scope of practice and continuity of care are probably not necessary and may seem condescending. **Focus:** Assignment, supervision

17. **Ans: 4** Current mood and behavior is the priority so that you will be able to make preparations for physical or chemical restraints, isolation or a private room, and staffing. The other questions are also relevant. However, be aware that if you are challenging the appropriateness of the psychiatric unit versus the trauma unit, you will probably have to contact the nursing supervisor, because the ED nurse will not be able to assist you with this issue. **Focus:** Prioritization

18. **Ans: 2, 4, 3, 6, 1, 5** The first step is to maintain an awareness of the ways that medication errors can occur. Check the original order for legibility and clarification. Consult a drug reference to determine if the patient's condition warrants the type of medication ordered and to see if *Klonopin* and *clonidine* are different names for the same drug. (Note: Medications become familiar. Experienced nurses will recognize that Klonopin [clonazepam] and clonidine are not the same drug and therefore may not consult a reference; however, all nurses should continue to look up new or unfamiliar drugs.) Call the physician if the order is not clear or if the medication does not seem appropriate for the patient's condition (physicians can get drug names confused, too). Advise the pharmacy about any errors or changes, so that the correct medication is delivered. Consider writing an incident report even though you did not make a medication error, so that system errors can be evaluated and prevented in the future. **Focus:** Prioritization

19. **Ans: 3** The patient is experiencing medication side effects. This condition is frightening and uncomfortable for the patient, but it is not usually harmful. Initiating swallow precautions or waiting for the spasms to pass delays the most appropriate intervention; intramuscular or IV administration of diphenhydramine will rapidly alleviate the symptoms. **Focus:** Prioritization

20. **Ans: 1, 4, 3, 2** The highest priority is patient 1, who has symptoms of neuroleptic malignant syndrome, which is rare but potentially fatal. This patient should be transferred to a medical unit. Patient 4 may have

agranulocytosis. The mortality rate is high, and interventions include discontinuing the medication, aggressively treating the infection, and providing protective isolation. Patient 3 has symptoms of tardive dyskinesia, which should be reported so that the medication can be discontinued. There is no known treatment, and discontinuation does not always relieve the problem. Patient 2 is showing anticholinergic effects, which can be treated symptomatically (i.e., provide sips of water or hard candy, encourage use of artificial tears, place a warm towel on the abdomen, give stool softeners, and encourage the use of sunglasses). **Focus:** Prioritization

21. **Ans: 3, 4, 1, 6, 5, 2** The least restrictive method is verbal intervention. The patient should be allowed to stay in public areas if possible, and then moved to isolated spaces. Finally, if nothing else works, the patient can be physically restrained for safety purposes. **Focus:** Prioritization

22. **Ans: 3** Although all unusual behavior requires ongoing assessment, intervention, and documentation, motor agitation presents the greatest safety issue because excessive physical activity such as running about or flailing the arms and legs creates a risk for injury to self and others and/or exhaustion (to the point of death). Avolition is a lack of energy in initiating activities. Echolalia is pathologically repeating other people's words or phrases. Stupor is a state in which the patient may remain motionless for a prolonged period. **Focus:** Prioritization

23. **Ans: 3** The health care team must always be vigilant for actual physical disease; however, the patient most likely has an undiagnosed somatoform disorder, which is a chronic and severe psychological condition in which the patient experiences physical symptoms but without apparent organic cause. Depression and anxiety are common among patients with somatoform disorders. Once physical disease has been ruled out, having emotional support from a consistent health care provider is often the most effective approach for somatoform disorders. Thus all options should eventually be considered. **Focus:** Prioritization

24. **Ans: 3, 4, 6** Anyone who was involved in the direct care of the patient should be invited to participate. The purpose of this root cause analysis is to review the event to identify behaviors, signs, or signals of risk for suicide. This information would be used to increase the staff's awareness to prevent future similar events. Inviting the wife and family is not appropriate, because the performance of the staff is internally reviewed to improve performance. The purpose is not to fix blame or to create a situation that engenders guilt for the wife or family (or the staff). Likewise, the purpose of the analysis is not to provide psychotherapy or support for the wife or family. (Referrals should be made for this.) **Focus:** Assignment

25. **Ans: 4** If the patient meets the criteria for admission to a medical-surgical unit, nutritional restoration is the primary concern. Concurrently, the health care team will assist the patient to achieve success in the other areas. **Focus:** Prioritization

26. **Ans: 2** The oral route is the least intrusive. In addition, the patient and family can participate in determining the food plan and food choices. The nasogastric and IV routes are options for patients who are in life-threatening situations. Rapid feeding via these routes increases the likelihood of refeeding syndrome. Hypodermoclysis is a subcutaneous method of delivering fluids or medications and is an unlikely choice for this patient. **Focus:** Prioritization

27. **Ans: 1** The UAP should be instructed to observe the amount of food eaten and ensure that the patient is not throwing the food out. After meals, observation is necessary to ensure that the patient does not induce vomiting. Ritualistic behaviors can be subtle or difficult to define. Observation for these behaviors cannot be delegated. Requests for special foods could be delaying tactics or attempts to manipulate the staff. The UAP should not be responsible for deciding if food requests are appropriate. Daily weights may not be ordered. In addition, repeatedly telling the patient that she is underweight is counterproductive, because she does not believe she is underweight. **Focus:** Delegation

28. **Ans: 4** Reminding the patient of a previous contractual agreement and her responsibility in meeting treatment goals is the best response. (For certain patients, allowing limited times for exercise may be part of the contract in the early phase, if the patient has been compulsively exercising.) Avoid opening opportunities for manipulation by allowing "a few more minutes" of exercise. Exploration of the purpose that exercise serves should be carried out by a psychotherapist. Power struggles over food should be avoided. Privileges may be forfeited if the behavior persists, but the response would be improved by stating specifically what privileges will be lost. **Focus:** Prioritization

29. **Ans: 2** The patient continues to refer to herself as "fatty" and still has a disturbed body image; however, she has appropriate knowledge and her self-esteem has improved. **Focus:** Prioritization

CASE STUDY 1: Chest Pressure, Indigestion, Nausea, and Vomiting, pages 99-100

1. **Ans: 4** Monitoring and recording intake and output are within the scope of practice for UAPs. Initiating telemetry, performing venipuncture, and obtaining ECGs require additional education and training. Attaching ECG leads may be done by UAPs in some facilities, as may venipuncture and ECG recording. However, the UAPs performing these tasks would

Answer Key

require additional specialized training. These actions are generally considered to be within the scope of practice of licensed nurses. **Focus:** Delegation

2. **Ans: 3**   Cardiac monitoring is the highest priority, because the client's heart rate is rapid and irregular and the client is experiencing chest pressure. The client is at risk for life-threatening dysrhythmias such as frequent premature ventricular contractions (PVCs). Measuring vital signs every 2 hours, checking levels of cardiac markers, and recording a 12-lead ECG every 6 hours are important, but cardiac monitoring takes precedence. **Focus:** Prioritization

3. **Ans: 1**   With frequent PVCs, the client is at risk for life-threatening dysrhythmias such as ventricular tachycardia or ventricular fibrillation. Amiodarone is an antidysrhythmic drug used to control ventricular dysrhythmias. Nitroglycerin and morphine can be given for chest pain relief. Atenolol is a beta-blocker, which can be used to control heart rate and decrease blood pressure. **Focus:** Prioritization

4. **Ans: 2**   A troponin T level of more than 0.20 ng/mL is an elevated level and indicates myocardial injury or infarction. Although the other laboratory values are all abnormal, none of them is life threatening. **Focus:** Prioritization

5. **Ans: 1**   Morphine sulfate has been ordered to relieve the chest discomfort that is common in the setting of acute myocardial infarction. Relief from the chest pain is the highest priority at this time. Ranitidine is a histamine$_2$ blocker used to prevent gastric ulcers. Scheduling an echocardiogram or drawing blood for coagulation studies, although important, will not help relieve chest discomfort. **Focus:** Prioritization

6. **Ans: 1, 2, 6**   Measuring vital signs, recording intake and output, and assisting clients with activities of daily living are all within the scope of practice of the UAP. Administration of IV drugs, venipuncture for laboratory tests, and assessment are beyond the scope of practice of UAPs. **Focus:** Delegation, supervision, assignment

7. **Ans: 4**   Measuring and recording vital sign values are within the scope of practice of the UAP. When the UAP makes a mistake, it is best to communicate specifically, stressing the importance of recording vital sign values after they have been obtained. Supervision should be done in a supportive rather than confrontational manner. Notifying the nurse manager is not appropriate at this time. Reprimanding the UAP in front of others also is not appropriate. **Focus:** Delegation, supervision

8. **Ans: 2**   Chest pain can be an indicator of additional myocardial muscle damage. Additional episodes of chest pain significantly affect the client's plan of care. Small increases in heart rate and blood pressure after activity are to be expected. The client's temperature, only 0.2° higher than at admission, is not a priority at this time. **Focus:** Prioritization, delegation, supervision

9. **Ans: 1**   HCTZ is a thiazide diuretic used to correct edema and lower blood pressure, and should be taken in the morning so that its diuretic effects do not keep the client up during the night. A side effect of HCTZ is loss of potassium, and clients may require potassium supplementation. Captopril is an angiotensin-converting enzyme inhibitor and will lower blood pressure. It is never appropriate to take twice the dose of this drug. **Focus:** Prioritization

10. **Ans: 1, 3, 4, 5, 6**   All of these interventions are within the scope of practice of an experienced LPN/LVN. You would be sure to instruct the LPN/LVN when to notify you or the health care provider of any abnormal findings. Preparing a teaching plan requires additional education and is more suited to the RN. Taking vital signs and reminding the client about bed rest could also be delegated to the UAP. **Focus:** Delegation, supervision

11. **Ans: 3**   The dressing should be left in place for at least the first day after the client is discharged to prevent dislodging the clot. Heavy lifting and exercise should be avoided for several days. A small hematoma or bruise is expected and is not abnormal. It is not necessary to keep the affected extremity straight after the client is off bed rest. **Focus:** Prioritization

12. **Ans: 4**   Normal sinus rhythm with a rate of 88 beats/min is a normal finding. There is no need to delay the client's discharge, give early medications, or draw additional cardiac markers. **Focus:** Prioritization

CASE STUDY 2: Dyspnea and Shortness of Breath, pages 101-102

1. **Ans: 2**   The patient's major problems at this time relate to airway and breathing. The patient's anxiety is most likely directly related to his breathing difficulty. An acid-base imbalance may result from the patient's breathing problem, but this is not the highest priority at the moment. **Focus:** Prioritization

2. **Ans: 1**   Baseline arterial blood gas results are important in planning the care of this patient. The unit clerk can schedule the pulmonary function tests and chest radiography. The albuterol therapy is a routine order. **Focus:** Prioritization

3. **Ans: 3**   The pH is on the low side of normal and the $Paco_2$ is elevated, which indicates an underlying respiratory acidosis. The HCO_3^- level is elevated, which indicates compensation. Both the Pao_2 and the oxygen saturation levels are low, which points to hypoxemia. These blood gas results are typically expected when a patient has a chronic respiratory problem such as COPD. **Focus:** Prioritization, knowledge

4. **Ans: 1, 2, 3, 6**   The patient's major problem at this time is impaired gas exchange with hypoxemia. Strategies to compensate include administration of low-flow oxygen as well as interventions to improve gas

exchange, such as having the patient cough and deep breathe and perform incentive spirometry. These strategies may improve the patient's condition and prevent the need to initiate a code and/or transfer to the ICU. A saline lock is a good idea, but giving the patient too much fluid may worsen his condition by producing a fluid overload. The patient's symptoms call for initiation of a rapid response to treat him now and prevent the need for a code. **Focus:** Prioritization

5. **Ans: 4**   Increasing oxygen flow for a patient based on a physician's order is within the scope of practice of LPNs/LVNs. UAPs may measure vital signs. Arterial draws for laboratory tests are not within the LPN/LVN's scope of practice. Hand-held nebulizers are usually operated by respiratory therapists. **Focus:** Delegation, supervision

6. **Ans: 1, 4, 6**   Assisting patients with activities of daily living such as toileting are within the scope of practice of UAPs. Once licensed nurses or respiratory therapists have taught the patient to use incentive spirometry, the UAP can play a role in reminding the patient to perform it. UAPs can participate in encouraging patients to drink adequate fluids. Assessing and teaching are not within the scope of practice of UAPs. Performing pulse oximetry could be appropriate for experienced UAPs once they have been taught how to use the pulse oximetry device to gather additional data. **Focus:** Delegation, supervision, assignment

7. **Ans: 3**   Barrel chest and clubbed fingers are signs of chronic COPD. The patient had a productive cough on admission to the hospital. Bilateral crackles are a new finding and indicate fluid-filled alveoli and pulmonary edema. Fluid in the alveoli affects gas exchange and can result in worsening arterial blood gas concentrations. **Focus:** Prioritization

8. **Ans: 1**   Furosemide is a loop diuretic. The uses of this drug include treatment of pulmonary edema. Intake and output records and daily weights are important in documenting the effectiveness of the medication. A side effect of this drug is hypokalemia, and some patients are also prescribed a potassium supplement when taking this medication. **Focus:** Prioritization

9. **Ans: 3**   The patient's temperature was elevated on admission. Further elevation indicates ongoing infection. The health care provider needs to be notified and an appropriate treatment plan started. All of the other pieces of information are important, but are not urgent. The patient's incontinence is not new. **Focus:** Supervision, prioritization

10. **Ans: 4**   The heart rate and blood pressure are slightly increased from admission and the respiratory rate is slightly decreased. The continued elevation in temperature indicates a probable respiratory tract infection that needs to be recognized and treated. **Focus:** Prioritization

11. **Ans: 2**   Discharge planning and IV administration of antibiotics are more appropriate to the scope of practice of the RN. However, in some states LPNs/LVNs with special training may administer IV antibiotics. (Check the regulations in your state.) Administering oral medications is appropriate to delegate to LPNs/LVNs. Although the LPN/LVN could weigh the patient, this intervention is appropriate to the scope of practice of the UAP. **Focus:** Delegation, supervision

12. **Ans: 4**   The patient is demonstrating improper use of the MDI by taking 2 puffs in rapid succession, which can lead to incorrect dosage and ineffective action of the albuterol. Teaching is the first priority. As you work with this patient, you may determine that he would benefit from the use of a spacer. Sitting up in a chair may also be useful, but these interventions are not the first priority. Notifying the provider that the patient needs to continue with nebulizer treatments is not within your scope of practice and does not address the problem, which is that the patient does not know how to properly use his MDI. **Focus:** Prioritization

13. **Ans: 1, 3, 4, 5**   A dietitian can help with the selection of foods that are easy to chew, do not form gas, and are high in calories and protein. Serum prealbumin levels are a good indicator of nutritional status and should be monitored. Small meals can help prevent meal-related dyspnea. Using a bronchodilator before meals will reduce bronchospasm. The second response does not demonstrate respect for the patient's role in his care. Dry foods stimulate coughing. **Focus:** Prioritization

14. **Ans: 3**   The patient with COPD often has chronic fatigue and needs help with activities. Teaching the patient not to rush through activities is important because rushing increases dyspnea, fatigue, and hypoxemia. Patients with COPD should be kept on low-flow oxygen because their stimulus to breathe is a low arterial oxygen level. **Focus:** Supervision, delegation, prioritization

CASE STUDY 3: Multiple Clients on a Medical-Surgical Unit, pages 103-104

1. **Ans: 1, 3, 4, 6**   It is important to recognize that the RN continues to be accountable for the care of all clients by this team. Appropriate client assignments for the LPN/LVN include clients whose conditions are stable and not complex. Ms. J is currently experiencing chest pain, and Ms. B is a complex new admission. **Focus:** Assignment, delegation, supervision

2. **Ans: 2**   Although it is important that the nurse see all of these clients, Ms. J's assessment takes priority. Her chest pain may indicate coronary artery blockage and acute heart attack. None of the other clients' needs is life-threatening. **Focus:** Prioritization

3. **Ans: 3**   Cardiac catheterization is usually accomplished by inserting a large-bore needle into the femoral

vein and/or artery. Clients are routinely restricted to bed rest for 4 to 6 hours after the procedure to prevent hemorrhage. Family members are usually permitted to visit as soon as the client returns to the room. **Focus:** Prioritization

4. **Ans: 5, 4, 1, 2, 4, 2, 4, 2, 4, 3**   The client should be placed on telemetry upon admission to the unit. When the client experiences chest pain, vital signs should be checked immediately, followed by the ECG. Nitroglycerin is usually tried before morphine to relieve the chest pain. Hypotension is a side effect of nitroglycerin. Blood pressure and heart rate are monitored whenever nitroglycerin is administered. When nitroglycerin fails to relieve chest pain, IV morphine is the next action, and the health care provider should be notified. **Focus:** Prioritization

5. **Ans: 4**   Assessment and teaching are more appropriate to the educational preparation of licensed nursing staff. Monitoring and recording intake and output are within the educational scope of the UAP. The UAP could perform pulse oximetry after undergoing orientation and being taught to use the device. **Focus:** Assignment, delegation, supervision

6. **Ans: 1**   A temperature elevation to 102° F is an indicator of an infectious process. The other criterion parameters are near normal, and assessment/evaluation would instead be based on abnormalities from each client's baseline. **Focus:** Delegation, supervision

7. **Ans: 3**   Acute chest pain can indicate myocardial ischemia, coronary artery blockage, and/or myocardial damage. The UAP's question should be Answered with the most accurate response. Although the unit may have protocols that the UAP should be familiar with, option 4 is not the most accurate response. **Focus:** Prioritization

8. **Ans: 2**   Assisting clients with activities of daily living (ADLs) such as feeding are most appropriate to the scope of practice of the UAP. **Focus:** Delegation, supervision, assignment

9. **Ans: 3**   The nurse should gather more information before notifying the health care provider. Pulse oximetry assessment provides information about the client's oxygenation status. Clients with chronic obstructive pulmonary disease (COPD) usually receive low-dose oxygen because their stimulus for breathing is a low oxygen level. Coughing and deep breathing help mobilize secretions. **Focus:** Prioritization

10. **Ans: 1**   This client's temperature elevation is most likely due to an infection. The health care provider must be notified to modify the client's plan of care. Administering acetaminophen and removing extra blankets may decrease the client's temperature, but they will not treat the infection. **Focus:** Prioritization

11. **Ans: 1**   The client's temperature elevation indicates an infectious process. For elderly clients with bladder infections, changes in level of consciousness are frequently a sign. **Focus:** Prioritization

12. **Ans: 2**   Assisting clients with ADLs is appropriate to the educational preparation and scope of practice of the UAP. Teaching, assessing, and administering medications fall within the scope of practice for licensed nurses. **Focus:** Delegation, supervision

13. **Ans: 2**   A common side effect of beta-adrenergic agonists such as albuterol is increased heart rate. Drugs such as albuterol are commonly prescribed for clients with COPD to use as needed to dilate the airways when experiencing shortness of breath. Although the other factors are important and may be related to the client's COPD, they may not have contributed to the increase in heart rate. **Focus:** Prioritization

14. **Ans: 4**   Standards of practice for the use of restraints require that nurses attempt alternative strategies before asking that a client be restrained. A physician's order is required for continued use of restraints but can be obtained after the fact if the client's actions endanger his or her well-being. **Focus:** Prioritization, delegation, supervision

15. **Ans: 3**   The UAP is new to the unit and may need assistance or instruction regarding the completion of this assignment. **Focus:** Delegation, supervision, assignment

16. **Ans: Right task, Right person, Right circumstances, Right direction/communication, Right supervision/evaluation**   According to the National Council of State Boards of Nursing, the Five Rights are essential for the process of delegation. The right task is assigned to the right person in the right circumstances. The RN then offers the right direction/communication, and right supervision/evaluation. **Focus:** Delegation, supervision, assignment

CASE STUDY 4: Shortness of Breath, Edema, and Decreased Urine Output, pages 105-106

1. **Ans: 2**   All of these findings are important, but only the presence of crackles in both lungs is urgent, because it signifies fluid-filled alveoli and interruption of adequate gas exchange and oxygenation, possibly pulmonary edema. The patient's peripheral edema is not new. The faint pulses are most likely due to the presence of peripheral edema. The dry and peeling skin is a result of chronic diabetes and merits careful monitoring to prevent infection. **Focus:** Prioritization

2. **Ans: 3**   Teaching, instructing, and assessing are all functions that require additional education and preparation. These interventions fall within the scope of the professional nurse. Providing the patient with ice for the urine collection and reminding the patient to collect her urine fit the scope of practice of the UAP. **Focus:** Delegation, supervision

3. **Ans: 1**   A patient with a serum potassium level of 7 to 8 mmol/L or higher is at risk for electrocardiographic changes and fatal dysrhythmias. The health care provider should be notified immediately about this potassium level. Although the serum creatinine and blood urea nitrogen levels are quite high, these levels are commonly reached before patients experience symptoms of CKD. The serum calcium level is low, but not life threatening. Keep in mind that there is an inverse relationship between calcium and phosphorus, so when calcium is low, expect phosphorus to be high. **Focus:** Prioritization

4. **Ans: 4**   Kayexalate removes potassium from the body by exchanging sodium for potassium in the large intestine. Diuretics such as furosemide generally do not work well in chronic kidney failure. The patient may need a calcium supplement and subcutaneous epoetin alfa; however, these drugs do nothing to decrease potassium levels. **Focus:** Prioritization

5. **Ans: 1**   Inserting a urinary catheter is within the scope of practice of LPNs/LVNs, and the LPN/LVN must be under the supervision of an RN. Planning care, teaching respiratory care techniques, and discussing options such as renal replacement therapies all generally require additional education and training. In many acute care hospitals, LPNs/LVNs auscultate breath sounds as a part of their observations, and RNs follow up with overall assessment and synthesis of data. These latter interventions are more appropriate to the scope of practice of the RN. **Focus:** Delegation, supervision

6. **Ans: 2**   Checking vital signs usually includes measuring oral body temperature. Because the patient just finished drinking fluids, an oral temperature measurement would be inaccurate at this time. All of the other actions are appropriate and within the scope of practice of the UAP. **Focus:** Delegation, supervision

7. **Ans: 1, 2, 3, 5**   The usual fluid restriction for patients with chronic kidney failure is 500 to 700 mL plus urine output. All of the other actions are appropriate for a patient with fluid overload. **Focus:** Prioritization

8. **Ans: 2**   Even after beginning HD, patients are still required to restrict fluid intake. In addition, patients on HD have nutritional restrictions (e.g., protein, potassium, phosphorus, sodium restrictions). All of the other patient statements indicate an appropriate understanding of HD. **Focus:** Prioritization

9. **Ans: 3**   Temporary dialysis lines are to be used only for HD. As supervising nurse, you should stop the new nurse before the temporary HD system is interrupted. Breaking into the system increases the risk for complications such as infection. The blood pressure should always be assessed on the nondialysis arm. Postoperative patients should always be monitored for bleeding. Oxycodone, when ordered by the provider, is an appropriate analgesic for moderate to moderately severe pain. **Focus:** Delegation, supervision

10. **Ans: 3**   Changes in level of consciousness during or after HD can signal dialysis disequilibrium syndrome, a life-threatening situation that requires early recognition and treatment with anticonvulsants. Decreases in weight and blood pressure are to be expected as a result of dialysis therapy. A small amount of drainage is common after HD. **Focus:** Prioritization

11. **Ans: 1**   Measuring vital signs and weighing the patient are within the education and scope of practice of the UAP. The UAP could remind the patient to request assistance when getting out of bed after the RN has instructed to patient to do so. Assessing the HD access site for bleeding, bruit, and thrill require additional education and skill and are appropriately performed by a licensed nurse. **Focus:** Delegation, supervision

12. **Ans: 4**   Epoetin alfa is used to treat anemia and is given two to three times a week. It is given by either the IV or subcutaneous route. Most commonly epoetin alfa is given subcutaneously. All of the other statements about CKD patient medications are accurate. **Focus:** Delegation, supervision

13. **Ans: 1**   Hyperacute rejection occurs within 48 hours after transplant surgery. Increased temperature, increased blood pressure, and pain at the transplant site are manifestations. **Focus:** Prioritization

14. **Ans: 4**   The treatment for hyperacute rejection is immediate removal of the transplanted kidney and return to dialysis. Increased doses of immunosuppressant drugs are used to treat acute rejection, conservative management is used for chronic rejection, and IV antibiotics are administered for infections. **Focus:** Prioritization

CASE STUDY 5: Diabetic Ketoacidosis, pages 107-108

1. **Ans: 1, 2, 5, 6, 7**   Onset of symptoms and the amount of fluid loss help to determine acuity. Pain assessment of the abdomen should be performed to obtain a baseline; his pain is probably associated with diabetic ketoacidosis (DKA), but infection or trauma could also be factors. The physician should know if Mr. D had insulin today. Information about allergies should be obtained for all clients regardless of the presenting complaint. Understanding why he did not see the physician and knowing his last blood glucose reading do not alter your priority actions at this point. **Focus:** Prioritization

2. **Ans: 4**   Mr. D should be taken to a treatment room where evaluation and treatment can begin immediately. Paging the ED physician to come to the triage area is not necessary unless the client becomes unresponsive in the triage area. Calling the parents is not necessary because Mr. D is old enough to provide consent himself. (If Mr. D were underage, the treatment would not be delayed if the parents were unavailable in an emergency

situation.) Calling the primary care physician is usually done by the ED physician after the preliminary workup is completed. (Policies for calling private physicians vary among institutions.) **Focus:** Prioritization

3. **Ans: 3** Mr. D is severely dehydrated and is at risk for hypovolemic shock and electrolyte imbalance. Although he is demonstrating Kussmaul respirations, this breathing pattern is the body's attempt to compensate for the acidosis. Anxiety and noncompliance are also relevant, but can be addressed after Mr. D's condition is stabilized. **Focus:** Prioritization

4. **Ans: 1, 2, 3, 5** Checking vital signs, bagging up belongings, and measuring and recording output are within the scope of duties for the UAP. Checking blood glucose level is accomplished with a fingerstick and UAPs, particularly in specialty areas such as the ED, will frequently have been trained to do this task, but this may vary from state to state and facility to facility. Information should not be released by the UAP because of confidentiality issues. The RN should decide how to convey information to friends and family. **Focus:** Delegation

5. **Ans: 3, 6** Subcutaneous insulin is not absorbed fast enough and is inappropriate for emergency situations. (IV insulin would be appropriate.) The client is likely to be on orders for nothing by mouth until the vomiting subsides. Fluid replacement will be by IV route during the acute period. **Focus:** Prioritization

6. **Ans: 1** Normal saline (0.9% sodium chloride) is the first fluid used to correct dehydration in most adults with DKA. Half-strength saline (0.45% sodium chloride) can be used for children or adults at risk for volume overload. Potassium supplements are added within 1 to 2 hours after starting insulin. Solutions of dextrose 5% are added to the therapy once the blood glucose level approaches 250 mg/dL. **Focus:** Prioritization

7. **Ans: 2** Initially in clients with DKA, serum potassium level is expected to be within normal limits or elevated; regardless of the laboratory value, however, there is an overall potassium deficit. After insulin therapy, hypokalemia is expected as the potassium shifts back into the cells; therefore, if potassium level is initially low, it will be even lower after therapy. **Focus:** Prioritization

8. **Ans: 2** Her calculations are incorrect. The pump should be set at 7 mL/hr.
155/2.2 = 70.4 kg; round to 70 kg
70 kg/x units : 1 kg/0.1 units = 7 units
100 units/100 mL = 1 unit/1 mL : 7 units/x mL = 7 mL
   Calling the physician is inappropriate; the nurse is responsible for calculating the pump settings. Insulin is a high-alert drug, and calculations must always be double-checked. When discrepancies are discovered, the source of error must be determined and corrected. **Focus:** Prioritization, supervision

9. **Ans: 3** Acknowledging and reflecting underlying feelings is therapeutic. Options 1 and 4 give unsolicited advice, and option 2 is a platitude that is not supported by firsthand knowledge of the mother-son relationship. **Focus:** Prioritization

10. **Ans: 1** First, the situation should be assessed to determine if a HIPAA (Health Insurance Portability and Accountability Act) violation has occurred. Client information should be released only to facilitate continuity of care (i.e., in a shift report) and only to those who are directly involved in the care. If HIPAA rules were violated, the incident would be reported to the nurse manager for potential complaints related to the UAP's actions and so that the UAP could receive the proper remediation. Giving positive feedback for sincere efforts to assist clients and families is appropriate, but guidelines must be recognized and followed. **Focus:** Supervision

11. **Ans: 2** Before potassium is administered, it is important to know that the kidneys are functioning. The other information is important but has less relevance to the potassium infusion. **Focus:** Prioritization

12. **Ans: 2** Ask the secretary to correct the omission by calling the admissions office right away. In this case, client care is more urgent than filing a complaint or determining why the secretary made the omission. If you have a good relationship with the ICU nurses, they will probably take the report; however, you retain responsibility for the client's care until the admission procedure and transfer are completed. **Focus:** Supervision

13. **Ans: 2** Ventricular dysrhythmias suggest hypokalemia, which is a significant cause of death in clients with DKA. One P wave should normally precede every QRS complex. Frequent QRS complexes will be present in tachycardia. An artifact is usually caused by loose leads or client movement. **Focus:** Prioritization

14. **Ans: 1, 4, 5, 6, 7** Other signs and symptoms of hypokalemia include paralytic ileus, nausea and vomiting, abdominal distention, confusion, and irritability. Seizures, hallucinations, and cold, clammy skin are more associated with hypoglycemia. **Focus:** Prioritization

15. **Ans: 1, 4, 5, 6** The UAP can direct family and visitors to appropriate waiting areas, obtain equipment, and measure vital signs. An RN or MD should accompany Mr. D to the ICU; the UAP can help, but should not independently transport clients to the ICU. The unit secretary usually prepares the papers, but the RN is responsible for ensuring that everything is in order. In specialty areas such as the ED, UAPs may receive additional training to connect clients' cardiac leads to the cardiac monitor; however, the RN is responsible for assessing the cardiac rhythm. **Focus:** Delegation

CASE STUDY 6: Home Health, pages 109-112

1. **Ans: 1, 4, 5, 6** Ms. A's dyspnea and increased use of oxygen require rapid assessment. Mr. I's sample for a

CBC must be drawn when the bone marrow is most suppressed to accurately assess the impact of chemotherapy on bone marrow function. Ms. R should be seen as soon as possible after discharge to determine the plan of care. Mr. W needs to receive the scheduled dose of risperidone. Mr. D and Ms. F do not have urgent needs, and these visits can be rescheduled for the following day. **Focus:** Prioritization

2. **Ans: 1**   Ms. A's increased shortness of breath indicates a need for rapid assessment. In addition, high oxygen flow rates can cause an increase in the partial pressure of carbon dioxide ($Paco_2$) and suppression of respiratory drive in patients with COPD, so Ms. A should be seen as soon as possible. The other patients can be scheduled according to criteria such as location or patient preference about visit time. **Focus:** Prioritization

3. **Ans: 4**   In the home health setting, the patient is in control of health management, so enlisting the patient's cooperation for the visit is essential. In this response, the nurse indicates that the patient has a choice about whether the visit is scheduled for today but educates the patient about why it is important that the visit occur as soon as possible. Because the initial visit requires a multidimensional assessment, it is usually quite lengthy. The patient's comments do not indicate a lack of need or desire for home health services. **Focus:** Prioritization

4. **Ans: 2**   The patient has symptoms and risk factors that could indicate that her oxygen saturation is either excessively high or too low, so checking oxygen saturation is the first action that should be taken. The other actions may also be appropriate, but assessment of oxygen saturation will determine which action should occur next. **Focus:** Prioritization

5. **Ans: 1**   The goal for oxygen saturation for a patient with COPD is usually 90% to 94% because high oxygen levels can lead to increases in $Paco_2$. The next step is to notify the HCP, who may want to admit the patient to the hospital or order arterial blood gas analysis. It will be important to discuss appropriate home oxygen use with the patient and her husband, but not until the immediate situation is resolved. **Focus:** Prioritization

6. **Ans: 3**   Although the risperidone is scheduled for today, because the medication is absorbed gradually, rescheduling the dose for tomorrow will not have an adverse impact on control of the patient's schizophrenia. The other patients have more urgent needs and should receive visits today. **Focus:** Prioritization

7. **Ans: 2**   The chest pressure indicates that Ms. R is experiencing myocardial ischemia and requires immediate assessment and intervention (such as administration of sublingual nitroglycerin). The shortness of breath requires further investigation and may be related to the chest pressure and myocardial ischemia. The other responses also indicate the need for further assessment and interventions, such as teaching, but do not require immediate action. **Focus:** Prioritization

8. **Ans: 3**   National guidelines for patients with stable angina indicate that, if the chest pain is improving after nitroglycerin administration, administration of another nitroglycerin tablet is the first action to take. Completing the admission assessment, having her rest, and notifying the HCP about her chest pain are also appropriate actions, but administration of another nitroglycerin tablet and resolution of the chest discomfort are the priorities. **Focus:** Prioritization

9. **Ans: 4, 5, 6**   Home health aide education and scope of practice include assisting with personal hygiene and obtaining routine data such as vital sign values and daily weights. It is the RN's responsibility to evaluate these data and plan individualized care using the data. Assessments, medication preparation, and patient teaching about medications require more education and broader scope of practice, and should be performed by the RN. **Focus:** Delegation

10. **Ans: 2**   The focus in home health nursing is empowering the patient and family members by teaching self-care. Ms. R's condition is not so unstable that she needs to be reassessed today, because her chest pain did resolve after she took two nitroglycerin tablets, she has taken her medications, and her daughter will be available and has been educated about how to manage if Ms. R's condition deteriorates. The patient's symptoms of chest pressure, crackles, and edema do indicate a need for reassessment the next day. Although the home health aide will visit, the education and role of the home health aide does not include evaluating the patient's response to the ordered therapies and planning changes in care based on the evaluation. **Focus:** Prioritization

11. **Ans: 2**   Because Mr. I is in the nadir period following his chemotherapy, he is at high risk for infection. Avoidance of any cross-contamination from Mr. D's leg infection is essential. **Focus:** Prioritization

12. **Ans: 4**   The initial assessment and development of the plan of care, including interventions such as oxygen therapy, are the responsibility of RN staff members. The RN with the most experience in caring for patients with emphysema is the on-call part-time RN. Some patient care activities are assigned to staff members from other disciplines, such as LPNs/LVNs and respiratory therapists, after the plan of care is developed by the RN. **Focus:** Assignment

13. **Ans: 3**   Immunosuppression decreases the patient's ability to mount a fever in response to infection, so that even a minor increase in temperature (especially in combination with symptoms such as lethargy and confusion) can be an indicator of a serious infection, including sepsis. The decreased right-sided breath sounds are consistent with the patient's diagnosis of lung cancer. The poor appetite and dry oral mucous membranes also require assessment and intervention, but infection is one of the most serious complications of chemotherapy. **Focus:** Prioritization

14. **Ans: 4**   Mr. I's immunosuppression, fever, and possible sepsis diagnosis indicate that he should be assessed immediately once he arrives in the ED, so that he will avoid exposure to other ED patients. In addition, the appropriate treatment for sepsis is rapid initiation of intravenous antibiotics (after appropriate culture results are obtained). The other information will also be helpful, but will not ensure that Mr. I is assessed and treated rapidly in the ED. **Focus:** Prioritization

15. **Ans: Elevated temperatures, blood glucose levels, and blood pressures**   The elevated temperatures and blood glucose levels suggest a possible infectious process and should be reported to the HCP so that interventions can be quickly implemented to prevent complications such as sepsis, diabetic ketoacidosis, or hyperglycemic hyperosmolar nonketotic coma. The blood pressures should also be reported, because current national guidelines indicate that blood pressure for diabetic patients should be maintained at a level of less than 130/80 to decrease cardiovascular risk. The pulse, respiratory rate, and weight do not indicate a need for a change in the patient's treatment. **Focus:** Prioritization

16. **Ans: 3, 2, 1, 4**   Mr. D's assessment suggests that he has an acute lower respiratory tract infection such as pneumonia. Since his oxygenation may be compromised, the first action should be to determine his oxygen saturation. National guidelines indicate that initiation of antibiotics is a priority whenever patients have an infection, but if cultures are prescribed, they should be obtained before starting antibiotic therapy. Teaching about self-care can be done after the other interventions are implemented. **Focus:** Prioritization

CASE STUDY 7: Spinal Cord Injury, pages 113-114

1. **Ans: 2**   The priority at this time, with a spinal cord injury (SCI) at the C4-C5 level, is airway and respiratory status. The cervical spine nerves C3 to C5 innervate the phrenic nerve, which controls the diaphragm. Careful and frequent assessments are necessary, and endotracheal intubation may be required to prevent respiratory arrest. The other three concerns are appropriate, but are not urgent like airway and respiratory status. **Focus:** Prioritization

2. **Ans: 2, 4**   The experienced UAP can make sure that the oxygen flow setting is correct and that the cannula is in place once instructed by the RN. The experienced UAP would also know how to measure oxygen saturation by pulse oximetry. The nurse retains responsibility for ensuring that the client's oxygen flow rate is correct and interpreting oxygen saturation measurements. Assessments, including auscultation, and client teaching require additional education, training, and skill, and are appropriate to the scope of practice of the RN. **Focus:** Delegation, supervision

3. **Ans: 3**   The nurse should notify the provider immediately. The client's symptoms indicate the strong possibility of impending respiratory arrest. This client probably needs endotracheal intubation and mechanical ventilation. **Focus:** Prioritization

4. **Ans: 1**   The traction weights must be hanging freely at all times to maintain the cervical traction and prevent further injury. The other options are appropriate for the care of a client with cervical tongs. **Focus:** Prioritization

5. **Ans: 1, 4**   A nursing student can administer medications and simple treatments such as cervical tong pin care. The nursing student should be mentored by the nurse when monitoring traction during client repositioning and performing neurologic assessments. Initiating the client's care plan is within the scope of practice for the professional RN. **Focus:** Delegation, supervision

6. **Ans: 1**   The experienced UAP has been taught how to reposition clients while maintaining proper body alignment. The nurse remains responsible for ensuring that this action is performed correctly. Inspecting a client's skin and administering medications requires additional education and skill, and are appropriately performed by licensed nurses. Performing range-of-motion exercises also requires additional education and skill and is appropriate to the scope of practice of licensed nurses and physical therapists. However, some UAPs are given extra training and are able to perform range-of-motion exercises for clients. The skill level and job descriptions of UAP team members should be checked to determine their ability to perform range-of-motion exercises. **Focus:** Delegation, supervision

7. **Ans: 3**   Mr. M has a level C4-C5 spinal injury. The best way to assess motor functions in a client with this injury is to apply downward pressure while the client shrugs his shoulders upward. Testing plantar flexion assesses S1-level injuries. Applying resistance when the client lifts the legs assesses injuries at the L2 to L4 level. Having a client grasp and form a fist assesses C8-level injuries. **Focus:** Prioritization

8. **Ans: 3**   The client should be encouraged to perform as much self-care as he is able, and the UAP should help with care the client is unable to complete. The client's wife should also be taught to encourage the client to do as much as possible for himself. **Focus:** Prioritization, delegation

9. **Ans: 1, 2, 3, 4, 5, 6**   Clients should be taught to drink 2000 to 2500 mL of fluid each day to prevent urinary tract infections and calculus formation. They may be taught to decrease the amount of fluid intake after 6:00 to 7:00 PM to decrease the need to void, or to self-catheterize in the middle of the night. The other points are appropriate for a bladder training program. **Focus:** Prioritization

10. **Ans: 2**   The first, third, and fourth statements are reasonable client goals for rehabilitation. The second statement probably represents an unrealistic expectation, and the client needs additional teaching about setting realistic goals for rehabilitation. **Focus:** Prioritization

CASE STUDY 8: Multiple Patients with Adrenal Gland Disorders, pages 115-116

1. **Ans: 3**   These signs and symptoms indicate adrenal crisis (addisonian crisis), or acute adrenocortical insufficiency—a life-threatening event in which the need for cortisol and aldosterone is greater than the available supply. The other actions are important and will likely be implemented rapidly, because a common cause of acute adrenal gland hypofunction is hemorrhage, but the health care provider must be notified immediately. **Focus:** Prioritization

2. **Ans: 1**   The patient is hypotensive and most likely hypovolemic. Because the patient already has an IV line, the IV fluids should be started first to address the primary problem. The second IV line and typing and cross matching need to be accomplished rapidly, and the blood sample may be drawn at the same time the second IV line is inserted. The patient needs cortisol replacement, but with nausea and vomiting present, the oral route is not the best option. **Focus:** Prioritization

3. **Ans: 2, 3, 4**   The patient is experiencing nausea and vomiting, so oral fluids are not appropriate at this time. The UAP can take frequent vital sign measurements, record intake and output, and weigh the patient. The nurse should instruct the UAP about what variations in vital signs must be reported. **Focus:** Delegation, supervision

4. **Ans: 1**   The manifestations the patient has developed are classic signs of hypoglycemia, a complication of adrenal gland hypofunction. The nurse should check the patient's glucose level. If it is low, the patient should receive some form of glucose, most likely dextrose 50% IV. **Focus:** Prioritization

5. **Ans: 4**   A patient with hypercortisolism is immunosuppressed because excess cortisol reduces the number of circulating lymphocytes and inhibits production of cytokines and inflammatory chemicals such as histamine. These patients are at greater risk for infection. **Focus:** Prioritization

6. **Ans: 1**   Women with hypercortisolism may report a history of cessation of menses. Increased androgen production can interrupt the normal hormone feedback mechanism for the ovary, which decreases the production of estrogens and progesterone and results in oligomenorrhea (scant or infrequent menses). **Focus:** Prioritization

7. **Ans: 1, 3, 4, 6**   A patient with Cushing disease typically has paperlike thin skin and weight gain as a result of an increase in total body fat caused by slow turnover of plasma fatty acids. Weight loss is to be expected in a patient with hypocortisolism (e.g., Addison disease). The other findings are typical of a patient with Cushing disease. **Focus:** Supervision, prioritization

8. **Ans: 3, 4**   The educational preparation of the LPN/LVN includes fingerstick glucose monitoring and administering subcutaneous medications. Assessing cardiac rhythms and reviewing laboratory results require additional education and skill, and are appropriate to the RN's scope of practice. **Focus:** Delegation, supervision

9. **Ans: 1, 3**   The UAP can provide articles for self-care and reinforce what the RN has already taught the patient. The UAP can also remind the patient about changing positions. Instructing and assessing are within the scope of practice of the professional nurse. **Focus:** Delegation, supervision

10. **Ans: 1, 3, 4, 5, 6**   Cortisol replacement drugs should be taken with meals or snacks, because the patient can develop gastrointestinal irritation when the drugs (cortisone, hydrocortisone [Cortef], prednisone [Deltasone], fludrocortisone [Florinef]) are taken on an empty stomach. All of the other teaching points are appropriate. **Focus:** Prioritization

11. **Ans: 1**   When a patient with possible pheochromocytoma is assessed, the abdomen should not be palpated, because this action could cause a sudden release of catecholamines and severe hypertension. None of the other assessments should have an adverse effect on this patient. **Focus:** Prioritization

12. **Ans: 3**   During the 3- to 4-day VMA testing period, medications usually withheld include aspirin and antihypertensive agents. Beta-blockers are avoided because these drugs may cause a rebound rise in blood pressure. All of the other instructions are appropriate for this diagnostic test. **Focus:** Delegation, supervision

13. **Ans: 2**   The UAP should remind the patient about elements of the care regimen that the nurse has already taught the patient. Assessing, instructing, and identifying stressful situations that may trigger a hypertensive crisis require additional education and skill appropriate to the scope of practice of the professional RN. **Focus:** Delegation, supervision

14. **Ans: 1, 4**   The new nurse graduate who has just completed orientation should be assigned patients whose conditions are relatively stable and not complex. The new graduate should be familiar with the adrenal surgery after completing her orientation and should be able to provide the teaching the patient needs. The patient with a low potassium level will need some form of potassium supplementation, which the new nurse should be able to administer. The patient in addisonian crisis should be assigned to an experienced nurse. The fearful, anxious patient would also benefit from being cared for by an experienced nurse. **Focus:** Assignment

CASE STUDY 9: Multiple Clients with Gastrointestinal Problems, pages 117-120

1. **Ans: 6** Mr. R has several prognostic factors that increase the risk for death: age older than 50 years, and increased WBC and blood glucose level. Shock can occur secondary to bleeding; release of kinins, which causes vasodilation; or release of enzymes into the circulation. **Focus:** Prioritization

2. **Ans: 1, 2, 4** Ms. H, Ms. D, and Mr. A are in the most stable condition and represent the least complex cases according to the shift report. Mr. R's confusion and belligerence will make pain management especially difficult. Because of his pancreatitis, his laboratory results and symptoms of worsening should be closely monitored. Ms. T is at risk for electrolyte imbalances, especially hypokalemia. She needs repetitive perineal hygiene and skin assessment. TPN and central line management requires additional skill. Mr. K is in stable condition, but because of the family dynamics his care should be handled by an experienced nurse. **Focus:** Assignment

3. **Ans: 1, 2, 3, 4** Measuring vital signs, performing hygienic care, and transporting are within the scope of the UAP's duties. The UAP should not remove the dressing. If the dressing needs to be removed, the nurse should remove it, conduct the wound assessment, clean the area, and redress as needed. **Focus:** Delegation

4. **Ans: 3, 4, 5** The UAP can report on changes in vital sign values; giving parameters for notification is better than asking for general reports on any changes. The UAP can report that a client is having pain but is not expected to assess that pain. All staff should be aware of when registered inpatients come and go on the unit and should keep each other advised. (Note: Clients should also be encouraged to tell someone if they are going off the unit.) Judging response to treatment and evaluating drainage are responsibilities of the RN. **Focus:** Delegation

5. **Ans: 2** When the shift report is incomplete, you can ask for any type of additional information. However, vital sign values and orders for medications can be obtained from the records if the off-going shift neglects to give that information. A current pain report can and should be obtained directly from the client. The physician's plan for procedures and diagnostic testing is frequently communicated verbally to the nursing staff, but the physician's written notes may be pending, especially if it is an emergency admission or if the physician is trying to complete morning rounds. **Focus:** Prioritization

6. **Ans: 3** Giving written information about gallbladder disease and options will help Ms. H to prepare any questions she might have for the physician. If diagnostic results are pending, calling the physician is premature. Describing the surgical procedure is inappropriate because there is more than one type of procedure, and the one to be used is still undetermined. Explaining postoperative care would be appropriate once the need for cholecystectomy has been verified by the physician. **Focus:** Prioritization

7. **Ans: 5** In the provision of routine care, clients who need extra time should be left until last, so that care for others is not delayed. Mr. K will require more time and assistance because of age and weakness. Also, you will have to determine which medications can be crushed for delivery via PEG tube. Dealing with Mr. K's family is also more time consuming. **Focus:** Prioritization

8. **Ans: 1, 2, 3, 6** Remind the student of several things: The flat palmar surface of the hand is better than the fingertips when palpating for distention. If the wall suction is activated, it will interfere with auscultating for bowel sounds. Asking about pain first will guide the physical assessment steps. The skin on the anterior chest under the clavicle is a better place to check for turgor than the lower abdomen, especially if abdominal distention is present. Checking the drainage and inspecting for peristaltic waves or distention are correct actions. **Focus:** Supervision

9. **Ans: 3** Having the UAP take the client's vital signs, record them, and report them to the nurse mimics what should happen on a routine day. It is likely that you will want to talk to the nursing instructor, the nursing student, the new nurse, and the UAP to make sure that similar incidents do not happen in the future. If the client is unstable, you might opt to take her vital signs and reassess her yourself, but this will undermine the new nurse. It is unlikely that you would have to write an incident report for this situation unless the client has been harmed. **Focus:** Prioritization, supervision

10. **Ans: 3** With continuous NG suction, there is a loss of sodium and potassium. Also, the loss of acid via suctioning will result in an increase in blood pH or metabolic alkalosis. Full assessment of laboratory data is always important when a change in status is noted, but the other values are less relevant to this client's NG therapy. **Focus:** Prioritization

11. **Ans: 4** Stopping the diarrhea is a priority for Ms. T. Chronic, frequent diarrhea is demoralizing, and fluid and electrolyte losses cause weakness. If the bowel is allowed to rest, the cramping will stop. The other options also provide accurate information, but the potential resolution of the most disturbing symptom will encourage her to continue. **Focus:** Prioritization

12. **Ans: 3** Sulfasalazine is potentially nephrotoxic. The other adverse effects are also possible, but are less serious. **Focus:** Prioritization

13. **Ans: 2** Explaining the physiologic reason helps the UAP to understand that rest is part of the therapy. Following physician's orders is important, but it is an inadequate explanation. Depression does not justify

bed rest. Using large words to explain common concepts should be avoided, regardless of the audience. **Focus:** Supervision

14. **Ans: 1**   If Mr. A is homeless, he will need instructions for adapting the dressing change procedures because of inconsistent access to hot water, soap, and adequate bathroom facilities. The social worker can be contacted for assistance with financial issues related to medication or transportation. Simplify written material and verbally reinforce it, and/or instruct Mr. A to have a friend read the information to him. **Focus:** Prioritization

15. **Ans: 3**   Washing the hands is the first basic step for dressing change. Helping Mr. A identify other ways to maintain asepsis would be more useful than stressing strict sterile technique. **Focus:** Prioritization

16. **Ans: 2**   Bowel sounds should resume in 24 hours; this signals GI system readiness. The client's subjective reports of hunger (or lack of hunger) should not dictate initiation of feedings. The pharmacy may label the formula according to the prescriber's order but will not determine the feeding schedule. **Focus:** Prioritization

17. **Ans: 1, 3, 4, 5**   Elderly clients are especially at risk for hyperglycemia, aspiration, diarrhea, and fluid overload. Hypotension is not a direct complication of enteral feedings. **Focus:** Prioritization, knowledge

18. **Ans: 4, 1, 3, 2**   Use therapeutic communication skills with Mr. R to convince him to return to his room. Assess his mental status related to decision making; he is at risk for injury and self-harm. Assess Ms. H's vomiting and give an antiemetic if appropriate. Assess what Mr. K's family needs from the physician and page the physician if appropriate. Remind Mr. A that he will be notified as soon as possible about discharge. (Tip: Discharge planning begins at the time of admission. During discharge teaching and early on the day of discharge, advise and remind clients that discharge requires several steps [i.e., physician's order; follow-up paperwork; consultation with the case manager, social services office, physical therapy department, etc.]. This information will help them to understand the need to wait and will reduce impatient inquiries.) **Focus:** Prioritization

19. **Ans: 4**   Helping her to prioritize will build skill and confidence. She feels upset, but she has not made any errors that have compromised client care. Sending her off the unit further delays care, leaves her without support, and hinders opportunities to problem solve. Asking the UAP to help her or helping her with select tasks is the second best choice because it demonstrates team support. Taking over one of her clients is not necessary unless care and safety are compromised. **Focus:** Supervision

20. **Ans: 1, 2, 3, 4**   The low calcium level and the falling hematocrit and Po_2, in combination with the elevated WBC and his age, are indicators of a high mortality

risk. High level of pain is not a prognostic factor, but severe unrelieved pain should always be reported. Blood type will not affect the physician's decisions about therapy. **Focus:** Prioritization

21. **Ans: 3, 4, 5, 1, 6, 7, 2**   Stay with the client, reestablish oxygen per nasal cannula, and have a colleague gather equipment. (Note: Check oxygen saturation with nasal cannula in place and replace with nonrebreather mask as needed.) Restart the IV infusion so that emergency fluids or drugs can be given. Check the blood glucose level to rule out a hypoglycemic reaction. Continuously monitor vital signs. If at all possible, reinsert the NG tube; however, this is not a lifesaving priority. **Focus:** Prioritization

22. **Ans: 3**   Mr. R has sufficient severe problems to warrant intensive care. The physician is responsible for the decision to transfer Mr. R; however, the nurse must recognize and advocate for clients who are decompensating. Ordering laboratory and other diagnostic testing may be warranted, and reestablishing NG suction is important, but ultimately the client should be transferred to the ICU. Surgery is unlikely until aggressive medical management measures are exhausted. **Focus:** Prioritization

23. **Ans: 1, 3, 5, 6, 7**   Transferring Mr. R to the ICU is a priority because his condition is unstable. Documentation must be completed, and totaling IV fluids is part of the complete documentation. Briefly assessing clients is a safety measure; client decompensation during shift change is not uncommon. Thanking ancillary staff is a team-building measure. Asking the UAP to measure vital signs for all the clients is unnecessary. If select clients are in unstable condition, or if there is a reason that the vital signs may have changed since the last routine reading, then remeasuring vital signs is appropriate. Asking the ED to hold the client until the next shift will displease the ED staff, but admission should be deferred to the oncoming shift unless there is adequate time to assess the client immediately on arrival and review the orders. (Note: Admitting a new client can take 30 minutes or more depending on the complexity of the orders, the acuity of the client's condition, and the facility's admission forms.) **Focus:** Prioritization

CASE STUDY 10: Multiple Patients with Pain,
pages 121-124

1. **Ans: 6, 3, 2, 1, 5**   Mr. A's respiratory status (i.e., rate, rhythm, pulse oximetry reading) should be quickly checked. Mr. O should be checked for shock symptoms, mental status changes, and escalating pain. Mr. L and Ms. R are both in relatively stable condition but need quick pain assessments and reassurance that their needs will be met. Ms. J and her family should

be approached last, because they need time and patience, and caregivers should not appear rushed. Mr. H is currently in the OR. **Focus:** Prioritization

2. **Ans: 1, 2, 4**   Ms. R and Mr. L have conditions that require pain medication but are less physiologically complex. Mr. H will be just out of surgery later in the shift, but hernia repairs are routine and reasonably predictable; this is a good postoperative case for a new RN. Mr. O will require careful assessment for slowly developing complications such as hemorrhage or peritonitis. Ms. J and her family will need support through anticipated grief and loss and complex decision making for hospice and end-of-life issues. Mr. A's respiratory status must be carefully monitored, and he has complex pain and care issues. **Focus:** Assignment

3. **Ans: 4**   Acknowledge loss and encourage the patient to talk about the past. During this discussion, you and she might find activities that could be adapted to her current situation. Try to avoid giving false reassurance, changing the subject, or switching the focus from her needs to your concerns. **Focus:** Prioritization

4. **Ans: 3**   The shower is preferred, because arthritis patients can have trouble getting in and out of the bathtub. An RN should suggest relaxation techniques and evaluate outcomes of therapies. **Focus:** Assignment

5. **Ans: 2**   Encourage staff members to deal directly with each other to define and resolve problems. If staff cannot resolve the problem among themselves or if the issue is a chronic problem, then the charge nurse or unit manager should intervene. Helping the new nurse to look at the chart should not be necessary at this point. Asking the patient does not address the problem of the missing documentation. Potentially, the new nurse could look at the PCA for a record of self-administered medication, but the machine does not replace good communication between staff members. In addition, the patient's response must be documented, even though he is self-administering the medication. **Focus:** Supervision

6. **Ans: 1, 2, 3, 5**   Helping with hygienic care and reinforcing instructions that have been explained by the RN are within the scope of practice of the UAP. Mr. H should not need any specialized equipment, so the UAP can prepare the bed and gather routine equipment, such as devices for measuring vital signs. The UAP can get coffee, but the nurse may also decide to encourage Ms. J's family to take occasional breaks off the floor. Also, sending one of the family members to get things is a way for the family to have an active role. Mr. O's skin care and assessment should be performed by the RN; the problem is extensive, and pain medication may need to be titrated. A nurse should assess Mr. A, because his oxygen saturation was decreasing during the night. **Focus:** Delegation

7. **Ans: 1, 3, 5**   Because communication is limited in unresponsive patients, all staff members should be watchful for signs. The RN should instruct the UAP on specific things. Reminding patients that staff are available to help relieve pain is appropriate. If the UAP suspects pain, asking the patient a direct "yes-or-no" question is appropriate; then the nurse can be notified. Assessing pain and evaluating outcomes are the responsibilities of the RN. (Note to student: Even if the patient says to the UAP, "The position change helps to relieve my pain" the nurse should still follow up and do a pain assessment.) **Focus:** Delegation

8. **Ans: 2, 1, 4, 3**   It is unlikely that Mr. O's pump will deliver excess medication; however, it is appropriate to discontinue the pump until its functioning can be completely checked. But do not forget to go back soon after and troubleshoot the problem with the pump. Mr. L is probably having ongoing pain issues, but loud calls for assistance must be investigated. Mr. A must be assessed for mental status changes related to hypoxia or encephalopathy. In addition, he needs help to clean up, to get back in bed, and to reposition the oxygen cannula. The other nurse could ask someone else to witness if necessary. **Focus:** Prioritization

9. **Ans: 3**   Mr. L is having an exacerbation of pain that is probably related to the movement of the kidney stone. This type of pain is severe, but usually Transient. If the bolus dose is inadequate, the physician could be notified for a dosage increase. Deep breathing may help somewhat, but the patient will have trouble focusing. Reminding him to use the PCA pump is not necessary at this point. **Focus:** Prioritization

10. **Ans: 4**   Use a matter-of-fact tone of voice to acknowledge his underlying problem (pain). Restarting the IV line addresses the immediate issue. Contacting the physician for oral medications might be considered if no one is able to restart the IV line. Calling the supervisor is a possibility if the patient continues to complain and wants to make a report. Defensive statements such as "It's not my fault" can make the situation worse. **Focus:** Prioritization

11. **Ans: 3**   Scant output suggests that the stone is lodged and obstructing the outflow of urine. This can result in damage to the kidney. Hematuria with or without pain can occur because the stone has irritated the tissue. Dull pain that radiates into the genitalia and urgency are common with kidney stones. **Focus:** Prioritization

12. **Ans: 3**   Elevating the injured extremity will minimize the swelling. If the leg swells, there is additional pressure on nerves. Moving the toes helps, but Mr. O may be too sleepy to consistently comply because of administered pain medication. Diversion therapy is less useful in the acute phase of injury and treatment. Placing the patient in high Fowler position will necessitate raising the leg to a higher and more uncomfortable position. **Focus:** Prioritization

13. **Ans: 1** Pain on passive motion is a sign of possible compartment syndrome. A sudden increase in pain is more associated with arterial obstruction. Itching is a frequent problem associated with a cast that can be relieved by blowing cool air under the cast. Absence of pain without medication could be related to maintaining elevation, ice application, and rest. **Focus:** Prioritization

14. **Ans: 3** Measure vital signs first and then report your findings to the physician. Mr. O is at risk for occult abdominal trauma, and your findings represent a change of status and could be signs of internal bleeding. **Focus:** Prioritization

15. **Ans: 2** Mr. H is anticipating that the pain is going to be worsened by activity. Giving medication 45 minutes before the activity assures him that the pain will be minimized. The second-best option is to reassure him that medication is available if he needs it. Around-the-clock medication and notification of the physician are not necessary at this point. **Focus:** Prioritization, knowledge

16. **Ans: 2** Obtain and administer the medication in the dosage and form in which it was ordered. You can call the provider if you are unable to read the order, or if you are seeking to have the order changed (i.e., the pharmacy does not have the medication). Asking preference for immediate versus controlled-release action is an inappropriate way to phrase the question to the patient. **Focus:** Prioritization

17. **Ans: 3** Mr. H may be experiencing urinary retention because of bladder atony related to the surgical procedure. A distended bladder can mimic hernia pain and cause significant discomfort, and Mr. H may not have the urge to void. Calling the physician and initiating "nothing by mouth" status are premature at this point. Reassurance may be somewhat comforting, but does not address the immediate symptom. **Focus:** Prioritization

18. **Ans: 4** Mr. A has complex needs. Although the staff get tired of hearing continual complaints, everyone should work together to try to solve the problem. Reminding staff that patients have a right to care is rhetorical and not very useful. Offering to care for Mr. A every day does not help the team to overcome bias or improve patient care. When feedback is given, statements that begin with "You should" should be avoided. **Focus:** Supervision

19. **Ans: 1. Physical therapist, 2. RN, 3. RN, 4. RN, 5. RN, 6. UAP, 7. UAP** TENS requires specialized equipment and training and should be handled by a physical therapist. An RN should give medications, answer questions, and assess for aggravating factors. Personal comfort items are permissible, but the RN should remind the family that belongings can get misplaced. The UAP is qualified to help with routine position changes and can reinforce instructions given by the RN. **Focus:** Assignment

20. **Ans: 2** First call the pharmacy and ask about compatibilities. If the solutions and medications are compatible, you can give them simultaneously. If there are incompatibilities, you may decide to give the morphine first, because this can be administered quickly and will give the patient immediate relief. Then you can call the physician for an order to stagger medication times or to establish a second IV site. (Note to student: You may encounter facilities or situations that allow the nurse to change medication times or to start a second peripheral IV site without a physician's order; however, medication and IV therapy generally require a physician's or health care provider's order. Follow policy and procedure manuals and ask charge nurse or supervisor for guidance.) **Focus:** Prioritization

21. **Ans: 4** Conduct additional pain assessment with vital sign measurement. This will determine what interventions are needed. **Focus:** Prioritization

22. **Ans: 2** If you decide to question the nurse or check on the patients, specific examples are more useful than vague generalizations. Specific examples will also help you determine whether there are extenuating circumstances that the UAP may be misinterpreting. Comments about patient care issues should not be ignored; all team members should be encouraged to watch out for the health and safety of patients. **Focus:** Supervision

23. **Ans: 1** A patient like Ms. J has taken opiates for a long time. Constipation is the only opioid side effect to which the patient does not develop tolerance. Respiratory depression, nausea, vomiting, and sedation may have occurred when Ms. J was first receiving opioids but are now less of a concern. **Focus:** Prioritization

24. **Ans: 3** Lorazepam is an anxiolytic. Naproxen is a nonsteroidal anti-inflammatory drug. Doxepin is used for depression or neuropathic pain. Dicyclomine is given to reduce smooth muscle spasms. **Focus:** Prioritization, knowledge

25. **Ans: 4** Communication skills are important in dealing with the family and the physician. If you have exhausted this route, the next step is to move up the chain of command. Calling another physician is not appropriate. If the son calls the physician, it may make the situation worse. You must function under the current orders and use additional nonpharmacologic measures until the issue is resolved. **Focus:** Prioritization

26. **Ans: 3** Help the nurse to prioritize what has to be done, and help her recognize what can and cannot be delegated. Offering help is appropriate if patient safety is compromised, and it does contribute to team building; however, it does not help her learn to organize her work. Letting her struggle is one method of learning, but new nurses deserve guidance and support. Help her to determine what tasks can be passed on to the next shift, and then she can discuss this during shift report. **Focus:** Supervision

Answer Key

27. **Ans: 1, 2, 4, 6** Emptying the trash, assisting patients with personal items, changing linens, and recording urine as output are within the scope of duties for the UAP. Helping patients, such as Ms. R change position in bed, is also appropriate. (There may be times when the nurse should change the patient's position if assessments of the skin or mobility are needed.) The nurse should assess Mr. L's back pain and need for additional medication. Mr. O's leg must be assessed by the nurse for perfusion; merely looking to see if the leg is elevated is insufficient. **Focus:** Delegation

28. **Ans: 2, 4, 5, 6** Electronic units are usually very effective in assisting the staff to keep track of dispensed doses; however, users must enter correct data and most systems have "workarounds" that negate safety measures. Try to gather as much information as you can and discuss the problem with the unit manager. This could be a case of theft, but it may also be a system error that needs to be corrected. It is not appropriate to draw patients into this problem, and forcing everyone to stay is pointless if you have already interviewed each individual. **Focus:** Supervision, prioritization

29. **Ans: 3, 4, 1, 5, 6, 2** The report should be succinct and organized, so that the listener will have a clear idea of who you are talking about, what the major issues are, what measures were done to address the issues, and what requires follow-up. The listener also needs the opportunity to clarify what you have said. This will increase mutual understanding. **Focus:** Prioritization

CASE STUDY 11: Multiple Clients with Cancer, pages 125-128

1. **Ans: 1, 2, 5, 6** When the client responds to a question, you gather information about ease of respirations and cerebral perfusion. Noting the presence of complex equipment will help in making assignments, particularly if the staff is inexperienced. Measuring vital signs, checking intake and output, and palpating for pain are not necessary during this brief assessment unless there is reason to suspect that the client is decompensating. (Note: Some nurses will briefly palpate the radial pulse to detect irregularities and assess peripheral perfusion.) **Focus:** Prioritization

2. **Ans: 3, 4** Mr. B and Ms. C are clients in relatively stable condition who would be capable of speaking with a nursing student for a prolonged time. Mr. N is also communicative and in stable condition, but limiting the number of people that enter the room is best practice for neutropenic clients. Mr. L has recently been transferred from the SICU. His tracheostomy tube with secretions and the nasogastric tube will make communication very tedious and overwhelming for him and the student. Mr. U needs frequent skilled assessment, and he is likely to be very uncomfortable, exhausted, and possibly dyspneic. Ms. G needs emotional support and preoperative teaching that are beyond the abilities of a first-semester student. **Focus:** Assignment, supervision

3. **Ans: 2** Staff and visitors with potentially communicable diseases should not enter Mr. N's protective environment. Pregnancy, inexperience, and fear do not automatically exclude staff members from this assignment. If the team leader has time and options for personnel, then opportunities for duty sharing for pregnant staff members and teaching for the inexperienced and fearful can be explored. **Focus:** Assignment, supervision

4. **Ans: 3** Acknowledge the student for taking responsibility for the error. Helping the student to feel comfortable in reporting errors rather than hiding mistakes is essential for client safety. Notifying the instructor, after acknowledging the student for taking responsibility, is appropriate so that the student can be counseled and procedures reviewed. All involved parties may elect to write separate incident reports. **Focus:** Supervision

5. **Ans: 2** Catheterizing this client increases the risk for infection, and the clean-catch method is adequate for a urinalysis. The other orders would be appropriate for this client. **Focus:** Prioritization

6. **Ans: 4** Increased secretions, difficulty swallowing, and loss of the protective epiglottis put Mr. L at risk for aspiration. The other diagnoses also apply to this client, but are of lower priority. **Focus:** Prioritization

7. **Ans: 1** Pulsation suggests that the tube may be malpositioned and pushing against the innominate artery. This is a medical emergency. Presence of food particles and difficulty with cough or expectoration suggest that cuff pressures should be monitored more closely. Increased secretions are expected in the postoperative period. **Focus:** Prioritization

8. **Ans: 3** The bag-valve mask (trade name: Ambu bag) will be the first thing that is needed if there is a problem with the tracheostomy equipment or with respiratory effort. With a tracheostomy, there should be no need for an endotracheal tube or a laryngeal scope. The insertion tray is also probably unnecessary, because the site should mature within 72 hours. **Focus:** Prioritization

9. **Ans: 2, 1, 3, 4, 6, 5** A Foley catheter with a drainage bag will be inserted. The tube is clamped distal to the injection port, then the BCG fluid is instilled through the catheter, and the catheter remains clamped for 2 hours. During those hours, Mr. B should be reminded to change position from side to side or prone to supine every 15 to 30 minutes. At the end of the 2 hours, the catheter is unclamped, and the fluid is drained. Two glasses of fluid are given to further flush the bladder. **Focus:** Prioritization

10. **Ans: 3** The toilet should be disinfected for 6 hours after discarding the fluid. The UAP should receive these specific instructions to safely manage this biohazard. Wearing a lead apron or sterile gloves is not necessary. **Focus:** Delegation, supervision

11. **Ans: 3** The goal is resumption of normal voiding within 3 days. Immediately after catheter removal and for 1 to 2 days thereafter, Mr. B may experience dysuria, urgency, and frequency. **Focus:** Prioritization

12. **Ans: 4, 2, 3, 5, 1** Mr. L is at risk for aspiration and an immediate airway obstruction if his tracheostomy tube is not suctioned. If a chest drainage system tips over, it is unlikely that anything untoward will occur; however, if the chest tube has been displaced, Mr. U is at risk for an open pneumothorax. The physician must be notified about Mr. N's fever so that therapy can be changed and cultures ordered to determine the source of infection. Ms. C must be assessed for signs of deep vein thrombosis. Mr. B needs reassurance that the dysuria is Transient and to be expected after intravesical therapy. **Focus:** Prioritization

13. **Ans: 1. UAP, 2. RN, 3. RN, 4. Wound, ostomy, continence nurse (WOCN), 5. WOCN** The UAP is able to assist Ms. C with hygienic care. The RN should explain the need for drains and give medications and assess outcomes. A WOCN will usually Answer initial questions about ostomy care and preventing complications for clients with new stomas. **Focus:** Assignment

14. **Ans: 4** Asking for extra help and delaying independent action is a type of regression that allows Ms. C to cope with the changes in self-image and bodily functions. The nurse should evaluate the situation daily to help Ms. C find alternative coping strategies. The other diagnoses may be relevant as her situation changes. **Focus:** Prioritization

15. **Ans: 4** Have her hold the clamp or do some other small task to engage her in participation. This creates the expectation that she can participate and will eventually handle the equipment. Verbally reexplaining the procedure and providing written material does reinforce the initial teaching, but being told will not help her master the psychomotor aspects. Having a family member or a staff member take over the procedure does not support the goal of eventual independence. **Focus:** Prioritization

16. **Ans: 3** Use 10 minutes to determine if Ms. C has an urgent need, but set some boundaries so that she will know what to expect. Making reference to other clients' needs is not appropriate. Telling her that she is okay minimizes her concerns. Calling a volunteer might be useful after you determine that her social needs could be met by a volunteer. **Focus:** Prioritization

17. **Ans: 1** Ms. G is demonstrating fear and anxiety related to uncertainty of the future. The other diagnoses are pertinent, but bringing the anxiety under control should precede giving her information, facilitating decision making, and dealing with body image. **Focus:** Prioritization

18. **Ans: 4** First acknowledge Ms. G's feelings and do additional assessment about "things" that you could help her with. It is natural for her to be anxious about the surgery, but there may be other issues (i.e., problems with family, money, work, etc.). The other options might be appropriate after the situation is assessed. **Focus:** Prioritization

19. **Ans: 1** All of the conditions warrant calling the physician. However, tracheal deviation is a symptom of tension pneumothorax, and the nurse may have to intervene before the physician can arrive or phone in orders. Dysrhythmias are one sign of tumor lysis syndrome secondary to hyperkalemia. Decreased urinary output for Mr. B is probably related to an obstruction, but other causes should be investigated. Ms. C is at risk for hemorrhage or peritonitis. **Focus:** Prioritization

20. **Ans: Any three of the following:** Tracheal deviation, severe dyspnea, extreme agitation, increased respiratory rate, increased pulse, progressive cyanosis, distended jugular veins, and lateral or medial shift in the point of maximum impulse. **Focus:** Prioritization

21. **Ans: 1** For Mr. U, the tension pneumothorax has most likely been induced iatrogenically by the covering of the chest wound. (For clients without open chest wounds, the priority action is performing a needle thoracotomy.) Initiating CPR is inappropriate at this point. Having the crash cart and intubation equipment nearby is a precaution, but should not delay other interventions. **Focus:** Prioritization

22. **Ans: 2, 1, 4, 3** Using the SBAR format, the nurse first identifies himself or herself, gives the client's name, and describes the current situation. Next, relevant background information, such as the client's diagnosis, medications, and laboratory data, is stated. The assessment includes both client assessment data that are of concern and the nurse's analysis of the situation. Finally, the nurse makes a recommendation indicating what action he or she thinks is needed. **Focus:** Prioritization

23. **Ans: 1, 2, 3, 4, 5, 8** Determining what tasks/duties are pending and seeking replacement coverage are all appropriate. Because she is new, reminding her about the workload and her probation are appropriate as verbal warnings. Any of us could have a personal emergency at any time; refusing to let her go or expecting disclosure of personal details could be carefully considered if her behavior is repetitive. **Focus:** Supervision, assignment

24. **Ans: 2** This is an opportunity to help the student find her own Answer. You can help her to work through her own feelings and to identify the boundaries of the nurse-client relationship. Redirecting the student back to the instructor, acknowledging the student's ability to establish a relationship, and giving direct advice about how to set boundaries are all possible choices in working with students, but not as

useful as helping students to identify their own best practices. **Focus:** Supervision

CASE STUDY 12: Gastrointestinal Bleeding, pages 129-130

1. **Ans: 3**   Vomiting of bright red blood is a sign of active bleeding. The patient's physical assessment findings and vital sign values are indicative of physiologic compensation for blood loss. Risk for aspiration is not an immediate concern because Mr. S is currently alert and there is no reason to suspect that his gag reflex is not intact. Anxiety and noncompliance can be addressed later. **Focus:** Prioritization

2. **Ans: 2, 3, 4, 5**   Mr. S is at risk for hypovolemic shock. Decreases in urine output or hemoglobin level and hematocrit should be monitored. Occult blood (Hemoccult) testing of emesis and stool should be performed to confirm upper and lower gastrointestinal bleeding. Semi- or high Fowler position is used to decrease risk for aspiration during vomiting and/or nasogastric tube (NG) tube insertion. A 22-gauge catheter is not the best choice for this patient. He may require a blood transfusion and/or large fluid volumes; 16- to 18-gauge catheters are better choices. Preparing the patient for surgery at this point is premature, because bleeding resolves spontaneously in most hospitalized patients. **Focus:** Prioritization

3. **Ans: 1**   Repeating vital sign measurements falls within the scope of the UAP's abilities. There is no indication that blood glucose level should be checked every 2 hours. Gathering certain types of equipment can be delegated. However, NG lavage is not a typical task for a UAP; if you delegate the gathering of equipment for this procedure, you will have to provide an itemized list. The UAP should not be responsible for notifying the family, even with the patient's permission. **Focus:** Delegation

4. **Ans: 1. UAP, paramedic, RN, or LPN/LVN, 2. Paramedic or RN, 3. RN, 4. LPN/LVN or RN, 5. RN, 6. Clergy or RN, 7. RN**   In an emergency situation, many team members will perform tasks simultaneously. There will be variation and overlap in the roles and duties of personnel according to the facility's policies. Any team member could apply the automatic blood pressure cuff; however, an experienced UAP will frequently do this task without being told to do so, because he or she knows that other team members must perform more complex procedures. Either an RN or a paramedic can insert peripheral IV lines. NG tube insertion and lavage should be done by the RN, because the initial gastric return and response to lavage should be continuously assessed. Foley insertion can be done by the LPN/LVN (also by the RN). (Note: Some institutions will allow UAPs with additional training to insert Foley catheters.) The RN is responsible for blood transfusions. Clergy (if available) can assist by comforting and supporting family members. If clergy is unavailable, the RN must assume this responsibility. Assessment should be performed by the RN. **Focus:** Assignment, delegation

5. **Ans: 3**   A tense, rigid abdomen could signal perforation, peritonitis, and/or a worsening hemorrhage. The other findings are relevant but are less immediately urgent. **Focus:** Prioritization

6. **Ans: 2, 1, 6, 7, 4, 3, 5**   Place the patient in high Fowler position to prevent aspiration. The length is measured for tip placement into the stomach. Check for the most patent nostril by inspecting or by occluding each nostril and checking for air flow. (Note: Checking for nostril patency could precede measuring the length of the tube.) Gently insert the tube into the most patent nostril. When the tube is just above the oropharynx, have the patient tip the chin down, then gently advance the tube. When the tip reaches the posterior pharynx, have the patient sip water. Swallowing closes the epiglottis and helps to prevent tracheal intubation. Checking placement is essential before instilling saline. **Focus:** Prioritization

7. **Ans: 4**   Page the physician and document your actions. The physician may opt to order restraints if the patient cannot make safe decisions. The physician may try to convince the patient to agree to the therapy or have the patient sign an AMA form if he continues to refuse treatment. The nursing supervisor and the patient advocate can be notified if the situation escalates. **Focus:** Prioritization

8. **Ans: 2**   To expedite the STAT order, draw the specimen yourself. (Note: In addition, you may delegate to the unit clerk the task of calling the laboratory and alerting them to the potential error in labeling.) The other options will only delay the STAT order. After Mr. S's condition is stabilized, tracking down the cause of the error will help prevent recurrences. **Focus:** Prioritization, supervision

9. **Ans: 1**   In a medical emergency, the patient can receive O-negative blood. An antibody reaction could result if type A or B blood is administered without typing and cross matching. **Focus:** Prioritization, knowledge

10. **Ans: 4, 5, 6, 1, 2, 3, 7, 8**   Inspect the bag. If the product appears unusable or if the bag is damaged, contact the blood bank for another unit. Checking labels and identification is essential. At the bedside, two licensed professionals should compare the bag and identification band. (Note: Priming of the tubing and filter could be done any time before starting the transfusion. Many nurses will perform this step while they are measuring vital signs using an automated blood pressure cuff. In an emergency situation, equipment preparation can be done while waiting for the unit to come from the blood bank.) Measuring vital signs immediately before starting

the transfusion provides a baseline in case of transfusion reaction. An acute reaction is most likely to result with transfusion of the first few milliliters of blood (or within 15 minutes). A delayed reaction may occur several days after the transfusion. Frequent measurement of vital signs (according to hospital policy) and complete documentation are standard requirements. **Focus:** Prioritization

11. **Ans: 2**   Denial is the most common defense mechanism seen among substance abusers. Option 1 represents rationalization, or giving reasons for behavior. Option 3 represents projection, which is a transfer of unacceptable behavior onto others. Option 4 represents suppression, which is a conscious awareness of and avoidance of dealing with the problem. **Focus:** Prioritization, knowledge

12. **Ans: 3**   Assess Mr. S's ability to make a clear and logical plan. He does have a right to leave and may have an acceptable alternative (i.e., he wants to go to another hospital or to call his family physician); however, if he is not able to make safe decisions for himself (or others) then you are obligated to act to ensure his safety. The use of "Why?" should be avoided, because it creates a defensive response. After assessing, you may decide that calling the wife and the physician are appropriate actions. **Focus:** Prioritization

13. **Ans: 1**   Watch for signs of neurologic irritability (i.e., psychological [anxiety, jumpiness, or nervousness] and physical [fine tremors, tachycardia, diaphoresis]). Delusions and seizure are later signs. Slurred speech is more frequently associated with alcohol intoxication. **Focus:** Prioritization

14. **Ans: 1, 2, 3, 5, 6**   Death can occur from myocardial infarction, fat embolism, peripheral vascular disease, aspiration pneumonia, electrolyte imbalance, sepsis, or suicide. Anaphylaxis would not ordinarily occur unless the patient was allergic to one of the treatments (i.e., drug allergy). **Focus:** Prioritization

15. **Ans: 2**   First assess the patient and try to determine exactly what occurred. You may decide to use the other options based on your assessment findings. **Focus:** Prioritization

CASE STUDY 13: Head and Leg Trauma and Shock, pages 131-134

1. **Ans: 4**   National guidelines for the emergency management of traumatic brain injury (TBI) indicate that the assessment of airway and breathing is the priority action for this client. Ms. A's slow and irregular respiratory rate is a risk factor for hypoxemia, which would decrease oxygen delivery to the brain as well as other vital organs and tissues. The other assessment information should also be obtained quickly, because Ms. A is at risk for hypothermia, blood loss associated with a possible left leg fracture, and aspiration. **Focus:** Prioritization

2. **Ans: 4**   The Glasgow Coma Scale (GCS) offers a standardized and objective way to assess and document LOC. Although the other responses also accurately describe the client's LOC, they do not provide objective data that can be readily used to determine changes in the client's neurologic status. **Focus:** Prioritization

3. **Ans: Decerebrate**   Stiff extension of the arms and legs is seen in decerebrate posturing, which indicates damage to the midbrain and brainstem. **Focus:** Prioritization

4. **Ans: 2, 3**   Ms. A's bradycardia and hypotension suggest that she is experiencing neurogenic shock in response to her head injury. It is also important to remember that, with any traumatic injury, hypovolemic shock caused by hemorrhage should be considered. In this case, Ms. A should be assessed for blood loss associated with her leg injury and for internal bleeding caused by blunt trauma to her chest and abdomen. **Focus:** Prioritization

5. **Ans: 4**   Lumbar puncture is contraindicated in a client who may have increased intracranial pressure (ICP), because it increases the risk for herniation of the brainstem through the foramen magnum at the base of the skull. Checking for a positive Babinski sign and obtaining an electrocardiogram are not priorities for this client, but would not place the client at any increased risk. Increasing the IV rate is appropriate based on the client's blood pressure. **Focus:** Prioritization

6. **Ans: 3**   The initial care of clients with traumatic injuries in the ED requires the expertise of an RN with extensive ED experience. Neither the agency RN nor the ICU RN will be familiar with the location of equipment and with the organization of care in your ED. Although the LPN has experience in the ED, the LPN/LVN scope of practice does not include the complex assessments and interventions that will be needed in caring for this client. (The LPN could be assigned to assist the RN caring for Ms. A.) **Focus:** Assignment

7. **Ans: 1**   The most important goal for an unconscious client who is vomiting is to prevent aspiration. Turning Ms. A to her side (while maintaining cervical spine stability through the use of the backboard and cervical collar) is the best method to ensure that she does not aspirate. Suctioning would also be utilized, but does not clear the airway as well as having the client positioned on her side. Hyperoxygenation may also be required for this client, but will not protect the airway while she is vomiting. A nasogastric (NG) tube is usually not inserted in clients with possible facial fractures. Insertion of an orogastric (OG) tube may be ordered, but would not protect from aspiration at the present time. **Focus:** Prioritization

8. **Ans: 2**   National advanced trauma life support guidelines indicate that a CT scan should be done as soon as possible after a closed head injury in order to determine the extent and types of injury and guide interventions, such as surgery. The other orders are also appropriate for the client, but do not need implementation as rapidly. **Focus:** Prioritization

9. **Ans: 4**   Ms. A's arterial blood gas results indicate uncompensated respiratory acidosis and hypoxemia. Because her respiratory drive is suppressed, she will need rapid intubation and ventilation using a mechanical positive-pressure ventilator. She may need surgery, in which case it would be appropriate to have blood available in the blood bank. Although ongoing monitoring of the magnesium level is indicated, the magnesium level is in the low-normal range, so administration of magnesium is not a priority at this time. Insulin would not typically be administered for a small glucose elevation such as this in a nonfasting client. **Focus:** Prioritization

10. **Ans: 1**   The client's fixed and dilated pupils, widened pulse pressure, and bradycardia are caused by increasing pressure on the brainstem and indicate that she is at risk for brainstem herniation, which would result in brain death. Immediate surgical intervention is needed to prevent this complication. She is at risk for the other complications, but they are not as life threatening. **Focus:** Prioritization

11. **Ans: 4**   Normal ICP is 0 to 15 mm Hg and cerebral perfusion pressure (CPP) should be at least 60 mm Hg or higher. CPP is calculated using the formula MAP − ICP = CPP. Ms. A's CPP is 58 mm Hg ($80 - 22 = 58$); interventions should be implemented immediately to decrease her ICP and improve CPP. The other data indicate a need for ongoing monitoring but do not require immediate intervention. **Focus:** Prioritization

12. **Ans: 1, 6, 7**   Evidence-based guidelines recommend the use of mannitol in clients who have TBI with increased ICP in order to reduce ICP and improve CPP. In hypotensive clients, CPP may also be improved by administering vasopressors to raise MAP. Positioning the head of the bed at 30 degrees also reduces cerebral edema by promoting venous drainage from the cerebral circulation. Although neurologic assessments such as checking the GCS score and observing pupil reaction to light are necessary, the stimulation caused by these interventions can increase ICP. Suctioning and repositioning also cause transient increases in ICP. It is important to monitor ICP, MAP, and CPP during these procedures and modify care to avoid unnecessary increases in ICP or decreases in CPP. **Focus:** Prioritization

13. **Ans: 1, 6, 7, 8**   Client data collection, collection of urine specimens, and administration of medications through an OG or NG tube are included in LPN/LVN education and scope of practice. An experienced LPN/LVN would be expected to report any changes in client status to the supervising RN. Usually repositioning a client would also be included in the LPN/LVN role; however, this client is at risk for increased ICP during positioning and should be monitored by the RN during and after repositioning. Assessments of breath sounds, neurologic status, and the endotracheal tube cuff in critically ill clients should be accomplished by an experienced RN. **Focus:** Delegation

14. **Ans: 1**   Lower-than-normal $Paco_2$ levels cause cerebral vasoconstriction and result in further cerebral hypoxia. The RN should notify the health care provider and anticipate a decrease in the ventilator rate. The oxygen percentage being delivered by the ventilator should be evaluated, since a lower fraction of inspired oxygen (Fio_2) may be adequate. However, the current Pao_2 will not have any adverse effect on cerebral perfusion. The decrease in HCO_3^- reflects a compensatory mechanism for the client's respiratory alkalosis and will resolve spontaneously when the $Paco_2$ level rises. **Focus:** Prioritization

15. **Ans: 3**   Ms. A's high urine output suggests that she has developed diabetes insipidus (DI), a common complication of intracranial surgery. Because DI can rapidly lead to dehydration in a client who is unable to take in oral fluids, the priority action here is to obtain an order to increase the IV rate. Continuing to monitor the output and checking the specific gravity would also be needed but would not correct the risk for dehydration. Because Ms. A's neurologic status is so poor, it is unlikely that changes in her neurologic status would be helpful in determining the effects of DI. **Focus:** Prioritization

16. **Ans: 4**   All of the orders contain abbreviations that, according to the Institute for Safe Medication Practices, may increase the chance for medication errors. The Joint Commission has also mandated that the abbreviation "U" (for units) should be included on hospital "Do Not Use" lists. **Focus:** Prioritization

17. **Ans: 2**   Gastric stress ulcers are a common complication of head injury unless histamine$_2$ (H_2) blockers (such as famotidine) or proton pump inhibitors (such as pantoprazole [Protonix]) are administered prophylactically. Administration of famotidine may decrease the risk of pneumonitis if aspiration occurs, minimize the effects of gastroesophageal reflux, and decrease stomach irritation, but none of the other responses addresses the use of H_2 blockade in head injury. **Focus:** Prioritization

18. **Ans: 2**   Because the client has just been repositioned, it is likely that the elevated ICP is caused by poor positioning. The head and neck should be maintained in good alignment, because neck flexion can cause venous obstruction and an increase in ICP. Administration of mannitol and further elevation of the head of the bed may be used to lower ICP if repositioning Ms. A's head and neck is ineffective. However, these measures should be used only if her MAP is high enough to maintain a CPP of 60 mm Hg. Checking Ms. A's pupils would not offer any additional information, and the stimulation may increase her ICP. **Focus:** Prioritization

19. **Ans: 1**   The assessment data suggest the development of compartment syndrome, an emergency that can lead to permanent neuromuscular damage within 4 to 6 hours without rapid treatment. Elevation of the

leg will further reduce blood flow to the leg. Continuing to monitor the leg without correcting the compartment syndrome will allow the ischemia to persist. Although restlessness may indicate pain in clients with intact neurologic function, Ms. A's neurologic status is severely compromised, and monitoring for restlessness will not be helpful in assessing for ischemic leg pain. **Focus:** Prioritization

20. **Ans: 2** When a client is unable to provide informed consent for a procedure, a close family member (who is likely to be most knowledgeable about the client's wishes) is able to give permission. Emergency procedures can take place without written consent for an unconscious or incompetent client when no family or legal representative is available to give permission. The nursing supervisor does not have the authority to consent to surgery for an unconscious client. **Focus:** Prioritization

CASE STUDY 14: Septic Shock, pages 135-138

1. **Ans: 2** The oxygen saturation indicates that the patient is severely hypoxic (despite an increased respiratory rate). Because this hypoxia will affect all other body systems, it should be treated immediately. The other orders also should be rapidly implemented, but they do not require action as urgently as the low oxygen saturation. **Focus:** Prioritization

2. **Ans: 2** A nonrebreather mask can provide a fraction of inspired oxygen (FIO_2) of close to 100%, which will be needed for this severely hypoxemic patient. Nasal cannulas deliver a maximum FIO_2 of 44%, simple face masks deliver an FIO_2 of up to 60%, and Venturi masks provide a maximum FIO_2 of 55%. **Focus:** Prioritization

3. **Ans: 1, 2, 6** Checking vital signs and urine output is included in UAP education. Experienced UAPs will know which patient information to report immediately to the supervising RN. UAPs working in the ED setting would also have been trained and know how to establish cardiac monitoring, although dysrhythmia analysis and treatment would be the responsibility of the RN. Obtaining and documenting assessments and starting an IV line should be done by the RN. **Focus:** Delegation

4. **Ans: 1** Although atrial fibrillation at rapid rates can cause a significant drop in cardiac output and blood pressure, the rate of 90 to 114 is not a likely cause of the patient's hypotension. Cardioversion or administration of antidysrhythmic medications such as amiodarone or metoprolol may be needed if the heart rate increases. Ongoing cardiac rhythm monitoring is necessary. **Focus:** Prioritization

5. **Ans: 2** The ABG values indicate that the patient is hypoxemic (low PaO_2 and oxygen saturation) and has a severe uncompensated respiratory acidosis (low pH and elevated $PaCO_2$). Because she is unable to maintain adequate oxygenation and ventilation independently, intubation and mechanical ventilation are indicated. Sodium bicarbonate is administered only if metabolic acidosis is present. Although the patient will need ongoing respiratory monitoring and may also benefit from albuterol therapy, these therapies are not adequate in a patient with these severe ABG abnormalities. **Focus:** Prioritization

6. **Ans: 5, 4, 3, 9, 6, 1, 7, 2, 8** The need for intubation should be explained to the patient and family. The patient should be placed supine with the head and neck in the "sniffing" position just before intubation, because lying flat usually increases dyspnea. The patient should be preoxygenated for 3 to 5 minutes before the intubation attempt. Inflation of the endotracheal tube cuff is needed for effective ventilation. Checking for exhaled carbon dioxide through continuous wave-form capnography is the most accurate way to assess endotracheal placement; the presence of bilateral breath sounds also is used to check placement. After the initial assessment of endotracheal placement is completed, the tube should be secured before obtaining a chest radiograph to confirm optimal placement. **Focus:** Prioritization

7. **Ans: 4** The low blood pressure indicates that systemic tissue perfusion will not be adequate, so measures to improve the blood pressure need to be implemented rapidly. The second priority is to treat the infection that is a likely cause of the temperature elevation and hypotension. The crackles heard in the patient's left lung do not need immediate intervention, because her oxygen saturation is 93%. The nonpalpable pedal pulses are associated with the hypotension and will improve if blood pressure is increased. **Focus:** Prioritization

8. **Ans: 1, 3, 4, 5, 6, 7** The decreased blood pressure and increased heart rate are indicators of shock. The elevation in temperature suggests that sepsis (and massive vasodilation) may be the cause of the shock. The blood-streaked and cloudy urine, and back and abdominal pain point to a urinary tract infection (UTI) and/or pyelonephritis as the cause of the sepsis. Diabetic patients are at increased risk for UTI and sepsis. Atrial fibrillation is not an indicator of sepsis and is unlikely to be the cause of Ms. D's hypotension. **Focus:** Prioritization

9. **Ans: 3, 4, 1, 5, 2** Guidelines from the national *Surviving Sepsis* campaign suggest that the first action should be fluid infusion, because Ms. D's minimal urine volume and history of not taking in fluids indicate that she is hypovolemic. In addition, sepsis is associated with massive vasodilation, which leads to hypotension and decreased tissue perfusion, so increasing the circulating volume is essential for this patient. The dopamine infusion should be started next to counteract the circulatory vasodilation. The blood for culture (and specimens for any other ordered cultures) should be obtained before the antibiotics are started. All of these orders should be implemented

rapidly, because septic shock quickly leads to multiple organ dysfunction syndrome, which is usually fatal. Acetaminophen can be given to decrease the patient's temperature, but the other actions have a higher priority. **Focus:** Prioritization

10. **Ans: 3** The most common complication of too-rapid IV infusion of fluids is volume overload leading to heart failure. Although peripheral edema, decreased urine output, and jugular venous distention may be indicators that heart failure is developing, they do not occur as rapidly as the backup of fluids into the pulmonary capillaries and then into the alveoli. **Focus:** Prioritization

11. **Ans: 1** The first action should be to evaluate the patient for symptoms of toxic effects of dopamine, because interventions may be needed to correct these. Dopamine is a high-alert medication, and dosage calculations should be double-checked by at least two licensed personnel; however, initial actions after a medication error should focus on evaluation of the patient. Notification of the HCP and appropriate documentation of the medication error are also needed, but should be done after evaluating the patient. **Focus:** Prioritization

12. **Ans: 4** High doses of dopamine are sympathomimetic and increase cardiac conduction and automaticity. The elevated heart rate for this patient will increase her cardiac workload and should be reported to the HCP. The blood pressure increase is a therapeutic effect of dopamine. The changes in respiratory rate and oxygen saturation require intervention, but would not be caused by dopamine infusion. **Focus:** Prioritization

13. **Ans: 1, 4** LPNs/LVNs are educated and licensed to perform tasks such as monitoring and documenting intake and output, bedside blood glucose monitoring, and administering insulin under the supervision of an RN. Although LPNs/LVNs can collect data about patients, actions such as administering IV antibiotics to critically-ill patients and monitoring for therapeutic and adverse effects of vasoactive medications require more education and RN-level skill. **Focus:** Delegation

14. **Ans: 3** The decrease in PA wedge pressure indicates that the patient is still hypovolemic and will need an increase in IV fluids. The arterial blood pressure is improved, and you already have an order to increase the dopamine if needed. The atrial fibrillation rate is not dangerously elevated. Although the patient's temperature still is elevated, it has decreased from the previous reading. **Focus:** Prioritization

15. **Ans: 2** The elevated glucose level will require that you administer the ordered insulin lispro using the hospital standard sliding-scale insulin orders. Potassium will move into cells along with glucose as insulin is administered, so the patient's potassium level does not require additional treatment. The other abnormalities indicate

the need for continued monitoring, but will not require any immediate action at this time. **Focus:** Prioritization

16. **Ans: 1** The travel RN has the required ICU experience to provide care in this complex case and has been working at the hospital long enough to be familiar with how to obtain supplies, communicate with other departments, and so on. The other nurses either lack experience in caring for critically-ill patients (the new graduate and the PACU nurse) or will not be able to offer the continuity of care that is desirable for the patient. **Focus:** Assignment

CASE STUDY 15: Heart Failure, pages 139-142

1. **Ans: 3** The Joint Commission mandates that "MS" as an abbreviation for morphine sulfate should be on all hospital "Do Not Use" lists, because this abbreviation can be interpreted as magnesium sulfate. Orders 1 and 4 also use abbreviations that the Institute for Safe Medication Practices suggests may lead to confusion, although these are still acceptable to The Joint Commission. The parameters for oxygen delivery could be stated in the order; however, the CCU policy will clarify this. **Focus:** Prioritization

2. **Ans: 3** Evidence-based guidelines for the treatment of acute heart failure indicate that oxygen administration to relieve symptoms of hypoxemia is a priority. The other actions are also appropriate, but not as the initial action. **Focus:** Prioritization

3. **Ans: 1** The client's symptoms of hypoxemia and pink frothy sputum and her history of increasing shortness of breath and mitral valve regurgitation suggest pulmonary edema (severe left ventricular failure) as a probable diagnosis. (She also has symptoms of right ventricular failure, but these are not as great a concern.) The client's history does not indicate that she has pulmonary hypertension, so cor pulmonale is not a likely concern. Myocardial infarction may be a precipitating cause for pulmonary edema, but the acute dyspnea is the first concern for treatment. Although hypoxemia occurs with a pulmonary embolus, crackles and frothy sputum are not consistent with this complication. **Focus:** Prioritization

4. **Ans: 2** The client is hypoxemic, so giving oxygen at the highest level possible is the priority. Activation of the Rapid Response Team and administration of morphine are also appropriate actions. Coughing and deep breathing are not likely to be helpful, because they will not clear fluid from the alveoli. **Focus:** Prioritization

5. **Ans: 4** The best clinical indicators of sudden changes in cardiac output are vital signs such as blood pressure, pulse rate, and respiratory rate. The other data may also be useful in determining the adequacy of perfusion, but they are not as important as the blood pressure and pulse rate. **Focus:** Prioritization

6. **Ans: 3**   Although the assessment indicates that a loop diuretic is indicated, before administering furosemide, it is essential to know the client's potassium level. Her PVCs indicate ventricular irritability, which can be caused by hypokalemia. Angiotensin-converting enzyme (ACE) inhibitors can increase potassium levels, so it is also essential to know the potassium level before giving the enalapril. The retention catheter is also appropriate for this client, but the priority is to ensure that her potassium level is within normal limits and then administer the diuretic to decrease her volume overload. **Focus:** Prioritization

7. **Ans: 4**   LPN/LVN education and scope of practice include insertion of catheters. Administering medications to clients in unstable condition is best accomplished by RNs who have experience in caring for critically-ill clients. Although some LPNs/LVNs may be able to perform venipuncture, obtaining a blood sample could be delegated to the laboratory staff so that the LPN/LVN can insert the catheter. **Focus:** Delegation

8. **Ans: 4**   Morphine is used in pulmonary edema for its effect as a venodilator, which decreases venous return to the heart and reduces ventricular preload. Although morphine is used to treat angina, this client has not reported chest pain. Morphine may decrease Ms. C's respiratory rate, but this is not a desired effect. Morphine may decrease the client's anxiety, but this is not the primary reason for administering it to clients with pulmonary edema. **Focus:** Prioritization

9. **Ans: 2**   KCl is infused at a rate no faster than 10 mEq/hr through a peripheral IV line, and no faster than 20 to 30 mEq/hr through a central catheter. Infusing KCl too rapidly (over 1 or 10 minutes) is contraindicated, since this may cause cardiac arrest. Administering KCl over 8 hours would delay the administration of the furosemide and also leave the client vulnerable to continued dysrhythmias. **Focus:** Prioritization

10. **Ans: 4**   Because Ms. C's major problem is pulmonary edema, the most useful information will be changes in her lung sounds. The other information is also helpful in assessing for volume overload, but not as pertinent to the diagnosis of pulmonary edema. **Focus:** Prioritization

11. **Ans: 2**   Because nesiritide causes vasodilation and diuresis, hypotension is the most common adverse effect. Systolic blood pressure of less than 90 mm Hg is a contraindication for nesiritide infusion. The other data will also be useful in determining whether the client's condition is improving or in assessing for adverse effects but are not as important as frequent blood pressure measurement. **Focus:** Prioritization

12. **Ans: 1**   An RN with experience on a coronary step-down unit would be familiar with the care of clients with left ventricular failure. You have not had an opportunity to evaluate the knowledge level of the agency RN; in addition, this RN will not be familiar with hospital or CCU policies, location of supplies, and so on. The experienced CCU nurse is caring for a client whose condition is potentially very unstable, which leaves little time to assess and intervene for Ms. C. The new graduate is not experienced enough to care for a client like Ms. C, whose condition still may deteriorate. The new graduate could be teamed with a more experienced nurse to learn more about the care of clients with severe left ventricular failure. **Focus:** Assignment

13. **Ans: 2**   Dysrhythmias and visual disturbances are symptoms of digoxin toxicity, a common problem in clients taking digoxin. Digoxin toxicity can lead to fatal dysrhythmias such as ventricular tachycardia and ventricular fibrillation, so measurement of the digoxin level should be ordered. The other findings would not be unusual in a client with chronic heart failure and mitral valve disease, although ongoing assessments are indicated. **Focus:** Prioritization

14. **Ans: 1, 5**   Because you are concerned that the client may have digoxin toxicity, you should hold the digoxin. Hypokalemia can contribute to the risk for digoxin toxicity, and Ms. C is not acutely short of breath, so the furosemide (which causes potassium loss) should also be held until you consult with Ms. C's physician. There are no indications that the other medications are causing any adverse effects, so they should all be administered. **Focus:** Prioritization

15. **Ans: 3, 4, 1, 2**   Using the SBAR format, the nurse first identifies himself or herself, gives the client's name, and describes the current situation. Next, relevant background information, such as the client's diagnosis, medications, and laboratory data, are stated. The assessment includes both client assessment data that are of concern and the nurse's analysis of the situation. Finally, the nurse makes a recommendation indicating what action he or she thinks is needed. **Focus:** Prioritization

16. **Ans: 1, 2, 5, 6**   National guidelines indicate that discharge instructions for clients with heart failure should address topics such as weight monitoring, diet, follow-up appointments, medications, activity levels, and what to do if symptoms recur. Daily weights are an excellent means of monitoring volume status. Clients should be taught to call the health care provider when symptoms first begin to worsen, rather than waiting until they need to be admitted to the hospital. ACE inhibitors such as captopril can cause orthostatic hypotension, so changing positions slowly is important to avoid dizziness and falls. Furosemide should not be taken in the evening, because it will affect sleep quality. High fluid intake can cause volume overload in clients with heart failure. **Focus:** Prioritization

17. **Ans: 1**   It is important that clients with heart failure be taught that, when therapy with beta-blockers is

started, symptoms such as fatigue may temporarily get worse. As the client takes the medication for a longer period, these symptoms should resolve. The client's bradycardia is also an expected effect of carvedilol. If clients are not told to expect these symptoms, they may discontinue the beta-blocking medications. The other actions are not indicated, based on Ms. C's assessment. **Focus:** Prioritization

CASE STUDY 16: Multiple Patients with Peripheral Vascular Disease, pages, 143-144

1. **Ans: 5, 4, 2, 6, 1, 3** The worsening back pain of Mr. S may signal an AAA that is enlarging, and he is at risk for rupture, which is urgent and immediately life threatening. Ms. Q's hypertension should be assessed next, because she is at risk for complications such as stroke. Next, Mr. R, the patient with the severe pain, should be assessed and given pain medication. Ms. A is scheduled for Doppler studies and may have questions and need teaching before the procedure. Ms. C, the patient with Raynaud disease, should be assessed next, although the symptoms she is reporting are typical of this problem. Finally, you should see Mr. Z to discuss arranging for someone to talk with him about smoking cessation. **Focus:** Prioritization

2. **Ans: 2** Palpation of the abdomen must be avoided, because the mass may be tender and there is risk of causing a rupture. Auscultating for a bruit and observing for pulsation are appropriate assessment techniques. Pain assessment is appropriate, because such patients typically experience steady, gnawing abdominal, flank, or back pain that is unaffected by movement and may last for hours or days. **Focus:** Supervision, prioritization

3. **Ans: 3** The patient's symptoms and your assessment findings indicate an AAA that may be expanding, and this places the patient at risk for rupture. This is an urgent situation, and the provider should be notified immediately. You should not place the patient in a high sitting position, because this may place added pressure on the patient's AAA, leading to rupture. **Focus:** Prioritization

4. **Ans: 1** LPN/LVN educational preparation includes inserting Foley catheters. In some states LPNs/LVNs can insert IV catheters and administer IV drugs, but this is not true of all states and facilities. To perform these actions, the LPN/LVN would need additional education and training. Check local, state, and facility policies. The UAP could be delegated to measure the patient's vital signs, with instructions from the nurse about what findings to report. **Focus:** Delegation, supervision

5. **Ans: 1, 2, 3** The nursing student should be able to provide teaching about simple concepts such as coughing and taking deep breaths, perform simple assessments such as measuring peripheral pulses, and administer oral medications, all under the supervision of the nurse. The nurse or someone with special training in performing venipuncture should draw blood for the laboratory tests. The patient may have questions about the surgery, so discussion about the reasons for surgery should be carried out by an experienced nurse. The nurse could mentor the student by allowing the student to be present during the discussion. **Focus:** Delegation, supervision

6. **Ans: 4** Postoperatively after AAA repair, bowel sounds are usually absent for 2 or 3 days, and patients have a nasogastric tube in place on low suction until bowel sounds return. The nurse should document the finding only and teach the student that this is to be expected and why. **Focus:** Delegation, supervision, prioritization

7. **Ans: 1** Administering the patient's blood pressure medications is aimed at correcting the problem. Getting the patient back into bed and reassessing the patient's blood pressure are appropriate actions but do not focus on the problem of lowering the patient's blood pressure. **Focus:** Supervision, delegation, prioritization

8. **Ans: 4** The nurse should intervene when the patient asks to have the docusate held, because opioids often cause side effects such as constipation. The patient must be taught about the importance of this medication in preventing unwanted side effects. If the patient has a good reason for refusing the docusate (e.g., he has been having episodes of diarrhea), then the nurse may hold the drug. The other actions are appropriate. Giving the pain medication before the dressing change will make the procedure less painful. **Focus:** Delegation, supervision

9. **Ans: 2, 3** Mr. Z is in stable condition, and the PACU nurse could begin educating him about smoking cessation. The PACU nurse is skilled at blood pressure monitoring and would have no difficulty meeting Ms. Q's needs for care. Ms. A and Ms. C need the care of a nurse who is experienced in caring for and educating patients with peripheral vascular disease to teach and Answer question. Mr. S's worsening back pain may indicate expansion of his AAA and he should be assigned to an experienced nurse. **Focus:** Assignment

10. **Ans: 1, 2, 3, 5** The underlying pathophysiology of Raynaud disease is vasospasm of the arterioles and arteries of the upper and lower extremities, usually unilaterally. All of the other teaching points are appropriate to share with a patient with Raynaud disease. **Focus:** Prioritization

11. **Ans: 3, 4, 5** The UAP can remind about and reinforce nursing care measures that have already been taught by the RN. Assisting patients to get out of bed is also within the scope of practice for UAPs. Assessing and inspecting the patient require additional education and

skills appropriate to the RN's scope of practice. **Focus:** Delegation, supervision

12. **Ans: 2**   Heparin at low doses interacts with antithrombin III to produce inhibition of clotting factors, which results in inhibition of fibrin formation. The drug does not "thin" a patient's blood or dissolve an existing clot. **Focus:** Prioritization

13. **Ans: 1**   The UAP's scope of practice and education include actions related to assisting patients with activities of daily living, such as ambulation. Monitoring, assessing, and providing instructions for the patient require additional education and skills, and are part of the RN's scope of practice. **Focus:** Delegation, supervision

14. **Ans: 1, 2, 4, 5**   Placing the patient in a supine position and elevating his foot places the extremity above heart level, which slows arterial blood flow to the foot and may lead to increased pain. All of the other actions are appropriate for a patient with Buerger disease. **Focus:** Prioritization

15. **Ans: 4**   Although all of these lipid profile findings are abnormal, the HDL cholesterol ("good cholesterol") level is much too low. A desirable HDL cholesterol level is 40 mg/dL in men and 50 mg/dL in women. The other results are of concern and must be attended to, but they are not as excessively abnormal as is the HDL level. **Focus:** Prioritization

CASE STUDY 17: Respiratory Difficulty After Surgery, pages 145-148

1. **Ans: 3**   The marked decrease in oxygen saturation over the last few hours indicates that Mr. E is developing respiratory complications that will require immediate nursing action. The other information also calls for assessment and possible intervention, but not as urgently as the change in his respiratory status. **Focus:** Prioritization

2. **Ans: 2**   Samples for measurement of antibiotic trough levels are drawn just before the next scheduled dose. Drawing the blood at 9:00 AM will give a slightly inaccurate trough level. Obtaining blood at 11:30 AM would be appropriate for assessing peak gentamicin level. **Focus:** Prioritization

3. **Ans: 2**   Oxygen saturations of less than 90% indicate hypoxemia, so the most important action is to improve oxygenation. Sitting in a chair usually improves gas exchange because the lungs can expand more easily. Mr. E's anxiety is due to hypoxemia, so morphine (which may suppress respiratory drive) is not an appropriate intervention to decrease anxiety. The assessment should be completed after interventions to improve oxygenation have been implemented. **Focus:** Prioritization

4. **Ans: 1**   The ABG results indicate that Mr. E is hypoxemic and has metabolic acidosis because of a cellular shift to the anaerobic metabolic pathway. These abnormalities should be corrected by increasing the Pao_2 level. The nonrebreather mask is capable of delivering fraction of inspired oxygen (Fio_2) levels of close to 100%. He is hyperventilating in response to hypoxemia, so administering morphine is not indicated. Although you will continue to monitor this client's respiratory status, monitoring alone is not enough at this time. **Focus:** Prioritization

5. **Ans: 3**   The increase in WBC count is an indicator of infection, a major concern in a client who has had a ruptured appendix. The WBC count may indicate that a change in antibiotic therapy is needed. The abnormalities in the other parameters indicate that ongoing CBC monitoring is necessary, but do not require any acute interventions. **Focus:** Prioritization

6. **Ans: 1**   An RN with experience in caring for pediatric clients would be familiar with the care of clients with infection and hyperglycemia, including blood glucose monitoring and administration of insulin. The new graduate does not have enough experience to care independently for a client who is still in somewhat unstable condition. Ms. O will require assessment and interventions before the on-call RN will be able to arrive. The agency RN will not be familiar with the location of supplies or with hospital policies, such as the standard sliding-scale insulin protocol. **Focus:** Assignment

7. **Ans: 4**   The client's symptom of worsening hypoxemia even with increases in supplemental oxygen occurring a few days after the initial injury (i.e., a ruptured appendix) are most consistent with ARDS. The other complications are possible diagnoses for this client, but are not as likely as ARDS. **Focus:** Prioritization

8. **Ans: 2, 4, 1, 3**   Using the SBAR format, the nurse first introduces himself or herself, then indicates the current client situation that requires intervention. The nurse then gives pertinent background information about the client. Next, the assessment and analysis of the client's problem are communicated. Finally, the nurse makes a recommendation for the needed action. **Focus:** Prioritization

9. **Ans: 1**   Improving Mr. E's oxygenation is the priority goal. BiPAP provides noninvasive positive-pressure ventilation, which can decrease the work of breathing and rapidly improve gas exchange. Intubation and mechanical ventilation may be needed for this client but will take longer to accomplish. Administering a bronchodilator and obtaining specimens for culture are also indicated but should be done after starting BiPAP ventilation. **Focus:** Prioritization

10. **Ans: 1**   Advanced cardiac life support guidelines indicate that a chest radiograph is the best choice to confirm ET tube placement 3 to 5 cm above the carina. The initial assessments performed after intubation are listening for bilateral breath sounds, checking

for carbon dioxide exhalation though continuous wave-form capnography, and observing for symmetrical chest wall movement with ventilation. Monitoring of oxygen saturation is useful in assessing response to treatment, but it is not the best indicator of correct ET tube placement, especially in severely hypoxemic clients. **Focus:** Prioritization

11. **Ans: 3**   Current evidence-based guidelines for mechanical ventilation in ARDS suggest a PaO_2 of 55 to 80 mm Hg as a goal; the FiO_2 should be decreased since exposure to high oxygen levels causes alveolar damage. Although the $PaCO_2$ is slightly elevated, mild hypercapnia is acceptable according to the most current research. Raising V_T will increase the chance for complications such as pneumothorax. The CMV mode is generally used for clients who are unconscious or paralyzed, because it allows the client no control of respirations and is very uncomfortable. **Focus:** Prioritization

12. **Ans: 1, 6, 7**   The PAWP and urine output suggest that Mr. E is hypovolemic, so increasing his IV fluid intake is essential. Nutritional interventions are important in critically-ill clients. Enteral feeding is the preferred method for administering nutrition, because nutrient metabolism is better and fewer complications occur than with total parenteral nutrition. Because Mr. E's temperature and WBC count are elevated despite receiving gentamicin and ceftriaxone, obtaining specimens for culture is appropriate. Furosemide administration would lead to further dehydration. The client's hypotension and tachycardia are most likely due to dehydration, so norepinephrine and diltiazem would not be ordered. Total parenteral nutrition is used when the enteral route is not possible. **Focus:** Prioritization

13. **Ans: 3**   Having a family member at the bedside will decrease the sense of isolation and anxiety that occurs in the ICU environment, especially in clients who cannot easily communicate because of intubation. The other methods listed may also be used. Restraints are sometimes needed in agitated or confused clients, although the need for restraints must be reevaluated frequently. Many clients do benefit from the use of antianxiety medications, although the use of neuromuscular blockade or paralysis is avoided unless absolutely necessary to improve ABG values. Reminding the client frequently not to pull at the ET tube may also be helpful. **Focus:** Prioritization

14. **Ans: 4**   The application of suction causes hypoxemia and trauma to the tracheal mucosa. Suction should only be applied to the catheter while it is being withdrawn to minimize these problems. Hyperoxygenation is necessary before performing suction for a client who is at risk for hypoxemia, although 5 minutes of hyperoxygenation is usually not necessary. Use of a closed-suction technique helps decrease the cost of suction catheters and is preferred

for clients receiving positive end-expiratory pressure (PEEP) ventilation, but an open-suction technique may also be used. Some clients may require sedatives or analgesics before suctioning, although these are not routinely given. **Focus:** Prioritization

15. **Ans: 3**   The current guidelines of the Centers for Disease Control and Prevention (CDC) indicate that keeping the head of the bed elevated will decrease gastric reflux and the risk for VAP. Current research does not support the need for changing ventilator tubing every 24 hours, and the CDC does not recommend this. Research has not established which method of giving enteral feedings (continuous or intermittent) is best for clients receiving mechanical ventilation. Continuous pulse oximetry may be used for this client, but will not decrease the risk for VAP. **Focus:** Prioritization

16. **Ans: 1, 3, 5**   LPN/LVN education covers skills such as providing oral care, monitoring NG tube feedings, and taking temperatures. Although a UAP might also be able to do some of these activities in a stable client, more education is needed to provide oral care or take temperatures in a client who is intubated and receiving mechanical ventilation. An experienced LPN/LVN would know which client data need to be reported to the supervising RN immediately. Positioning a client is also included in LPN/LVN education; however, placing a client with an ET tube and multiple hemodynamic monitoring lines in a prone position requires multiple staff members and should be supervised by the RN caring for the client. ET tube suctioning may be delegated to an experienced LPN/LVN in some settings, but in a client in unstable condition, suctioning should be done by the RN. Education and hemodynamic monitoring are RN-level responsibilities. **Focus:** Delegation

17. **Ans: 1**   When an alarm sounds, the initial action should be to assess the client. In this situation, the assessment of breath sounds, chest movement, and respiratory effort should indicate which respiratory complication the client may be experiencing. Depending on the assessment findings, the other actions may also be necessary. **Focus:** Prioritization

18. **Ans: 2**   The absence of breath sounds on the right and the high pressures needed to ventilate the client suggest a tension pneumothorax caused by barotrauma associated with positive-pressure ventilation and the use of PEEP. Displacement of the ET tube into one side or extubation also may lead to decreased breath sounds, but the ET tube position would change with these. Aspiration pneumonia is a common complication but does not present with a sudden onset and absent breath sounds. **Focus:** Prioritization

19. **Ans: 3**   With a tension pneumothorax, there are usually only a few milliliters of blood in the collection chamber, because there is no blood or fluid trapped in the pleural space. The presence of 100 mL of blood

indicates that there may have been trauma to the lung during the chest tube insertion. The other data are expected with chest tube insertion and pneumothorax. The air leak should be monitored, and analgesics should be used to control the pain Mr. E is experiencing. **Focus:** Prioritization

20. **Ans: 4** Mr. E has multiple risk factors for acute kidney failure, including his dehydration and use of the potentially nephrotoxic antibiotic gentamicin. Acute kidney injury is one of the common complications of ARDS. The other laboratory values are also abnormal but do not indicate a need for a change in therapy at present. **Focus:** Prioritization

CASE STUDY 18: Long-Term Care, pages 149-152

1. **Ans: 1, 4, 6** Although aspects of care for all six patients could be assigned to the UAPs, Mr. B, Ms. L, and Ms. Q all need assistance with ADLs, which fall within the scope of practice of the UAP. Ms. R's change in level of consciousness needs to be assessed, because this is a change from her baseline. Many aspects of Mr. K's care can be assigned to a UAP, but his tube feeding and care need the attention of a nurse. Mr. W's difficulty with breathing also requires assessment, because this is a change from his baseline. **Focus:** Assignment

2. **Ans: 3** Mr. W is having difficulty breathing, which could be life threatening. Ms. R needs to be assessed second to determine the reason for her confusion. None of the other patients' conditions are life threatening or unstable. **Focus:** Prioritization

3. **Ans: 2** This is an oral feeding that is within the scope of practice of an LPN/LVN. A UAP's scope of practice includes assisting a patient to ambulate and reminding a patient to use the bathroom. Assessing Mr. W's oxygenation status is more appropriately done by an RN. **Focus:** Delegation

4. **Ans: 1** Checking oxygen saturation via pulse oximetry will give you important information about Mr. W's oxygenation status and a possible reason for why he is experiencing difficulty breathing. Although checking blood pressure, urine output, and heart rate are important, they do not take first priority at this time. **Focus:** Prioritization

5. **Ans: 4** The priority concern for Mr. W at this time is difficulty breathing. He may be at risk for fluid excess because of his kidney failure, and this would be his second priority. He does not report chest pain. Decreased peripheral perfusion is not a priority at this time. **Focus:** Prioritization

6. **Ans: 4** Mr. W has crackles, a productive cough, and decreased gas exchange. The provider needs to be notified, because these signs and symptoms may indicate a respiratory infection that needs to be treated. Patients with COPD should receive low-flow oxygen (3 L/min or less), because their stimulus to breathe is a low oxygen

level. The patient is already having shortness of breath, which may be worsened with attempts to suction or to lay the patient flat in bed. **Focus:** Prioritization

7. **Ans: 2** All of the nursing responsibilities associated with the provider's orders are within the scope of practice of an LPN/LVN, but some, such as giving medications, are not within the scope of a UAP. You can direct the LPN/LVN to keep you updated regarding Mr. W's condition. As the nursing supervisor, you are responsible for ensuring that all of the patient care is provided during your shift. **Focus:** Delegation, assignment

8. **Ans: 4** The changes in Ms. R's urine, presence of an indwelling catheter, and fecal incontinence point to a urinary tract infection (UTI). In older adults, sudden confusion is a sign of UTI. Although the other three nursing diagnoses are applicable to this patient, the priority is recognizing and treating the infection. The confusion and communication issues should resolve when the infection is treated. Keeping Ms. R clean and dry to prevent skin breakdown is the second priority. **Focus:** Prioritization

9. **Ans: 1, 4, 5, 6, 7** All of these orders are within the scope of practice of a UAP except giving medications. **Focus:** Assignment

10. **Ans: 2, 3** Although all of these provider and nursing orders fall within the scope of practice of an LPN/LVN, all but giving medications can be assigned to a UAP. Administering medications is usually not within the scope of practice of a UAP. In some states, long-term care facilities employ medication UAPs. However, these UAPs must complete a special state-approved program and must demonstrate competency to take a pulse and measure blood pressure. **Focus:** Assignment, delegation

11. **Ans: 3** The patient is much improved. A pulse oximetry reading of 90% is acceptable for a patient with COPD, and the oxygen flow does not need to be changed. Waking the patient every hour for incentive spirometry is counterproductive, because the patient will not get the rest he needs. **Focus:** Prioritization

12. **Ans: 4** Your priority at this time is to assess the patient, because you need to know why Mr. B does not want to get up and walk before you take action. Pain may be the reason, but you do not know that until you assess the patient. Patients do have the right to refuse treatment, but the purpose of Mr. B's admission is rehabilitation so that he can go home, and early ambulation is important in the prevention of respiratory complications. The first priority is assessment to gather more information. **Focus:** Prioritization

13. **Ans: 1, 3, 5, 6** Mr. B does need to get up and walk. Administering his PRN pain medication may facilitate this. It is important to be attentive to the underlying problem and to strategize how to ensure that he receives appropriate rest, which will aid his recovery.

If he is unaware of the respiratory risks associated with failing to ambulate, it is an opportunity to teach him about this. It is not appropriate to belittle Mr. B's concerns by reminding him of the other patients' needs. Although you may want to talk with the UAP about getting more information and allowing patients to rest, there may be times when it is important to awaken patients from naps. **Focus:** Prioritization

14. **Ans: 2** A fairly common side effect of calcium therapy is gastrointestinal upset with nausea and vomiting, and giving this drug with food can minimize or eliminate this side effect. Although Ms. Q is at risk for fractures, this Answer does not focus on the problem. Giving the drug on an empty stomach will most likely make the nausea and vomiting worse. Holding the dose does not focus on the problem. **Focus:** Prioritization

15. **Ans: 3** Ms. L is pleasantly confused and should respond better to a gentle reorientation than to a loud, stern reprimand. The priority is ensuring that Mr. K's tube feeding is restarted; then the LPN/LVN could escort Ms. L back to her room, or assign this to the UAP. When Ms. L is being reoriented, the LPN/LVN should remind her that she is a patient. The fourth response could sound disrespectful toward Ms. L. **Focus:** Prioritization, assignment

16. **Ans: 4** Mr. K's living will is a legal document and must be respected. You should assess his status and check his advance directive document to make sure it is current, then respect his wishes. You would call the provider with notification of the patient's death. You should take his mother into a quiet room, calmly remind her of his wishes, have someone stay with her, and ask if there is someone you can call for her (e.g., a spiritual advisor or another family member). **Focus:** Prioritization

---

CASE STUDY 19: Multiple Pediatric Clients in a Clinic Setting, pages 153-156

1. **Ans: 1. APN student or pediatrician, 2. RN and GN, 3. LPN/LVN, RN, or GN, 4. UAP, 5. Social worker, 6. UAP, 7. RN, pediatrician, GN, and APN student, 8. Pediatrician** The APN student should perform the well-baby physical examinations under the supervision of a pediatrician (who could also perform this task). The RN should perform triage and mentor the GN in this task. LPN/LVN skills are appropriate for giving routine immunizations; the RN or GN could also perform this duty. Obtaining height and weight should be delegated to the UAP. The pediatric social worker would be the best person to ensure that the play area is stocked and organized. Play therapy equipment is specialized, and even simple elements such as the organization of the furniture can affect the therapeutic aspects of

play. Stocking the treatment rooms should be delegated to the UAP. The RN and pediatrician each perform physical assessments of all walk-in clients. The RN should also mentor the GN in this task. The APN student could also do this under the supervision of the pediatrician. The pediatrician must perform clinical supervision of the APN student. **Focus:** Assignment, delegation, supervision

2. **Ans: 2** First the nurse should assess the mother's decision and her level of knowledge. She may not understand the pharmacology of immunization or the child may have had a problem with previous immunizations. She has agreed to immunizations in the past, but now something has changed her mind. Other options may be appropriate depending on the assessment findings. **Focus:** Prioritization

3. **Ans: 2** Assess the child to gain additional information about illness. Acute febrile illness is generally considered a contraindication for administering immunizing agents because side effects are additive to existing illness and the symptoms of the two will be confused. Notifying the pediatrician, advising the mother, rescheduling the appointment, administering an antipyretic, and giving fluid may be appropriate, but these actions should follow evaluation of the febrile condition. **Focus:** Prioritization

4. **Ans: 3** Inconsolable crying for 2 hours is excessive, prolonged, and abnormal. Instruct the parent to call 911. The swelling can be treated with ice packs. Vomiting can be a sign of increased intracranial pressure, but fewer than three episodes is usually associated with minor injuries. A laceration on the forehead needs suturing, which should be done within several hours to prevent infection and reduce scarring, but the more pressing issue is to reaffirm with the caller that the bleeding is controlled. **Focus:** Prioritization

5. **Ans: 4** Additional psychosocial and physical assessment is needed to intervene properly. The other three options may be appropriate after initial assessment is completed. **Focus:** Prioritization

6. **Ans: 2** The priority is oxygenation. The other diagnoses are appropriate, but less urgent. **Focus:** Prioritization

7. **Ans: 3** Agitation and sweating are signs of severe respiratory distress. In addition, the child is attempting to maximize the thoracic cavity and to oxygenate more effectively by sitting upright and hunching forward. **Focus:** Prioritization

8. **Ans: 1** Increased respiratory rate and decreased breath sounds are ominous signs suggesting that the airways are obstructed. Respiratory arrest is imminent. A productive cough warrants close observation, because the client is at risk for mucus plugs and bronchial spasm, which could cause an obstruction. Other symptoms such as itching, restlessness, and wheezing accompany exacerbation of asthma and require attention, but are less urgent. **Focus:** Prioritization

9. **Ans: 6, 3, 1, 5, 2, 4, 7** Administer humidified oxygen while you are preparing the albuterol treatment. (If the albuterol is immediately available, you should give the treatment first and then administer the oxygen after the treatment is completed.) In acute exacerbations of asthma, short-acting beta$_2$ agonists are given, followed by corticosteroid therapy. A chest radiograph and CBC are appropriate to demonstrate underlying pathology such as infection that may contribute to the episode. Arrangements should be made to transfer the client to the hospital after the client's condition has been stabilized. Measuring peak flow rates to determine personal best is part of long-term management and client education. Radioallergosorbent testing can be scheduled on an outpatient basis. **Focus:** Prioritization

10. **Ans: 1. Pediatrician, 2. RN, 3. Unit secretary, 4. UAP, 5. Pediatrician, 6. RN and pediatrician, 7. RN or LPN/LVN, 8. UAP** The pediatrician must give the physician-to-physician report. The RN must give the nursing report. The unit secretary can notify radiology about the need for a copy of the chest x-ray. The UAP can help collect personal items, but the RN should delegate and give instructions. The pediatrician must determine the stability of the client's condition. The RN and pediatrician must do independent summaries of the client's condition. The pediatrician may rely on the RN's report of ongoing response to treatments. The RN can check the patency of the IV line, or the LPN/LVN can be assigned this task. (Note: There is variation in the scope of practice of LPNs/LVNs according to states' nurse practice acts. Policies can also vary among facilities within the same state.) The UAP can help the client transfer, but the RN must know that the UAP has had proper training in transfer techniques to prevent injury to self or client. **Focus:** Supervision, assignment, delegation

11. **Ans: 4, 1, 2, 3** James's condition is the most critical. He has airway compromise that could suddenly turn into a complete airway obstruction. Daisy is the next in priority. Although she is conscious, she cannot be allowed to continue unattended for a long period. At a minimum, delegate performing a blood glucose check to the LPN/LVN (or a UAP if appropriate training has been given) with instructions that the results be reported to you immediately. Sarah, Sam, and Ms. A have complex social circumstances that will be very time consuming to address; however, this family is a flight risk. Quickly check on the A family and alert all staff members about the need to support this family. Terry has a treatable ear infection; treatment and education are relatively straightforward. Then go back and do an in-depth assessment of the A family. **Focus:** Prioritization

12. **Ans: 2** James has symptoms of epiglottitis and is at high risk for an airway obstruction. The other diagnoses are relevant, but have lower priority. **Focus:** Prioritization

13. **Ans: 2** The child has an immediate need for oxygen. An upright position facilitates breathing, and parental comfort minimizes agitation and crying, which would increase oxygen consumption. Inspecting the throat is contraindicated because the procedure could exacerbate airway obstruction. Intubation equipment should always be available, but is not needed yet. (Note: If the clinic were attached to a hospital, you could alert the operating room about the need for a potential emergency intubation and/or tracheostomy.) Reassuring the parents that the condition will resolve spontaneously is inappropriate. **Focus:** Prioritization

14. **Ans: 3** In addition to the APN and the pediatrician, the best combination would be the experienced RN and GN. The child is acutely ill and may require immediate intervention for airway management. This is an opportunity for the experienced RN to closely supervise and mentor the GN. In the initial care of this child, there are few tasks that can be delegated to the UAP, and the expertise of the LPN/LVN is best utilized to monitor and assess other clients in more stable condition. **Focus:** Supervision, assignment

15. **Ans: 3** In a clinic setting, calling 911 is the best and safest option. Directing the parent to drive would be considered dangerous malpractice. There is a wide variation in skill set among ambulance drivers, whereas advanced EMS paramedics that respond to 911 calls are routinely trained to intubate. Although the pediatrician is qualified to intubate, this is not a typical task in a clinic setting, and prophylactically intubating the child at this point would be inappropriate. **Focus:** Prioritization

16. **Ans: 4** Based on the available information, you would suspect and confirm hypoglycemia and then give food or fluids to prevent complications. According to the American Diabetes Association, milk is better than juice because blood glucose level is stabilized by the lactose, fat, and protein. The mother should be notified and advised to come to the clinic; however, emergency treatments would not be delayed if she cannot be located. Asking the child to describe how she feels is appropriate, but taking time to elicit details of history from a 4-year-old with hypoglycemia is not a good use of time in the immediate situation. The physician should be alerted about the child's condition; however, oxygen is not needed, and it is unlikely that IV access is required at this time. **Focus:** Prioritization

17. **Ans: 4** The mother is very emotional, and she must be allowed to express her feelings first. In addition, accusing others of "not taking care of her" suggests that the mother may be using the defense mechanism of projection (transferring feelings and inadequacies of self onto others). Her anger and fear may be related to guilt for not appropriately informing the neighbor about the child's health condition. You could consider using the other three options after you have allowed

the mother to express herself and have further assessed the situation. **Focus:** Prioritization

18. **Ans: 1**   Acute otitis media is painful. Symptoms are relieved with acetaminophen (Tylenol) and application of a warm, moist towel to the outer ear. Other diagnoses are pertinent, but less urgent. **Focus:** Prioritization

19. **Ans: 3**   The LPN/LVN should perform an irrigation of the ear canal. Teaching of the parents should be done by the RN. "Watchful waiting" is not an appropriate medical approach for a child under 2 years of age because of the immaturity of the immune system. An order for an antihistamine, a decongestant, and a steroid should be questioned by the RN, because these are not recommended for the treatment of acute otitis media. **Focus:** Assignment

20. **Ans: 4**   In pediatrics, RNs will frequently calculate the dosage independently of the physician as a safety measure. Having another RN double-check the order and the math is not mandatory, but it is a common practice and adds an additional safety check. Once the error is validated, bring it to the attention of the pediatrician. Options 1 and 2 are incorrect because the dosage is too high. Option 3 is a possibility, but in this case the pharmacist is unlikely to have additional information that will clarify this order. (Note: 20 to 40 mg/kg/24 hr in four divided doses is not the most common way to see this dosage range, but examine the math closely: 20 to 40 mg/kg/24 hr in four divided doses is the same as 5 to 10 mg/kg/dose if given every 6 hours.) **Focus:** Prioritization

21. **Ans: 3**   Remind the GN that the infant is refusing to suck and that therefore administering oral medication may be challenging. Mixing medication with applesauce is appropriate in some circumstances, but for this client the volume of 3 oz is excessive. In addition, applesauce may or may not have been introduced into the diet, and it is inappropriate to introduce new foods during an illness. **Focus:** Supervision

22. **Ans: 3**   The priority for this family is safety and avoidance of injury. Both children have physical needs that are not being met. The infant may already have an arm injury. Ms. A's comment suggests that she does not have an understanding of appropriate developmental behavior for children, and there is concern about her ability to make safe judgments for herself and the children. The other diagnoses are also relevant for this family. **Focus:** Prioritization

23. **Ans: 1. RN, 2. RN and social worker, 3. All team members, 4. Social worker, RN, 5. UAP, 6. UAP, 7. LPN/LVN or RN, 8. UAP**   The RN must perform the initial physical assessment; it cannot be delegated. The RN and pediatric social worker both need to obtain an initial history. There is some overlap in history taking; however, in addition to the psychosocial circumstances, the RN needs to evaluate mechanism of injury to anticipate the extent and type of injuries and the potential for complications. All professional caregivers should observe for signs of abuse. The UAP will have less formal training in this area, but his or her input is still valuable. Any caregiver can contact Child Protective Services; however, in this case, the social worker is present and is the most appropriate person. If a social worker were not available, then the RN should assume this responsibility. The UAP can hold one child, accompany the infant to radiology, and assist the toddler to eat. The LPN/LVN can be assigned to give medication; the RN could also administer it. **Focus:** Delegation, assignment

24. **Ans: 4**   Try to use therapeutic communication first. An AMA form is not appropriate in this situation, because the mother's ability to make good judgments and to care for her children is a concern. The pediatrician should be notified, because the mother may respond to the physician's advice if she will not listen to anyone else. Threatening to call the police is likely to increase the mother's agitation and fears. **Focus:** Prioritization

CASE STUDY 20: Multiple Patients with Mental Health Disorders, pages 157-162

1. **Ans: Mr. D and Ms. G**   Mr. D has major depression, and Ms. G has dementia and depression. These two patients will require physical care and verbal coaching. The medical-surgical nurse would be most familiar with the care and conditions of these two patients. **Focus:** Assignment

2. **Ans: Ms. B, Ms. M, and Mr. S**   Ms. B, with a borderline personality disorder, and Ms. M, with manic behavior, need continuous and firm limit setting from an experienced and preferably a female nurse. They may be excessively argumentative or manipulative. Mr. S shows bizarre behavior, but he has a chronic condition. **Focus:** Assignment

3. **Ans: Mr. P and Mr. V**   Mr. P, who has paranoid schizophrenia, and Mr. V, who is actively suicidal, have the most acute conditions and therefore should be assigned to an experienced RN. **Focus:** Assignment

4. **Ans: Mr. D**   Mr. D needs assistance and encouragement to meet hygienic needs, and he can understand and follow instructions. Ms. B and Ms. M can accomplish their own hygienic care, but specific boundaries may need to be set about dressing appropriately. Mr. P could be easily provoked because of his paranoia. Mr. S has severe communication barriers that a new assistant may not understand. Mr. V is on suicide precautions. Ms. G could also be assigned to the assistant; however, patients with dementia do better if they have the same caregiver whenever possible. **Focus:** Assignment

5. **Ans: Ms. M and Mr. V**   Students generally prefer to complete this type of assignment with patients who are willing and able to carry on a reasonably coherent conversation. Ms. M (manic behavior) is probably the best choice, because she is likely to seek out the student (or any other person who enters the unit) and initiate a conversation. Mr. V (suicidal thoughts) would benefit from the attention that a student could give him, but the assigned mental health assistant and the student must be aware that the patient is on continuous one-to-one observation and that the presence of the student does not replace the observations made by the staff. Mr. D (depression) could Answer questions appropriately, but his energy will not sustain a prolonged interview. Ms. B (borderline personality disorder) is likely to seek out the student; however, special attention from a young male is not likely to be part of her treatment plan. Mr. P (paranoid schizophrenia) is likely to refuse an interview or will have a low tolerance for interaction. Mr. S (disorganized schizophrenia) provides an interesting opportunity for observing symptoms, but he is not a good historian, and chart data may be limited. Ms. G (dementia) would be an interesting choice for a mental status examination; however, she is not a good historian, and prolonged questioning is likely to increase her restlessness and agitation. **Focus:** Supervision

6. **Ans: 2**   Your first action would be to assess the patient for current mental status and for safety and comfort related to use of restraints. Additional information is necessary to validate the need for medications and restraints, and to determine if other interventions were tried before resorting to chemical and/or physical restraints. Based on your assessment of the patient and situation, you may decide to use the other three options. **Focus:** Prioritization, supervision

7. **Ans: 2**   Although minimizing clutter is important, rearranging furniture and belongings can increase confusion. Options 1, 2, and 4 are appropriate interventions to use with a patient who has dementia. **Focus:** Supervision

8. **Ans: 4**   AMA policies may vary, and transfer to specialty facilities can be complex and time consuming. Explain to the patient and/or family that leaving against advice may actually delay geropsychiatric placement, because the patient's place on waiting lists may be lost or a relationship may have to be established with another referring provider. The health care provider writes the order for transfer but is usually not involved in making the administrative arrangements. False reassurance to placate the daughter is not the best approach. Once the AMA policy is verified, the daughter can be assisted in filling out the appropriate AMA forms if she still wants to take her mother home. **Focus:** Prioritization

9. **Ans: 4**   Support the therapeutic milieu by demonstrating to all the patients that the psychiatric unit has social norms. Instructing Ms. M to stop interrupting is a concrete direction that delineates expected group behavior. Escorting her out may be the easiest solution, but parameters for behavior (i.e., raise your hand if you want to speak) and consequences (i.e., if you interrupt one more time you will have to leave) should be clarified first. The scenario suggests that the social worker is not able to control Ms. M. Frequently, the co-leader assists with individual behavioral management while the leader keeps the group on task. Ideally, these roles are discussed beforehand. Encouragement of confrontation could be used in a small group therapy session to teach patients to directly express and respond to one another; however, in this meeting having Ms. B defend herself is likely to lead to a loud and unproductive public screaming match. **Focus:** Prioritization

10. **Ans: 1**   Assess the patient for behaviors that would warrant seclusion (i.e., represent a danger to self or to others), then discuss your concerns with the provider. If seclusion is punitive, there is a potential for violation of rights, regardless of whether the order is verbal or written. Although patients do need limit setting and clear boundaries, you must intervene in the "least restrictive" manner. After additional assessment, you may decide that documentation, seclusion, and continued care are options. However, you may also decide that you need to go up the chain of command to prevent future similar incidents. **Focus:** Prioritization

11. **Ans: 2**   When the sodium level is low, the body retains lithium, so there is an increased risk for lithium toxicity. The chloride and potassium levels are within normal limits. The glucose level would be considered elevated if the patient has not eaten within the past several hours. **Focus:** Prioritization

12. **Ans: 1**   Have the student contact the instructor. An incident report should be filed so that a detailed record is available for review. The instructor can debrief the student, who is likely to be upset, and there may be unintentional elements of his behavior that triggered Ms. B's response. Ms. B should have an opportunity to talk about the incident also, but do not create a situation in which you find yourself having to defend one against the other. You should write an incident report that is separate and independent from the student's account. The incident is unlikely to be reported directly to the board of nursing, but it could go to peer review if the student's behavior appears to be questionable. **Focus:** Supervision

13. **Ans: 3**   Acknowledging feelings is therapeutic; at the same time, you are not necessarily confirming or denying the veracity of Ms. B's statements. Explain that any verbalizations of potential harm must be shared with the physician and psychiatric team. Rather than spend additional time with

Ms. B, gently inform her that you will contact the appropriate team members for follow-up. (The problem may be real, but Ms. B also has a long history of manipulating for attention.) Physical assessment will not provide any evidence of rape, but a rape crisis counselor could be contacted for long-term follow-up. **Focus:** Prioritization

14. **Ans: 1. Psychiatrist, 2. RN, 3. RN, 4. Mental health assistant, 5. RN, 6. Nurse anesthetist, 7. Mental health assistant, 8. RN, 9. Mental health assistant** The psychiatrist is responsible for obtaining informed consent. The RN is responsible for patient education and ensuring that all pre-procedural and post-procedural orders are completed. Under appropriate supervision, a mental health assistant can assist patients to prepare for the procedure by removing and storing personal items. Also, assistants can take vital signs and assist with meals. The nurse anesthetist should administer anesthesia. **Focus:** Delegation, assignment

15. **Ans: 4** The patient is expressing a delusion of grandeur and religiosity with clang associations. Acknowledge the underlying "healthy" intent and express appreciation for the gesture. Addressing the patient as Jesus supports the delusion, while contradicting the delusion is thought to have a reinforcing effect. Redirecting to concrete, here-and-now topics is appropriate after you have acknowledged the underlying feelings. Redirection is also appropriate when the patient is repetitive with delusional content. **Focus:** Prioritization

16. **Ans: 2** With thought disorder patients, use short, simple questions that are easy to understand and respond to. If this particular patient can state his name in response to the question, it would be a therapeutic accomplishment because of his severe thought disorder. The other options show interest in the patient, but it is unlikely that this patient could sustain the concentration required to play cards, to sit for 15 minutes, or to recall the events preceding hospitalization. **Focus:** Prioritization

17. **Ans: 1. Mental health assistant, 2. LPN/LVN and RN, 3. RN, 4. All team members, 5. RN, 6. Mental health assistant, 7. RN, 8. RN** The mental health assistant can assist with hygiene. The RN can delegate one-to-one observation to the mental health assistant but must supervise and give specific instructions. The RN or LPN/LVN could also do one-to-one observation; however, the task is usually delegated because the patient cannot be left alone, even for a few minutes, and the observation may be needed for hours or even several days. An LPN/LVN or RN can give medication. The RN is responsible for teaching, ensuring safety, and evaluating. Searching the patient's belongings should not be delegated; the task requires clinical judgment about potential for self-harm. All team members should use good communication techniques.

(Note: The nursing student could be involved in any of these actions with proper supervision but is never expected to take full responsibility for any of these tasks.) **Focus:** Delegation, assignment

18. **Ans: 2** Although Mr. P is paranoid, even psychiatric patients may be able to recognize their own medications. As with any patient, you should double-check the physician's order first to see if there has been an error. You could compare the order with the medication reconciliation list (if it is available) to see if the current order matches what the patient has taken in the past. The other options could be used after the medication order is clarified. **Focus:** Prioritization

19. **Ans: 4** The patient is in the pre-assaultive stage. Use a calm tone of voice and explain what you expect him to do. This will help him to gain control and convey that you respect his ability to participate in his own behavior control. Options 2 and 3 may be necessary after the verbal intervention. If at all possible, avoid sudden or quick actions, which could be interpreted as physical aggression. **Focus:** Prioritization

20. **Ans: 3** Give the assistant specific instructions to point out that the food is wrapped and sealed. Following him around the day room is not a good strategy, because it is likely to increase his suspicions and make him more anxious. Observing his interactions and checking his belongings for dangerous items should be performed by the RN. **Focus:** Delegation

21. **Ans: 1. RN, 2. Mental health assistant, 3. LPN/LVN, Mental health assistant, 4. LPN/LVN or RN, 5. RN, 6. Mental health assistant** The mental health assistant can assist Mr. D with hygienic care and redirect Ms. G away from the door. Remember to tell the assistant that Ms. G is at risk for falls. The LPN/LVN is the best team member to intervene with Ms. M, set boundaries, and direct her to dress appropriately. The mental health assistant could also direct Ms. M with appropriate clothing, but the therapeutic intervention of setting boundaries and linking immediate behavior to consequences should be done by an RN or LPN/LVN. Administering oral medications is within the scope of practice of the LPN/LVN. Psychiatric patients are routinely observed for "pouching" pills in the buccal area. The RN could also perform this task, but the LPN/LVN is a better choice because the RN should attend to more acute patients. The RN should assess Ms. B for suicide risk. Suicide precautions with one-to-one observation must be initiated. The psychiatrist must be notified, and the incident must be carefully documented. The RN should assess Mr. V for suicidal thoughts. Writing letters could be a positive and therapeutic action; however, letters may also contain evidence of final goodbyes. **Focus:** Delegation, assignment

22. **Ans: 7, 5, 2, 1, 4, 6, 3** Using the SBAR format, the nurse first identifies himself or herself, gives the patient's name, and describes the current situation. Next,

give relevant background information, such as the patient's diagnosis, medications, and laboratory data. The assessment includes both patient assessment data that are of concern and the nurse's analysis of the situation. Finally, the nurse makes a recommendation indicating what action he or she thinks is needed. **Focus:** Prioritization

23. **Ans: 2** You should talk to her first to give a verbal warning; she must acknowledge that she understands the call-in parameters. Explain that this type of behavior jeopardizes her probation status and that next time the incident will go into writing. Forcing an employee to come in during illness is not good for the other employees or the patients. You may have to tell the oncoming nurse about the short staffing, but make every effort to find a replacement. Working short-staffed is not safe or pleasant for anyone. **Focus:** Supervision, assignment

24. **Ans: 1, 2, 3, 5** Tasks 1, 2, 3, and 5 should be delegated to the mental health assistants. Shift change is a hectic time and you are trying to leave the unit in good order for the oncoming shift. Mr. S should not go to the gift shop today, he is still too disorganized. The nurse should take responsibility to talk to Ms. M. It was not a good day for this patient because she had several incidents of confrontation. For today, it is better not to touch Mr. P's belongings, especially if the clutter is not a safety issue; just leave them alone until his anxiety and suspicions are better controlled. **Focus:** Prioritization

25. **Ans: 1, 2, 4, 6, 8** Tasks 1, 4, and 8 are necessary tasks to provide a thorough shift-change report. Having some knowledge about the new patient (task 2) is useful in making assignments for the next shift. Task 6 should be done routinely for team building and morale. Tasks 3 and 7 are likely to require lengthy discussions and should be left for the next business day, when social services personnel will be available to assist the nursing staff and the family with these issues. Task 5 will be addressed by getting a report from the staff nurses who have been assigned to care for individual patients. **Focus:** Prioritization

CASE STUDY 21: Childbearing, pages 163-166

1. **Ans: 1, 2, 3, 4** Ms. N began prenatal care late at 24 weeks. She needs to know the danger signs and how to contact her provider if they occur. She should be offered assistance with smoking cessation, because smoking is a known risk factor for prematurity, low infant birth weight, perinatal infant death, and sudden infant death syndrome. Undertaking interventions now can help the pregnant woman to quit or reduce smoking and impact outcomes. Educating in the basics of nutrition is also a high priority, because Ms. N is 24 weeks pregnant, admits to a poor diet, and has gained excess weight in her pregnancy. Getting a flu shot in flu season is recommended for pregnant women. Pain relief would not be considered a priority topic because the client is only at 24 weeks gestation and has higher priority issues to address at this time; pain relief education can be addressed later. **Focus:** Prioritization

2. **Ans: 1** Chlamydia infection is associated with preterm labor and birth and with neonatal infection, and thus should be treated in pregnancy. Azithromycin is safe in pregnancy and is effective in curing chlamydia infection. **Focus:** Prioritization

3. **Ans: 2** Stress has been linked to preterm delivery and low birth weight of infants and should be addressed by the nurse as a serious risk factor. A 3-hour glucose tolerance test requires fasting even in pregnancy. Colposcopy is a procedure for assessing the cervix; it does not treat HPV infection. The presence of HPV is not an indication for cesarean section. **Focus:** Prioritization

4. **Ans: 3** This report summarizes in SBAR format the priority information that the ED RN needs to know to provide good care to this client at this time. Option 1 gives no background information. Option 2 gives nonpriority information, includes inaccurate information regarding family history, omits priority information, and includes no recommendation. Option 4 inappropriately gives a diagnosis, and the recommendation may not be appropriate. **Focus:** Prioritization

5. **Ans: 4, 1, 3, 2, 5** This ordering is based on client and staff safety. The agitated and angry man is a safety threat to the client and possibly to the staff, and dealing with him needs to be the first priority. The woman's report of bleeding and cramping are a safety threat to the fetus and so must be assessed quickly by measuring vital signs and applying a fetal monitor. The physician should be notified so that an examination can be performed promptly. Once the immediate safety of the mother and fetus are ensured, it would be appropriate to obtain a more thorough history. A social work consult would be indicated, but should be deferred until assessment is complete. **Focus:** Prioritization

6. **Ans: 3** Betamethasone administration is an evidence-based intervention that has been shown to decrease many neonatal complications such as respiratory distress, neonatal death, necrotizing enterocolitis, and cerebral vascular hemorrhage in the case of preterm delivery. This practice supports the Perinatal Core Measure of increasing the percentage of women at risk of preterm delivery who are given antenatal steroids. The nifedipine is used in this situation as a tocolytic to reduce uterine contractions. **Focus:** Prioritization

7. **Ans: 3** Scheduling a follow-up appointment is within the scope of practice of a nursing assistant. Options 1 and 2 are important client education tasks that the RN must perform. Option 4 requires professional collaboration between the RN and the social worker. **Focus:** Delegation

8. **Ans: 2** Ferrous sulfate should be taken with water or juice. Milk can slow the absorption of iron. The other statements are appropriate. **Focus:** Supervision

9. **Ans 2, 3, 4, 5:** These are all necessary data for the RN to have before recommending that the client either wait at home or come to the hospital. The RN must consider the client's history, current symptoms, and practical matters such as distance to the hospital, available transportation, and traffic conditions before giving guidance. Whether the client took her vitamin and iron today would not be priority information at this time. **Focus:** Prioritization

10. **Ans: 2** Options 1, 3, and 4 do not represent abnormal conditions in labor. Option 2, however, indicates more bleeding than normal in labor. It could be a sign of placental abruption or placenta previa and should be evaluated promptly. **Focus:** Prioritization

11. **Ans: 1, 3, 4** The elevated blood pressure should prompt the RN to ask questions regarding symptoms of preeclampsia. The symptoms in options 1, 3, and 4 are characteristic of preeclampsia. Those in options 2 and 5 are not. **Focus:** Prioritization

12. **Ans: 2, 3, 1, 4** After rupture of the membranes, it is a priority to assess fetal heart tones, because the intrauterine contents shift and there may be compression or prolapse of the umbilical cord. The presence of meconium in the fluid may indicate fetal hypoxia and thus also indicates the need for assessment of fetal heart tones. After heart tones are assessed, the provider should be notified of the presence of meconium in the fluid. The infant bed should be prepared in anticipation of a possible need for suctioning or intubation of the neonate at delivery because of the presence of meconium. Finally, Ms. N should be assessed to determine what the contraction pattern is and how she is coping, because the contractions may become more intense following rupture of the membranes. The prioritization is based on client safety and requires the nurse to know the implications of meconium-stained fluid and to anticipate changes in the plan of care because of it. **Focus:** Prioritization

13. **Ans: 1** Because Ms. N's labor is progressing rapidly and she is nearing delivery, an opioid would not be an optimal choice at this time. Although butorphanol is associated with less respiratory depression than other opioids, if it is given close to delivery it can cause respiratory depression in the neonate at birth. This medication would be more appropriately used earlier in labor if desired. The other choices are appropriate nursing actions for the pain and distress of this stage of labor. **Focus:** Supervision

14. **Ans: 2, 3, 5, 4, 1** The American Academy of Pediatrics and the American Heart Association publish guidelines for neonatal resuscitation that are updated regularly. The first action with this newborn is to move him to a prewarmed table in the delivery room.

Provision of warmth avoids the added challenge of cold stress for the newborn. The airway is opened by placing the infant in a supine position with the head very slightly extended. Because this newborn is depressed *and* had meconium-stained amniotic fluid, endotracheal suctioning is the next action. Following suction, the infant is stimulated by gently slapping the soles of the feet and/or rubbing the back. If the infant remains apneic or with a heart rate less than 100 beats/min, positive-pressure ventilation with bag and mask is initiated. The steps of resuscitation should be done rapidly and in the correct order. All resuscitation equipment should be prepared for each delivery in case of need. Gloves should be worn and all equipment should be clean or sterile as indicated to support the Perinatal Core Measure of reducing health care–associated bloodstream infections in newborns. **Focus:** Prioritization

15. **Ans: 4** The heart rate and respiratory rate, and findings of peripheral cyanosis are normal in the first hour of life. Central cyanosis, however, may suggest a cardiac or respiratory abnormality and must be evaluated. **Focus:** Prioritization

16. **Ans: 3, 4, 5, 1, 2** The first assessment is of the airway and respirations. Next, suctioning is performed if indicated. The heart rate is then assessed. Placement of identification bands is important for newborn security, but assessing and ensuring the physical stability of the infant in a systematic way is the first priority. Intramuscular administration of vitamin K is recommended for the newborn, but this can be done after the initial assessments and proper identification of the newborn. **Focus:** Prioritization

17. **Ans: 2, 3** Early skin-to-skin contact and early breast feeding are associated with breast feeding success. This supports the Perinatal Core Measure of increasing the percentage of newborns who are fed breast milk only. It is not recommended to give sterile water to a breast-feeding infant or to limit nursing time. **Focus:** Prioritization

18. **Ans: 3** Asthma is a relative contraindication to the use of carboprost due to its potential to cause bronchospasm. There are other appropriate drugs for postpartum hemorrhage that can be used in place of carboprost, such as misoprostol. **Focus:** Prioritization

19. **Ans: 2, 3** Assessing and massaging the uterine fundus help to prevent further hemorrhage by contracting the uterus firmly, which decreases the rapid blood loss present with uterine atony. If the maternal bladder is full, it can prevent effective contraction of the uterus, leading to uterine atony and continued blood loss. The nurse should encourage the mother to void frequently and, if she is unable to do so, bladder catheterization would be indicated. Checking vital signs and providing a high-iron diet are appropriate, but do not stop the bleeding. Maternal position is unrelated to hemorrhage. **Focus:** Prioritization

20. **Ans: 2** The statement that something is "gushing" would prompt the RN to assess immediately for further postpartum hemorrhage. The other reported symptoms are nonemergent and can be evaluated on the postpartum unit. **Focus:** Prioritization

21. **Ans: 2** Tachycardia is an early sign of possible hypovolemia from hemorrhage. Hypotension, mental status changes, and decreased urine output are later signs. The relative hypervolemia in pregnancy allows the mother to tolerate normal blood loss at delivery with relatively little change in vital signs. The RN must be alert to early signs of hypovolemia and assess promptly for excessive blood loss. **Focus:** Prioritization

DEFINITIONS

Prioritization: Deciding which needs or problems require immediate action and which ones could tolerate a delay in response until a later time because they are not urgent.[*]

Delegation: Transferring to a competent individual the authority to perform a selected nursing task in a selected situation. The nurse retains the accountability for the delegation.[†]

Assignment: The distribution of work that each staff member is responsible for during a given shift or work period.[‡]

THE FIVE RIGHTS OF DELEGATION[†§]

Right circumstances
Right task
Right person
Right direction and communication
Right supervision

THE FOUR Cs OF COMMUNICATION

Instructions and ongoing direction must be:
Clear
Concise
Correct
Complete

[*]Silvestri L: *Saunders comprehensive review for the NCLEX-RN® Examination,* ed 5, St Louis, 2011, Saunders.
[†]National Council of State Boards of Nursing: Delegation: concepts and decision-making process, *Issues,* December, pp. 1-4, 1995.
[‡]National Council of State Boards of Nursing: Business book: NCSBN annual meeting: mission possible: building a safer nursing workforce through regulatory excellence, 2005.
[§]Hansten R, Jackson M: *Clinical delegation skills: a handbook for professional practice,* ed 4, Sudbury, MA, 2009, Jones & Bartlett.